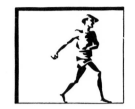

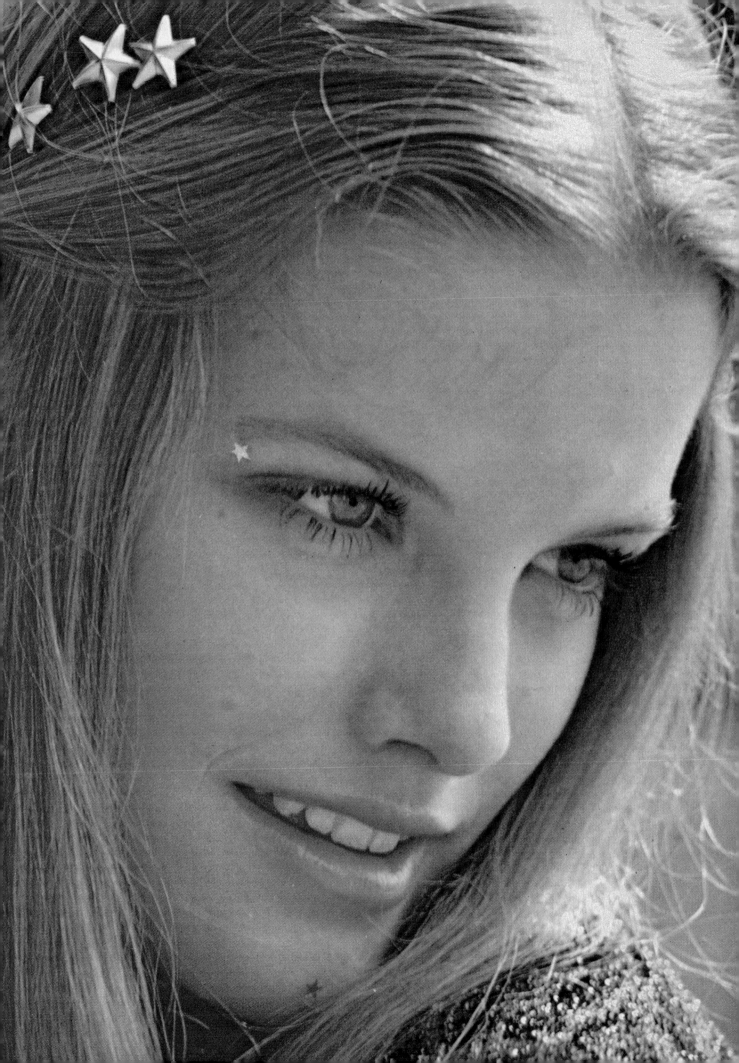

GLAMOUR'S BEAUTY & HEALTH & BOOK

By the Editors of Glamour Magazine

Simon and Schuster
New York

Copyright © 1968, 1969, 1970, 1971, 1972
by the Condé Nast Publications Inc.
All rights reserved
including the right of reproduction
in whole or in part in any form.
Published by Simon and Schuster
Rockefeller Center, 630 Fifth Avenue
New York, New York 10020

First printing

SBN 671-21200-1
Library of Congress Catalog Card Number: 65-23243
Manufactured in the United States of America

Editor: Phyllis Starr Wilson
Design: Miki Denhof
Layout preparation: Libra Graphic Services
Typography and black and white photographic preparation:
Ruttle, Shaw & Wetherill, Inc.
Color preparation, presswork and binding:
R. R. Donnelley & Sons Company

Photographs:

Michael Avedon
William Connors
John Cowan
Jim Dorrance
Van Glintenkamp
Claude Guillaumin
S. Hatami
Mark Hispard
Frank Horvat
Saul Leiter
Frances McLaughlin-Gill

Kenn Mori
Helmut Newton
Edward Oleksak
Gianni Penati
Rico Puhlman
Mike Reinhardt
Jerry Salvati
John Stember
Otto Stupakoff
J. P. Zachariasen

Drawings:

Sheile Camera
Richard Giglio
Elizabeth Jorg

Judy Markham
Philippe Weisbecker
Tad Yamashiro

CONTENTS

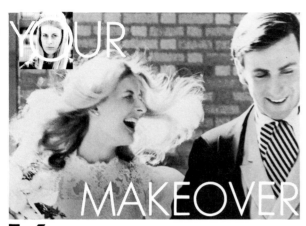
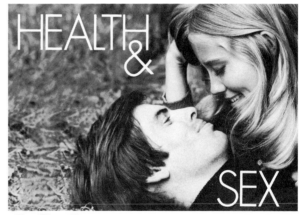
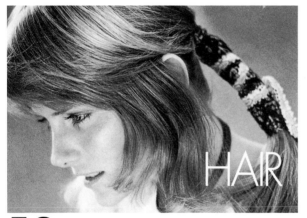
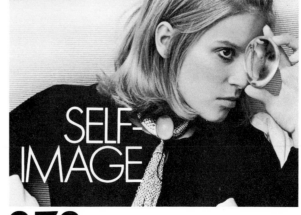
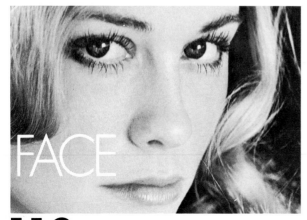
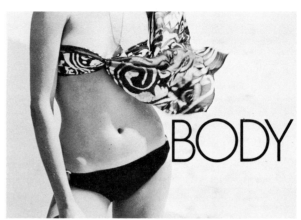

CONTENTS

YOUR MAKEOVER

HAIR

FACE

BODY

HEALTH & SEX

SELF-IMAGE

INDEX

THE MAKING OF A BEAUTY

Today a beautiful girl is less a result of nature than of her own technique and her awareness of what medicine, science and cosmetics can do for her. Even as short a time as six or seven years back if hair was fine and thin, you learned to live with it; now you give it body out of a bottle. If skin was drab, you could coat it with a heavy foundation to change its color, but you couldn't achieve the transparent healthy blush you can today with sheer gels and liquid colors.

Now that you can buy natural beauty at any drugstore counter, girls have to compete with not only born beauties but with a population of beautiful non-beauties whose looks are self-made, individual, unstereotyped, an outer expression or mark of the interior self. You can't do it without knowing yourself and realizing that even what is bad about your looks is *yours*, unique in the way it is put with the rest of your features to make you. A strong long nose, for instance, with the right haircut, the right eye makeup, the right clothes can become a very identifiable beauty mark, or if it is too strong and too long it can be shaded down, distracted from with contour makeup, or even reshaped by surgery if necessary.

 None of this can be achieved without feeling. In a way you have to be in love with yourself and your looks, which may seem a bit smug, but love transforms. Not always at first, but in time. If you are concerned enough about your looks, if you care for them—which is what this book tells you exactly how to do—eventually you will be transformed into a beauty. You might have to care even enough to undergo a kind of do-it-yourself analysis of your looks, and, as a psychiatrist said recently, any successful analysis takes a patient endowed with a lot of energy and will. The aim of this book is to help you make a successful analysis, a realistic evaluation of your good and bad features, in order to make something uniquely, attractively yours out of them. Because that is the only way to stand out in an age when everyone can be beautiful. You have to be willing to search for the look that really expresses the idea of what you want to be and the reality of what you can be. There will be setbacks—you will have to expect them. The success of any analysis and makeover depends primarily on finding your own beauty identity, then emphasizing it. The identity isn't always evident at first sight, recognizable at a glance; but once it is found there is no chance of missing it; it is YOU.

As you begin to discover your own look, the results will show. Other people will notice you—and that is a very important part of self-realization. No one lives in such complete self-confidence that she can do without recognition and affirmation. Even the most self-assured beauties know that. In fact, one put it this way: "Even before I was born my mother thought I was beautiful. She wouldn't accept anything else, so I had no choice but to submit to her. By her stubbornness she helped me to think I was beautiful. Actually I wasn't, but I learned to be." Very few girls have mothers like that, but it is not impossible for you to learn to have confidence in your looks. GLAMOUR has helped hundreds of young women to do this in our makeover series, and the editors hope that this book will help thousands more to do their own makeovers and find their own best possible look.

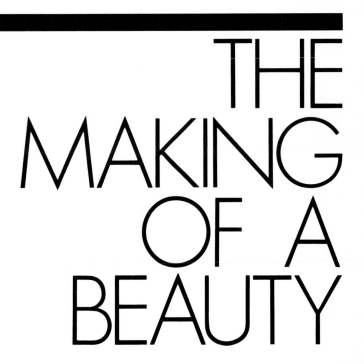

THE
MAKING
OF A
BEAUTY

BEAU
&HE

GLAMOUR'S BEAUTY HEALTH BOOK

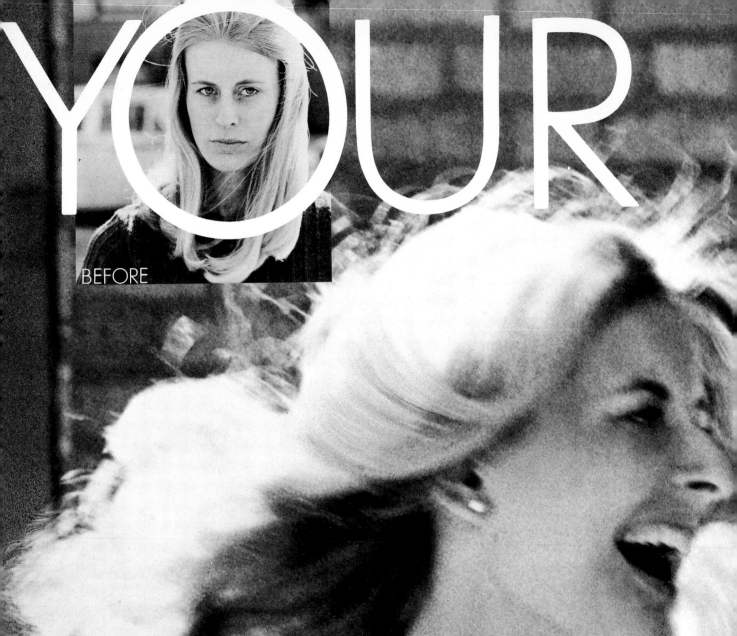

YOUR

BEFORE

YOUR MAK

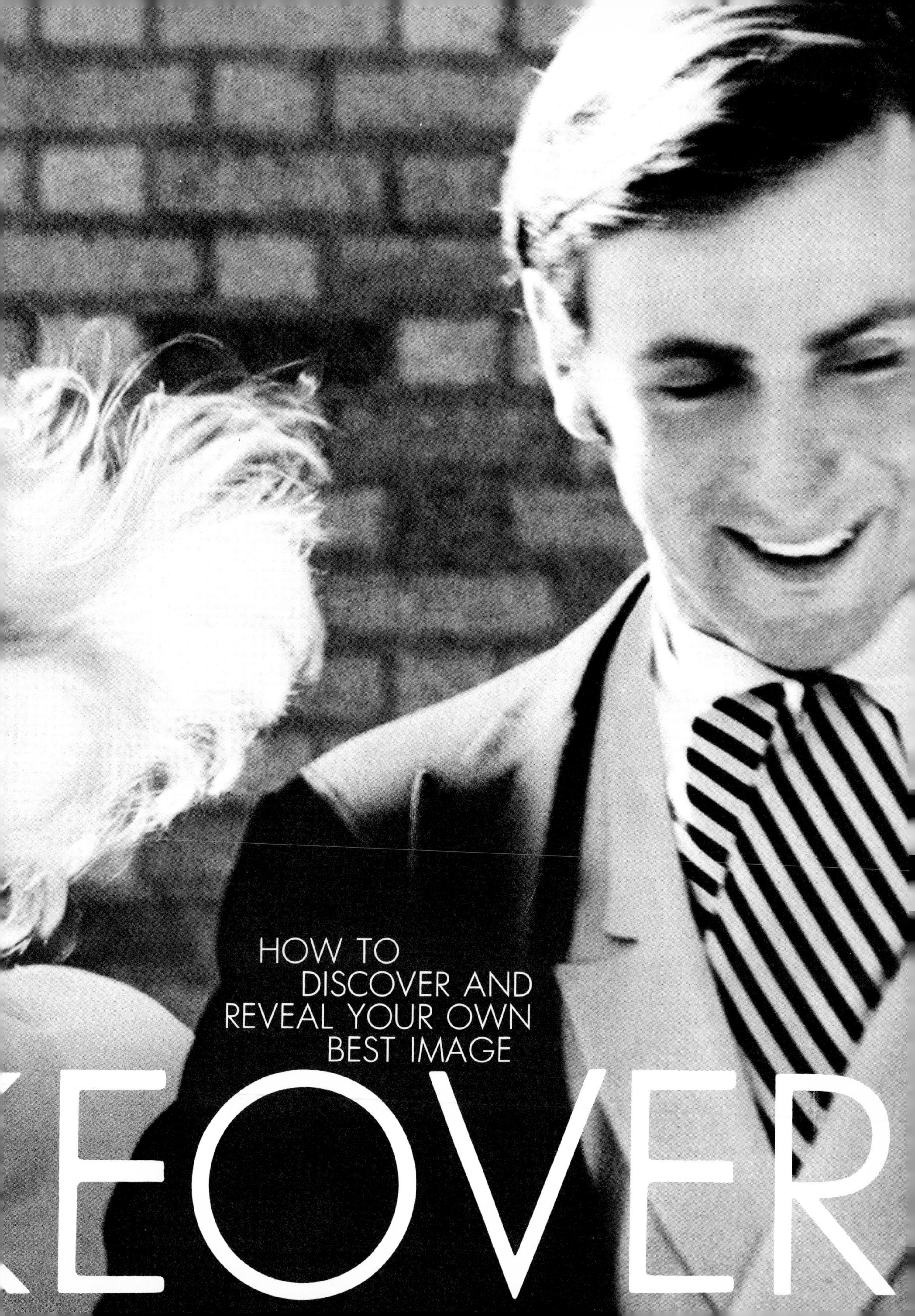

HOW TO
DISCOVER AND
REVEAL YOUR OWN
BEST IMAGE

EOVER

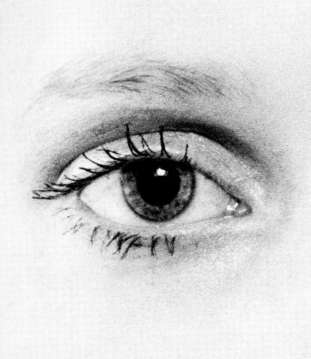
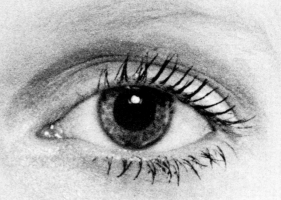

YOUR MAKEOVER

DO-IT-
YOURSELF

A makeover is basically a self-analysis of your looks, a realistic evaluation of your good and bad features in order to make the best you can of them, something uniquely yours and uniquely attractive. Each of the following lifestyle makeovers on real girls, not models, and each chapter in this book are set up to help you to do just that. Each chapter in a way is a step in your own do-it-yourself five-part makeover.

STEP 1 **HAIR**

Let's start with hair, because that is where one of the quickest and most satisfying changes can take place. Provided your hair is in good condition, you can sit right down before your mirror and start your hair makeover now . . . by asking yourself the seven questions that come up next. (If your hair isn't in good condition, read how to remedy that in Chapter II – Hair.)

A lot of the responsibility for a great haircut or styling falls on you, no matter who does the cutting. That statement comes from one of the best, if not the best, hairdresser in the country – Kenneth Battelle of the famous Kenneth Salon in New York. He suggested the questions and says that if you answer them realistically you're half way there to a great cut. Do this before you decide on a style or pick a hairdresser. (Exception: doing your own hair-cutting is the one thing in this do-it-yourself make-over that you cannot actually do yourself.)

1. *What texture is my hair—fine, medium, or coarse?* Most girls know, but if you're in doubt here's a helpful guide: If your hair has the texture of silk thread, tends to be fly-away, doesn't hold a set well, it's probably fine. If it's more like regular cotton thread, holds a set and in general behaves itself, it's medium textured. If your hair has the texture of darning thread, is sometimes unruly and hard to curl, it's probably coarse.

Along with texture, concern yourself with body or bulk. Is your hair thick, thin, or medium? Kenneth actually describes body as the amount of

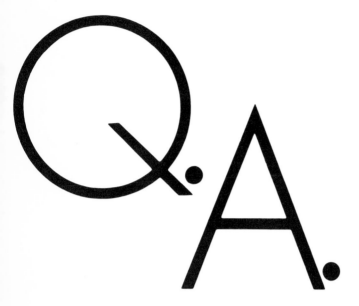

hairs on your head—if they're massed it's thick, sparse it's thin—plus the texture.

After you've established texture and body follow these tips:

Fine hair is usually thin in addition to being fine and really shouldn't be much more than chin length to look its best. It should be blunt cut and is easier to live with when it's all one length. Layering is not a particularly good choice.

Medium-textured hair with medium body can take just about any kind of styling you want unless it is very curly. Very curly hair, no matter what it's texture and bulk, shouldn't be cut super short—unless you want a Natural. Curly hair tends to curl up tightly in humid weather and you end up looking like a skin head.

Coarse thick hair is the hardest to generalize about. As a rule Kenneth says he would not advise thinning or tapering the ends but admits there could be exceptions. A long blunt cut is often the best bet because the length tends to weigh the hair down and the blunt edges help hold it in place. Talk this over with your hairdresser—don't just jump into thinning and tapering.

2. *How much time can I spend on my hair?* Be honest. If you haven't the time or temperament to set your hair daily, don't pick a complicated curly style that needs setting. Pick either a straightish blunt cut if you have no curl, or a layered one that you can wash and blow dry. (For this it doesn't matter whether your hair is moderately curly or straight, although a little wave helps.) Make the hairdresser aware of your time and temperament requirements.

3. *Am I handy with my hair?* Some girls just aren't. They can't even manage a neat pony tail or a few electric rollers. If that's you, settle for the simplest styling possible. Tell the hairdresser to keep in mind that you want a minimum of fussing and keep it in mind yourself, too, when you finally make your style choice.

4. *Do I get bored quickly with one look?* If so find a look that's versatile. In general, long hair tends to be more versatile than short. You can choose between wearing it up or down, and you can change the look by parting it differently.

5. *What kind of climate do I live in?* If you live in a muggy, tropical climate or a cold, damp one, your hair responds drastically. Curly hair can get bushy and out of hand while straight hair can go limp. In either of these climates, the more natural and basic the style the better it will hold. Anything forced into an unnatural shape will collapse.

6. *Am I realistic about what my hair will do?* This is probably the most important question of all. If you see yourself in a wild curly tangle you admired on some model and you've got fine straight hair—you're in for trouble. And if you think the right haircut is going to transform your curly hair into the superstraight kind you've seen on some girls, you're just dreaming. Haircuts can't work magic, they can only let you make the very best of what you've got—but that may be a lot more than you've been doing.

7. *What things have I tried in the past that definitely didn't work?* Bangs, layered hair, very short hair? If you're going to try any of these again, be sure you have a good reason for believing they'll work this time. You don't want to fall into the same trap twice.

The answers to these questions aren't meant to lead you to one instant perfect hairstyle, but they should give you a very good idea of what will work and what won't.

Don't

One big don't from Kenneth: Don't go to any hairdresser cold with no idea of what you want. Even a genius can't know what's right for you unless you help him.

Four basic cuts

Here are what Kenneth considers the four best cuts for most heads. None is so extreme that it will be out of date in a few months; they're all good solid classics that lend themselves to many variations.

1. The most basic cut is hair that's blunt cut

to one length all around the head. It can be any length from chin to shoulder or longer. It can be varied with bangs, a side or center part.

2. Another good cut is one that's blunt cut to one length, but the back is shorter than the sides. One variation of this cut could be hair that's cropped short and close to the nape of the neck in the back with chin length hair at the front and sides. The same cut might also be shoulder length in back with slightly longer front and sides. You can see the possibilities here.

3. The third cut is the opposite of the second. The sides are cut shorter than the back. For example, the front and side pieces might be cut chin length while the back is left shoulder length. Or part of the front section could be cut like long bangs, about eye level, and the rest cut shoulder length or left very long.

4. The fourth cut is a real layered one. There can be as many layers as you and your hairdresser decide you want, but the essentials—at least to Kenneth—are blunt cutting of the layers and uniformity of length for each layer. If one layer is three inches long, all the layers should be three inches. (All hairdressers do not agree with this, some believe in tapered cutting and layers of different length.) Kenneth's reasoning—tapering ends with a razor takes away some of the hair's body; ununiform layer lengths—say with very short ones cut on top and very long ones cut on bottom—give hair a straggly appearance instead of a full healthy look.

Unless you're going in for something mad and special, most towns of reasonable size have several good hairdressers to choose from. What's important for you is finding one who is familiar with the look you want. To be sure he or she is, go to one who has cut a friend's hair successfully in the style you want. Be sure to mention your friend's name or describe her to the hairdresser. This helps him immediately to recognize what style you're after. Or a picture of a style you like is an equal help.

Kenneth suggests you actually make two appointments a week apart and tell the hairdresser that you'll be back in a week's time for a second appointment. The first appointment should include a talk based on the questions you've answered above about how your hair behaves and so forth. Then discuss the style you want and get an opinion on whether he or she thinks it's a good choice. If the hairdresser doesn't feel it's right for your hair, take his advice and work out something more compatible but in the same feeling.

The second appointment is your chance to adjust anything you don't like after living with your new haircut a week. But most of all it should be a session on how to live with the new style—how to maintain it between visits, how to set it if it needs it or how to blow it dry plus any tips you can pick up that will make living with it easy.

By the time your second appointment is over so is your basic hair makeover. All you need to know now is how to keep it looking great for the rest of your life, how to solve any problems that may arise, and a lot more things like how to wear it wet when you've just come from swimming. All these you'll find in Chapter II.

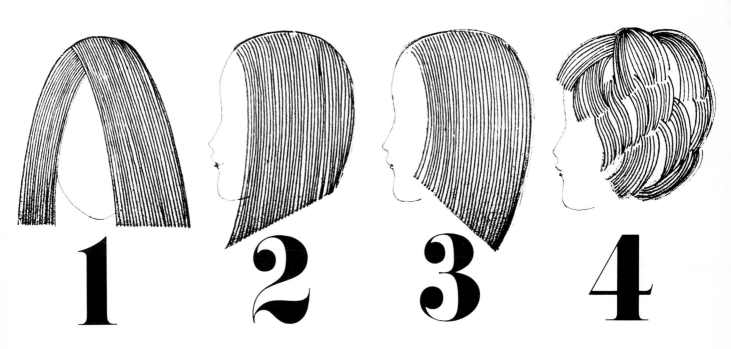

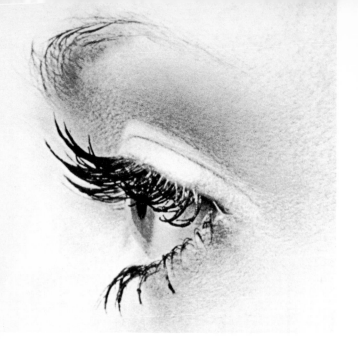

STEPS 4 & 5
HEALTH, SEX AND SELF-IMAGE

Since health, both physical and emotional, affects looks so drastically, the last two phases of your makeover deal with all the facts and some of the fictions about it. There are straightforward discussions with doctors and psychiatrists about gynecological problems young women have, about childbirth, about drugs, sexuality and the various lifestyles that are developing so rapidly in the seventies.

You may feel after reading these chapters that your image of yourself is a little blurred and needs defining, or that your attitudes about sex, marriage, career, and family require some readjustment. There are suggestions for doing that defining and adjusting by yourself, as well as for getting professional help in areas where you need it.

The editors of GLAMOUR think that this book will not only help you to makeover your looks but it may just about change your life by bringing about deeper insights into your way of thinking and feeling about yourself and other people. The new lifestyle makeovers that follow, makeovers that prepare a girl to meet the really important changes in her life—from single to married, college to career, young wife to mother, married to divorced, etc.— will be an enormous help. They are crammed with tips for making you more beautiful and your living more simple in our complex society.

STEP 2 **FACE**

To analyze your face, first isolate it for study by removing all makeup and brushing your hair back behind your ears. Your face—even if you have a skin problem that needs clearing up—is another place where you can see the immediate results of a makeover. It's a wonderful psychological boost to see what you can do in just the first half hour before your mirror. Really scrutinize your face objectively. Decide quite mercilessly what your best and worst features are, then turn to page 126 in Chapter III. There you'll find how to use makeup to expose only the best of you, to emphasize your best features so cleverly that they make the lesser ones fade into the background. You'll discover too a special section on correcting eye shapes with makeup, because eyes after all are the real focal points of beauty on any face. Actually there is a complete encyclopedia of everything you need to know about treating skin problems, changing skin tones, in brief about bringing the whole battery of modern cosmetic and medical technology to the aid of your facial makeover.

STEP 3 **BODY**

There are two easy quick tests to make of your body proportions to see if and what needs to be made over or shaped up. One is the Proportions Test on page 166, Chapter IV, to find which spots on your body are in trouble, hips, backside, tummy, whatever; and the other is the Pinch Test, page 168, to measure overall overweight. Take both of these. If they reveal that you have a body problem, then read on in Chapter IV to find out how to solve it. There are crash diets, long term diets, psychological aids, exercises for every kind of person from the laziest to the most active girls, and exercises for every trouble spot.

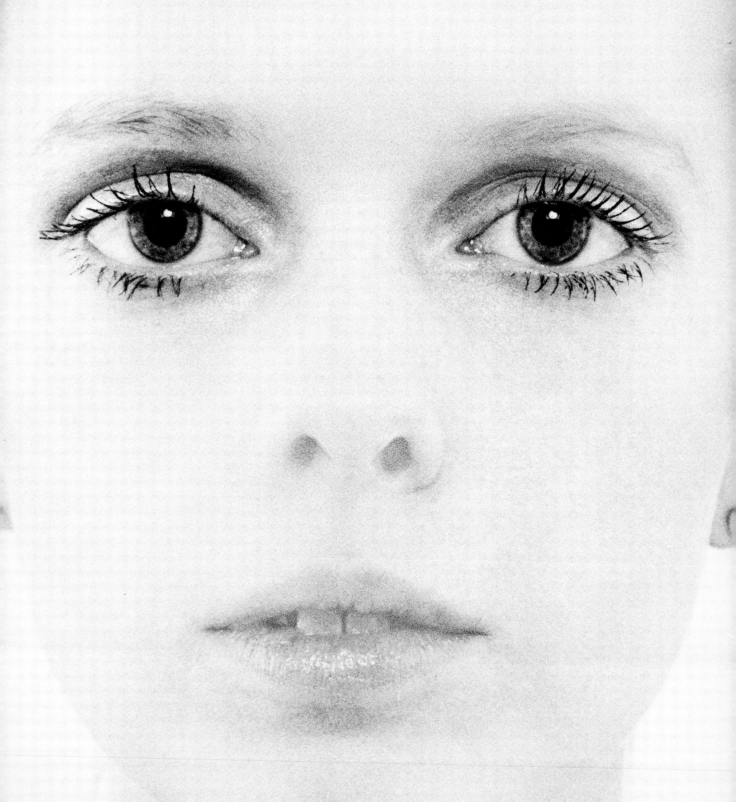

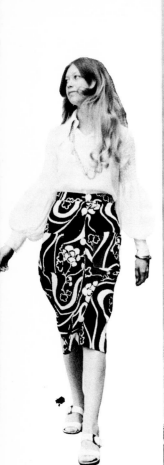

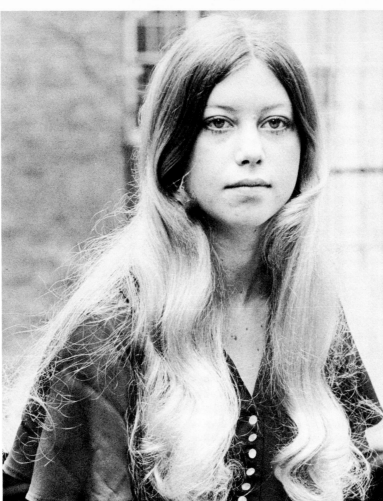

BEFORE

Lifestyle
makeover

HIGH SCHOOL
TO COLLEGE

Whether it's just a slight refresher course or a real cram session, practically every girl needs to do some boning up on her beauty know-how before starting college. Jane Carlough, the girl in this makeover, knew the look she wanted — easy, unfussy but together; she just needed some help to pull it off. There's also the problem of scheduling the time you have to spend on your college look — and the 8-minute beauty cram program we gave Jane to follow for her first year on campus is charted out in detail on the next pages. Jane's hair, like so many girls', had been lightened at home. This do-it-yourself project backfired when her hair started to break. She stopped the lightening and so was face to face with six inches of brown roots. She was also styling her hair so that it emphasized her too-round face, as you can see in the before photograph above.

Hair solution: A simple light streaking job is often the answer to lightened hair that's growing out. Light streaking only has to be done about three times a year instead of the almost monthly touch-ups required for all-over blonde coloring. The streaks blended in beautifully with Jane's brown hair and made the demarcation between the brown top and blonde bottom scarcely noticeable. Eventually when her hair has grown out completely Jane can stop the streaking altogether, if she likes, without any obvious gap. Our beauty editors took Jane to the Kenneth Salon in New York for her streaking and also a new styling. You can see how little was really changed but what a great difference it made to the contour of her face. Jane's hair was trimmed and shaped all around, and the shorter front pieces of hair shortened still further so that they would fall into the slightest curls or waves over her round cheeks, thereby slimming them instead of exposing them. We also showed Jane how to wear her hair up for a change, opposite page top, with the little tendrils curling into her cheeks and the back hair swirled up in a bun.

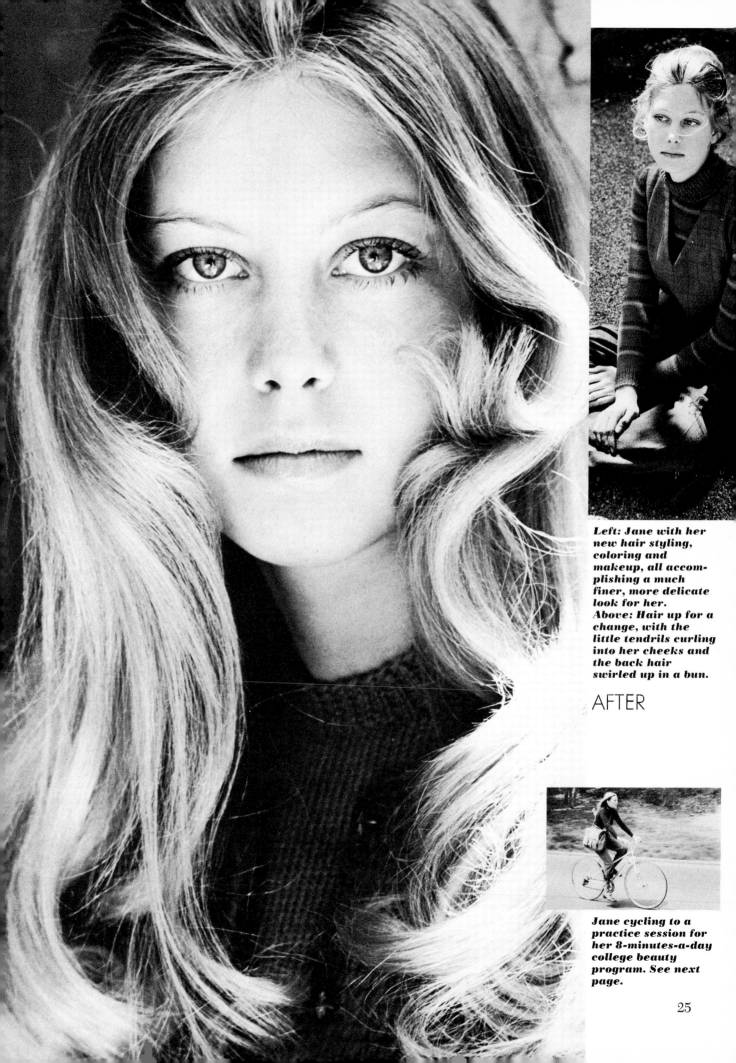

Left: Jane with her
new hair styling,
coloring and
makeup, all accom-
plishing a much
finer, more delicate
look for her.
Above: Hair up for a
change, with the
little tendrils curling
into her cheeks and
the back hair
swirled up in a bun.

AFTER

Jane cycling to a
practice session for
her 8-minutes-a-day
college beauty
program. See next
page.

BEFORE

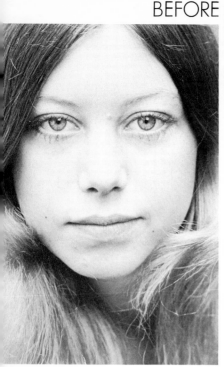

AFTER

Makeup solution: To further slim Jane's face we suggested she play up her eyes, drawing attention away from the cheeks. The play-up—a pale lime transparent shadow that made her blue eyes bluer, and lots of mascara on the top and bottom lashes to frame them. Jane also switched to a tawny pink transparent moisturizer base to warm her pale skin and added a pink blusher to define her cheekbones, again drawing the emphasis from the roundness of her cheeks.

8 minutes a day cram beauty program

For a smooth, straight flow of hair, wrap-set it in six minutes. Shampoo and towel-dry, comb snarl-free. Center and quarter part it from ear to ear, *see sketch opposite.*
Wrap hair clockwise. To begin wrapping, pick up section 1 and comb it across the center part into section 2. Keep smoothing and combing. Now start to wrap section 2 (with section 1 already wrapped into it) into section 3. Keep combing so that hair is smooth. Comb section 3 into 4. When all the hair is wrapped, anchor with bobby pins and let dry. You can pin as you work if that is easier. Practice will make you a pro.

		MON.	TUES.	WED.	THURS.	FRI.	SAT.	SUN.
MAKEUP		**3 minutes daily** Moisturizer Blusher Mascara on lash tips Lipgloss					**Festive addition: 3-minute face** plus 1 extra minute for eye shadow	
EXERCISE		**1 minute** Posture exercise						
HAIR		**6 minutes** Head wrap (after shampoo)				**6 minutes** Head wrap (after shampoo)	**4 minutes** Set hair in electric rollers	
BODY		**4 minutes** 3-minute leg shave 1-minute body moisturizing after bath				**4 minutes** 3-minute leg shave 1-minute body moisturizing after bath	**6 minutes** Buff finger and toe nails while hair rollers cool	
TOTAL		14 min.	3 min.	3 min.	3 min.	13 min.	14 min.	3 min.

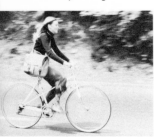

The heart of this cram routine, which we suggested Jane Carlough follow for her first year at college, is planning. Everything has its time allowance and time of the week. The schedule above organizes a girl's beauty time into an average of just eight neat minutes a day—some days a little more, others, less. The big point is not to put off what you should do today. Try this plan to keep your looks in shape and the time that you spend on them at a minimum.

26

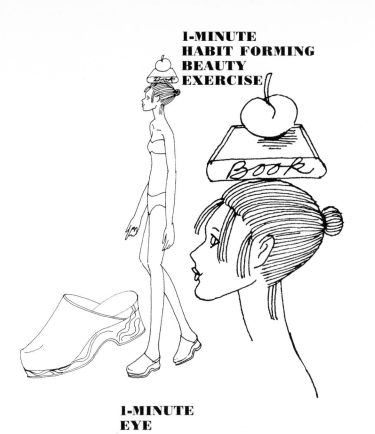

1-MINUTE
HABIT FORMING
BEAUTY
EXERCISE

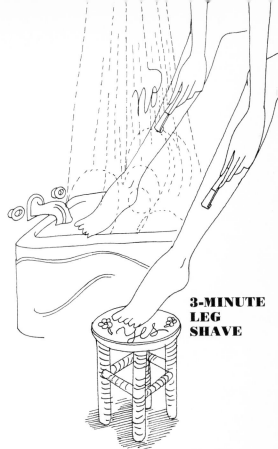

3-MINUTE
LEG
SHAVE

1-MINUTE
EYE

Highlighter

Shadow

To do the 3-minute make-up: Start with a moisturizer —tinted, if you like, for extra color. A generous smoothing will keep skin glowing, help prevent dryness, too. Next comes blusher. Pick a cream or gel that is see-through, and it's almost impossible to overdo. Add lots of lipgloss alone or over color. Flick the lashes with mascara and that's all there is to it. For special times, concentrate one minute more on your eyes. Mascara every lash more generously than usual, top and bottom. Use any transparent pastel shadow to circle the eye—*see diagram left*—and a pale highlighter under the brow.

To do the 1-minute exercise: Stand chin up, shoulders down and back, tummy tight and behind tucked in. Concentrate on every muscle. See if you can balance a book on your head, and try walking around in clogs with wooden soles that your feet muscles have to grasp in order to keep them on.

Leg shaving tip: Shave legs *before* you shower. This way the water and soap from your shower won't have a chance to soften your skin to the point where it's easily nicked. Just be sure you use soap or some other shaving preparation first.

6 MINUTES
TO SHINING
STRAIGHT
HAIR

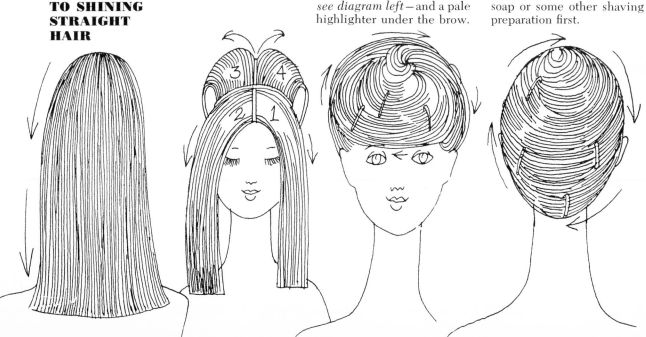

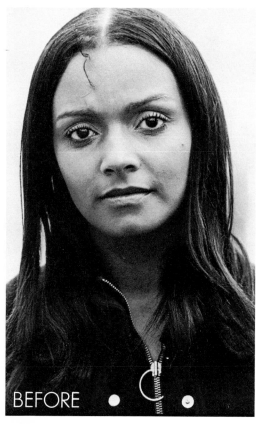

BEFORE

Lifestyle makeover

HOW TO TAKE YOUR LOOKS FROM COLLEGE TO JOB

If you're about to move into your first post-college job or if you're working now and balancing college at the same time, like Wynona Blackman here, things will run a lot smoother if you makeover your looks to suit your current lifestyle. What you need especially if you're working in a large city is a crash makeover program to pick up some of the loose beauty ends that usually aren't noticed on campus but show up in an office—plus a daily up-keep routine that takes only a matter of minutes. While Wynona was taking night courses in psychology in New York, she had a collection of part-time and free-lance jobs to help pay her tuition. Since she was constantly shuttling between class

and office she needed a makeup that was natural but not too bare-faced and that took the barest minimum of time to put on and keep on. She needed a basic wardrobe of things she could do with her hair under different situations—hair was her biggest beauty problem—you'll read more about it on the following pages. Part I in Wynona's makeover was a beauty analysis by our editors. Plusses: Her beautiful golden brown skin, hand-somely shaped lips and big direct tender dark eyes. Minuses: Hair weakened and straggly from straight-ening, a minor scar on her forehead that she was calling attention to by trying to hide, deep-color circles under her eyes.

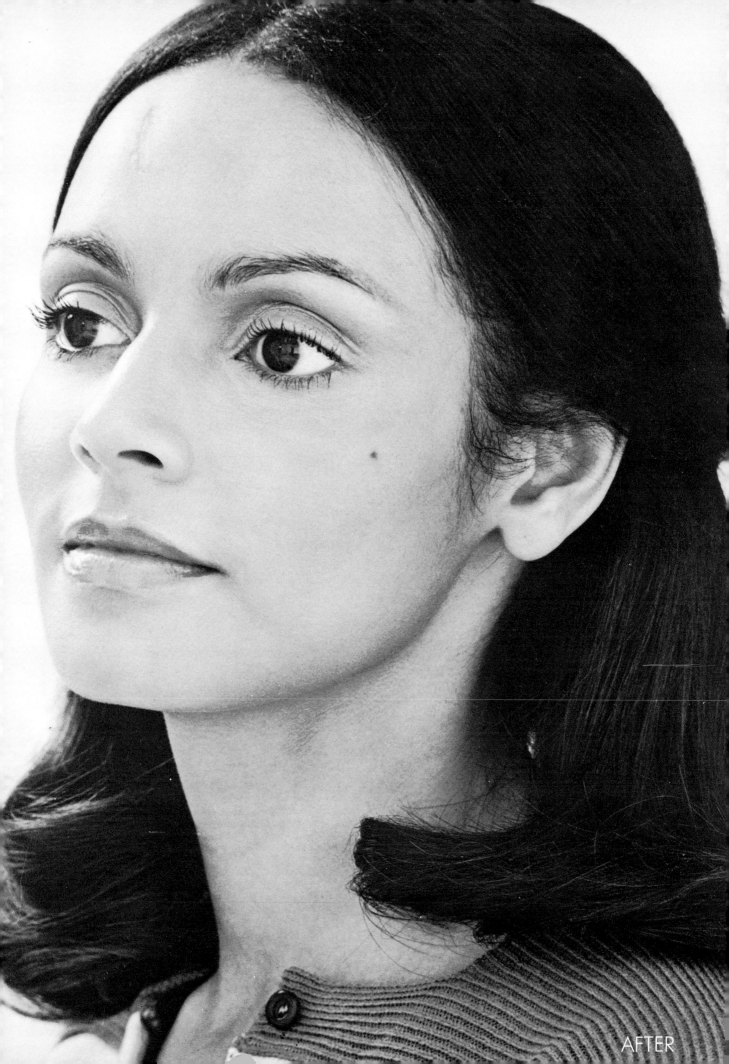

AFTER

4-minute makeup

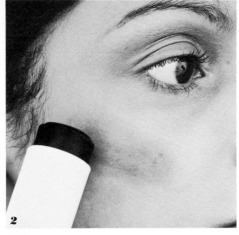

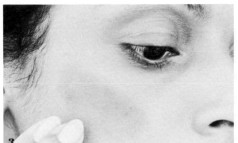

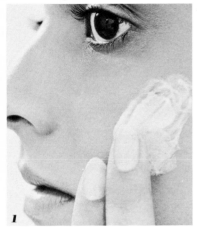

1

2

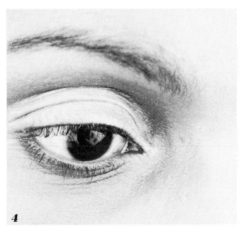

3

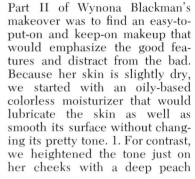

4

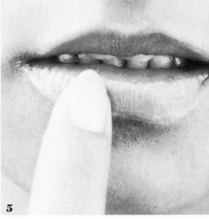

5

Part II of Wynona Blackman's makeover was to find an easy-to-put-on and keep-on makeup that would emphasize the good features and distract from the bad. Because her skin is slightly dry, we started with an oily-based colorless moisturizer that would lubricate the skin as well as smooth its surface without changing its pretty tone. 1. For contrast, we heightened the tone just on her cheeks with a deep peach transparent gel. 2, 3. If you have dark-toned skin, always pick your blusher in a strong rose or peach, not a bronze or tan that will get lost, and use it intensely, perhaps even blending in a second coat. 4. Then to lighten the circles around Wynona's eyes we at first suggested a pale coverup but this only put them in a pasty light. The solution was to shadow the entire upper eyelid and just under the lid—with a color. We chose mauve. Color put under the lower lid actually shows up as color instead of looking pasty. Also a little colorless gloss, which we suggested for over the eyebone, attracts light. 5. Next, her lips. Wynona had been using a transparent winey red stain to bring them out because she knew they were a good feature. But instead of highlighting, the dark stain with her dark skin tone made the lips recede. We suggested clear gloss—see results, *left*.

BEFORE

AFTER

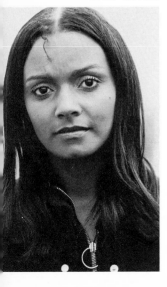

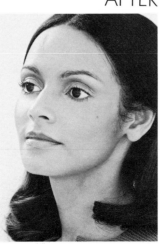

COLLEGE
TO JOB

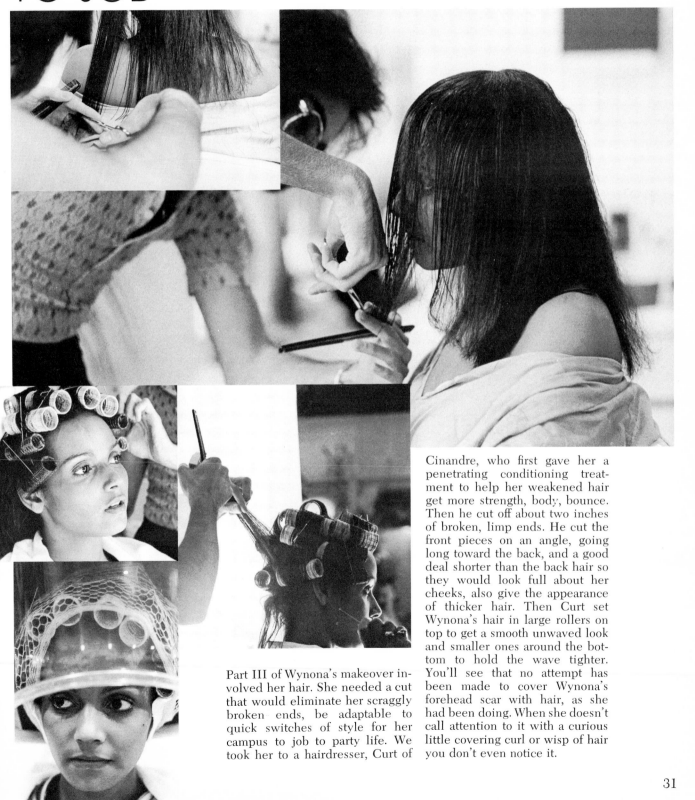

Part III of Wynona's makeover involved her hair. She needed a cut that would eliminate her scraggly broken ends, be adaptable to quick switches of style for her campus to job to party life. We took her to a hairdresser, Curt of

Cinandre, who first gave her a penetrating conditioning treatment to help her weakened hair get more strength, body, bounce. Then he cut off about two inches of broken, limp ends. He cut the front pieces on an angle, going long toward the back, and a good deal shorter than the back hair so they would look full about her cheeks, also give the appearance of thicker hair. Then Curt set Wynona's hair in large rollers on top to get a smooth unwaved look and smaller ones around the bottom to hold the wave tighter. You'll see that no attempt has been made to cover Wynona's forehead scar with hair, as she had been doing. When she doesn't call attention to it with a curious little covering curl or wisp of hair you don't even notice it.

Shuttling between jobs, classes and dates, sometimes with no chance to go home to freshen up, Wynona needs her own capsule portable makeup kit—so does any girl. We got it down to these essentials: stick of transparent gel blusher for cheek touch-ups, small powder compact to cover any shine, cotton swabs to remove makeup smudges, lipgloss, eye shadow and mascara. We also suggested that she keep a few staples in a desk drawer; paper-thin linen facial blotters, emery boards, makeup brushes, liquid makeup remover, moisturizer for face and hands, and a cologne atomizer.

COLLEGE

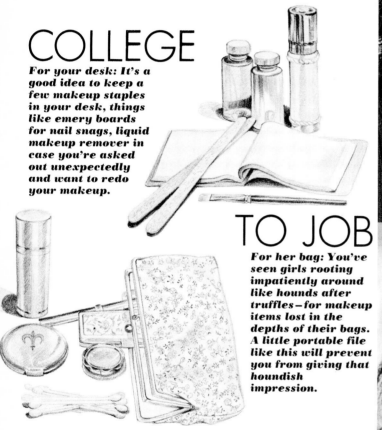

For your desk: It's a good idea to keep a few makeup staples in your desk, things like emery boards for nail snags, liquid makeup remover in case you're asked out unexpectedly and want to redo your makeup.

TO JOB

For her bag: You've seen girls rooting impatiently around like hounds after truffles—for makeup items lost in the depths of their bags. A little portable file like this will prevent you from giving that houndish impression.

Her organized makeup plan

Top right: This head was done by adding two small hairpieces, little clump just over the ears, after side parting hair in front, center parting it in back and catching it into two pony tails at the ears. Each tail is held with a coated elastic band, to protect Wynona's brittle hair, and a section of her own hair, about a pencil's thickness is wrapped around the band to hide it. The look is easy and fun for campus.

Bottom right: This head is soft and casual enough for campus and also for Wynona's part time jobs. It is the brush out for the set you saw done step by step on the preceding page.

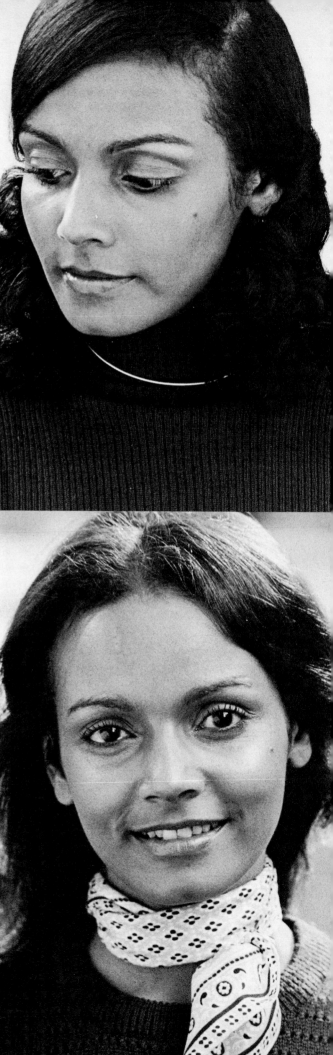

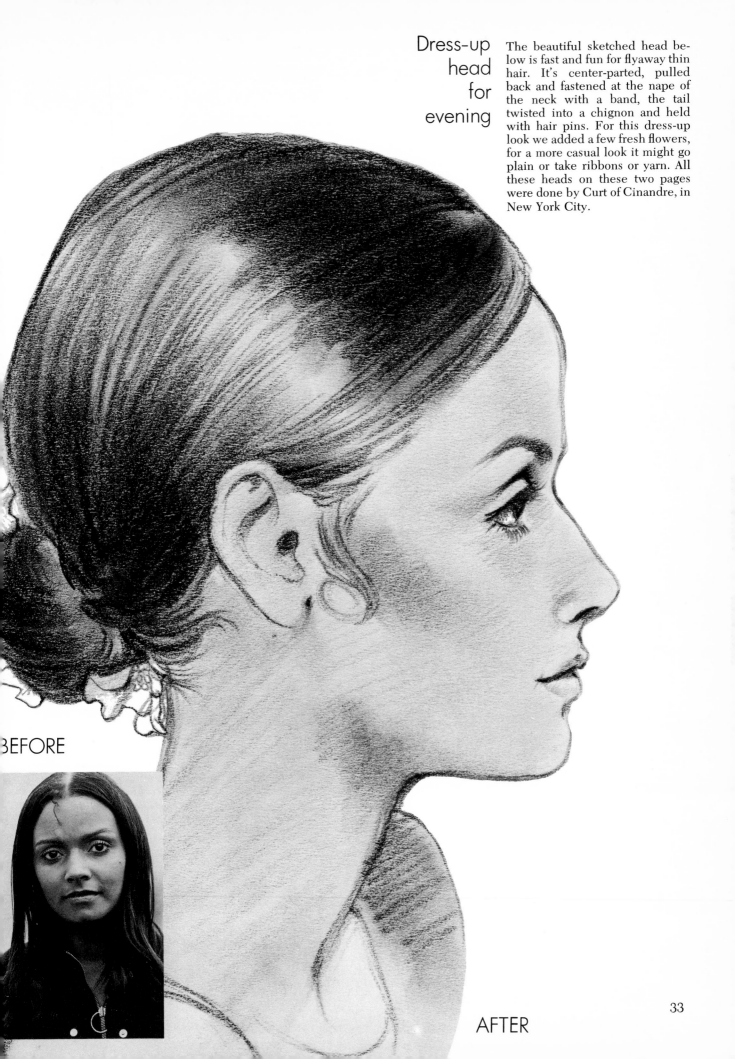

Dress-up head for evening

The beautiful sketched head below is fast and fun for flyaway thin hair. It's center-parted, pulled back and fastened at the nape of the neck with a band, the tail twisted into a chignon and held with hair pins. For this dress-up look we added a few fresh flowers, for a more casual look it might go plain or take ribbons or yarn. All these heads on these two pages were done by Curt of Cinandre, in New York City.

BEFORE

AFTER

33

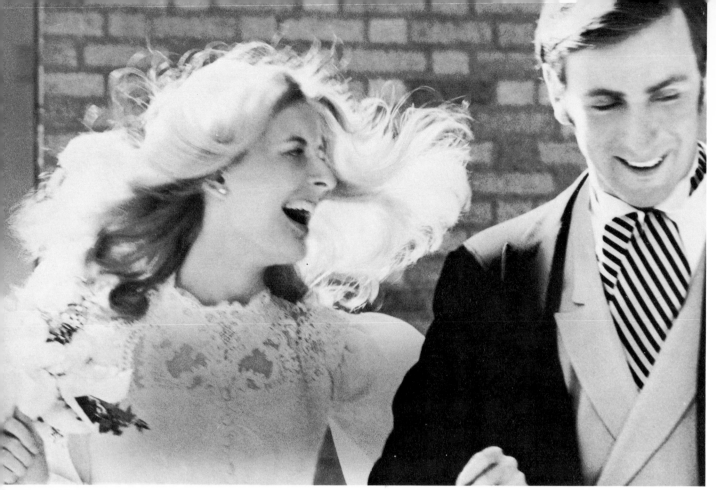

A lifestyle makeover prepares a girl to meet a real change in her life. It anticipates the bumps and gives her the means to get over them with ease and assurance. Take the switch from singledom to marriage—ecstasy and agony. No one is spared "wedding nerves" and Susan Wellacott—*above* with her new husband, Thomas Coyne—was no exception. But her GLAMOUR lifestyle makeover taught her to challenge the nerves before they really got to her. Susie started a crash program of organizing herself to choose china, buy gifts for her bridesmaids, put her new wardrobe together—all on her lunch hour. Actually it sounds wild, but continuing to work (Susie is an assistant editor) right up to the wedding is one of the smartest things a girl can do—time-, money- and nerve-wise. Our beauty editors also pointed out it was time for Susie to work out a new beauty routine. She'll have much less time to fuss with her hair and makeup, so a new schedule was planned including no-roller setting (Susie doesn't want her husband to see her in rollers) and a natural makeup that only takes minutes. See next pages.

SINGLE-TO- MARRIED SWITCH

Lifestyle makeover

The sensational swing of hair, *far right*, not only looks marvelous, it's a snap to keep up. It's the result of a haircut and drying technique that frees Susie from the old roller routine. Now she can just blow her hair dry in minutes. She has a new makeup plan, too, that gives her the soft pinked look here—all part of the switch to a new lifestyle. Hair *above* and *far right* by Maury Hopson.

34

BEFORE   AFTER

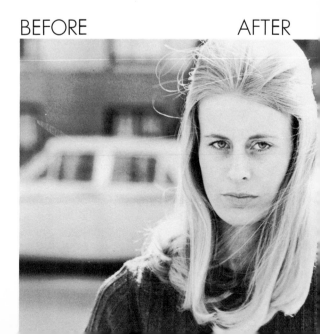

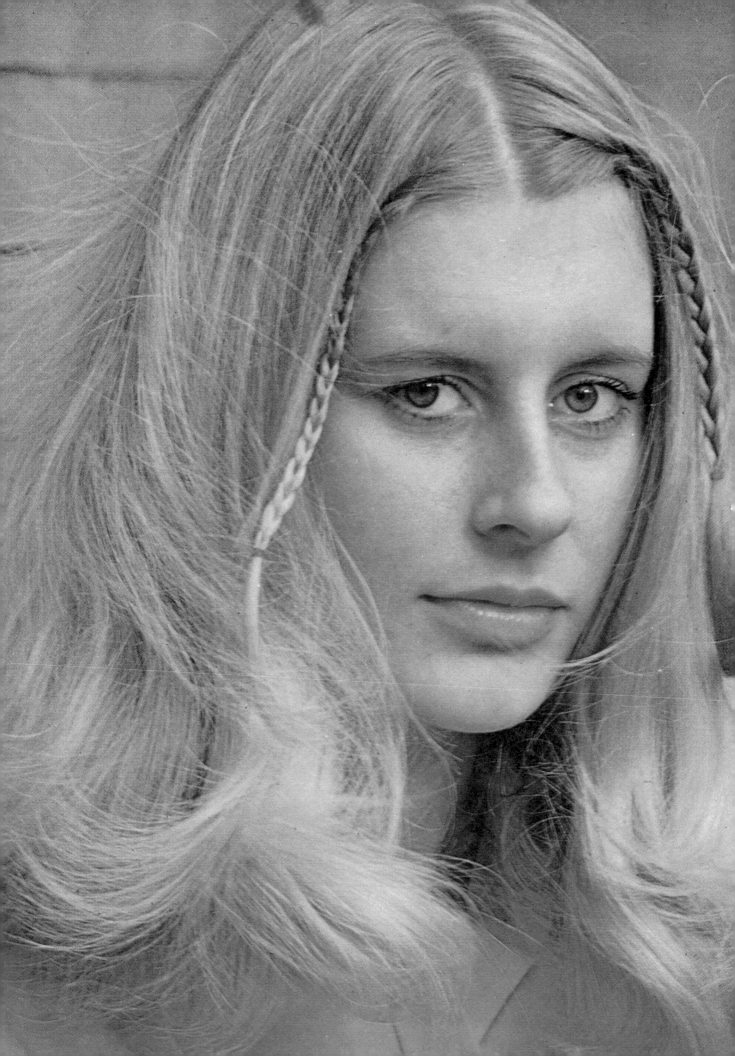

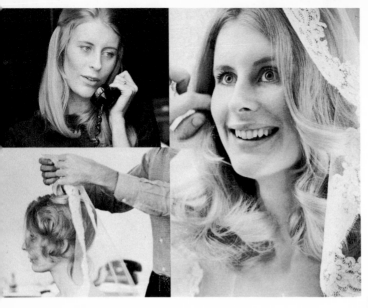

SINGLE-TO-MARRIED LIFESTYLE

More hair freedom

Hair was Susie's big problem—it's curly and tends to be unruly after it's washed. GLAMOUR suggested she have a micro-layer cut (top layer is cut slightly shorter than the bottom for more swing and control) and that she experiment with hairstyles and her wedding headpiece well in advance. The cut is so sensational she doesn't need to set her hair anymore. She just blows it dry by using a hand hair dryer plus a brush. The principle of blowing hair dry is to use the brush to smooth the hair and give it a line as it dries. Cutting the very front pieces of Susie's hair chin-length reduced their tendency to kink up after shampooing and gave her the flexibility to try the new looks too, *opposite*. Susie's one big splurge was to have her hairdresser Maury Hopson come to her home an hour or so before the wedding to help her arrange hair and headpiece together. She felt it was well worth the price and a perfect last-minute tranquilizer for wedding nerves.

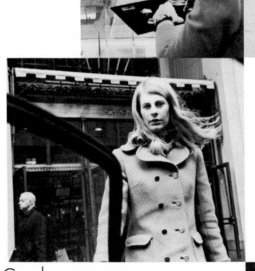

Crash program for lunch hours

Susie resolved not to let all the things she wanted to get done before her wedding throw her into panic. So once a week, usually Sunday evening, she sat down and organized what she wanted to get done during that week's five lunch hours. That's how she managed to pick a wedding dress, buy attendants' gifts, select a china pattern and dozens of other things without feeling pressured.

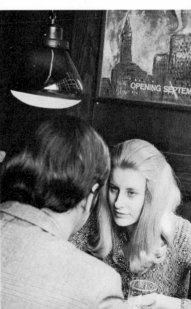

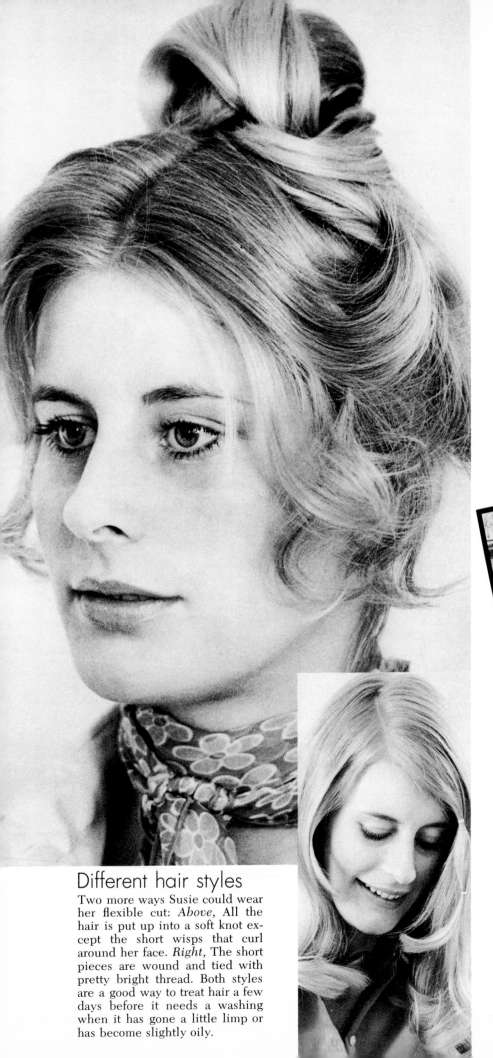

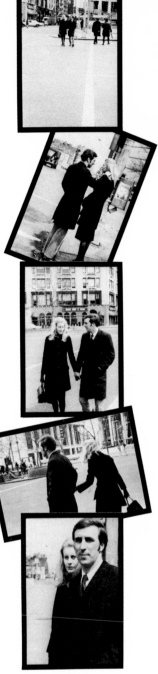

Different hair styles

Two more ways Susie could wear her flexible cut: *Above,* All the hair is put up into a soft knot except the short wisps that curl around her face. *Right,* The short pieces are wound and tied with pretty bright thread. Both styles are a good way to treat hair a few days before it needs a washing when it has gone a little limp or has become slightly oily.

Time for fun too

Even though Susie did fill most of her lunches with errands, she always left at least one noon free to be with Tom for a leisurely lunch together, *opposite page left,* or a quick lunch and walk, *above.* "Leaving no time for some fun together just before the wedding can start a marriage off on a somewhat tense footing," said Susie.

37

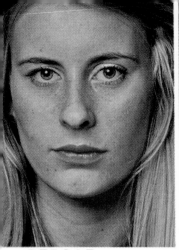

BEFORE

If there's one thing that gets scarce in the switch from a single lifestyle to a married one, it's time. One of the big musts for Susan Wellacott was a quick natural makeup plan to use for everyday and with some special touches — for evening. The "instant natural face" GLAMOUR gave Susie here looked so smashing she used it for her wedding day. Above, 1, Susie's blonde hair and slightly sallow skin seemed to melt into each other. For a natural pink look, we used a very pink mauve under makeup moisturizer all over the face and throat, 2 & 3, then a slick of deep blushed rose on the cheeks, 4.

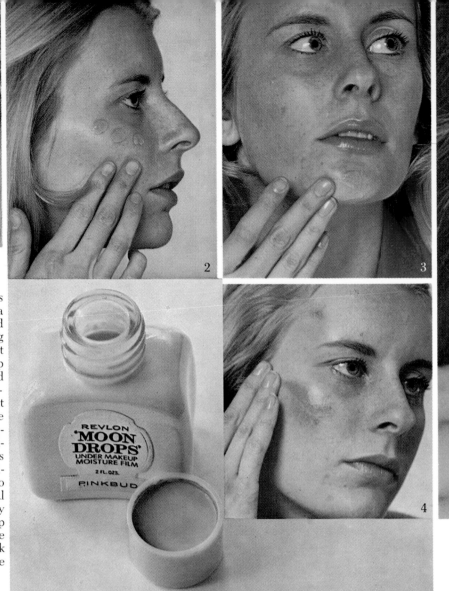

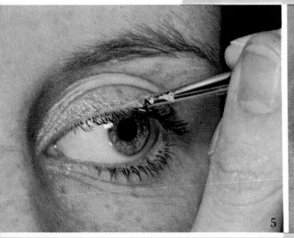

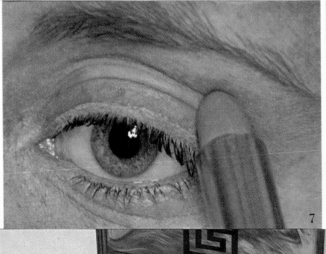

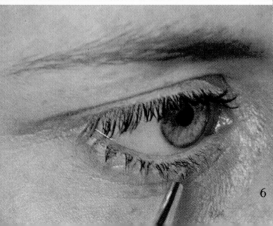

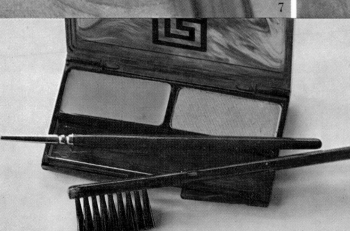

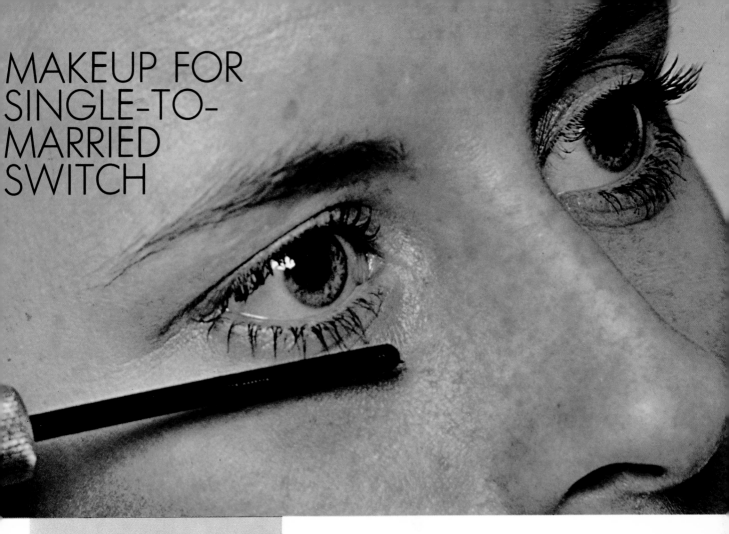

MAKEUP FOR SINGLE-TO-MARRIED SWITCH

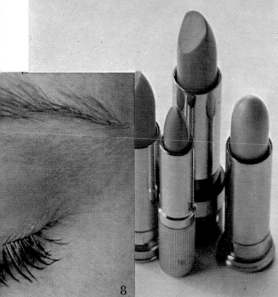

8

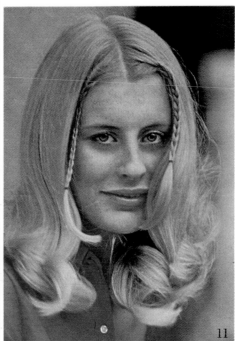

11
AFTER

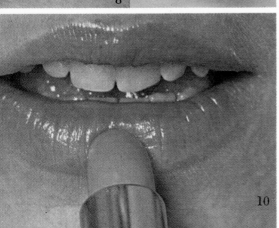

10

The softest line of color plus transparent shadow brings the eyes into focus here. To make Susie's pale blue eyes seem a more intense blue, the thinnest line of bright blue frost cake liner is drawn on the upper lid at the base of the lashes, 5. In 6, the same color is softly dotted below lower lashes. Since blue shadow above the eyes made Susie's look gray, we advised a delicate lavender stick shadow blended over the lid up to the brow bone, 7. Her brows were brushed with a soft brow brush to give them form and shape. For thick, full-looking lashes, lots of black mascara from a wand was stroked on top and bottom lashes, 9. The result, 8, is a completely natural eye. To finish the "instant natural face," Susie applied a bit of apricot lipstick, 10, plus lots of colorless lipgloss that adds a sexy sheen, 11. Another way for Susy to wear her microlayered new haircut.

BEFORE

Judy had let her hair go, seldom had time for even the barest makeup in the morning, so that casual for her sometimes slipped into haphazard.

FROM CAREER WIFE TO MOTHER

This makeover doesn't start with the usual ticking off of good and bad features, although, of course, that's involved, too. It starts instead with a long, honest look at exactly how many things you have to do each day and how much time you can afford to spend on each one. Judy Conze, the young woman in this makeover, had just added some important elements to her daily life: a new baby, a house in the suburbs instead of a city apartment to take care of, more shopping—and not just a walk around the corner but a drive to the nearest shopping center— plus two trips a day to pick up and deliver her husband to the train. In short, Judy needed help, and that's where GLAMOUR's beauty editors took over. We introduced her to some new time-saving ideas, like hair styles for electric rollers and a special kitchen makeup kit. To see how it was all done have a look at the following pages.

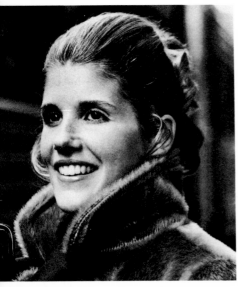

AFTER

Judy with her hair swept casually back to meet her husband at the train in the evening, a quick little hairdo that any hairdresser could show you how to adapt to your own hair texture and style, either without a hairpiece if your own is long enough, or with one if it isn't.

AFTER

A polished Judy and her daughter, Nichola

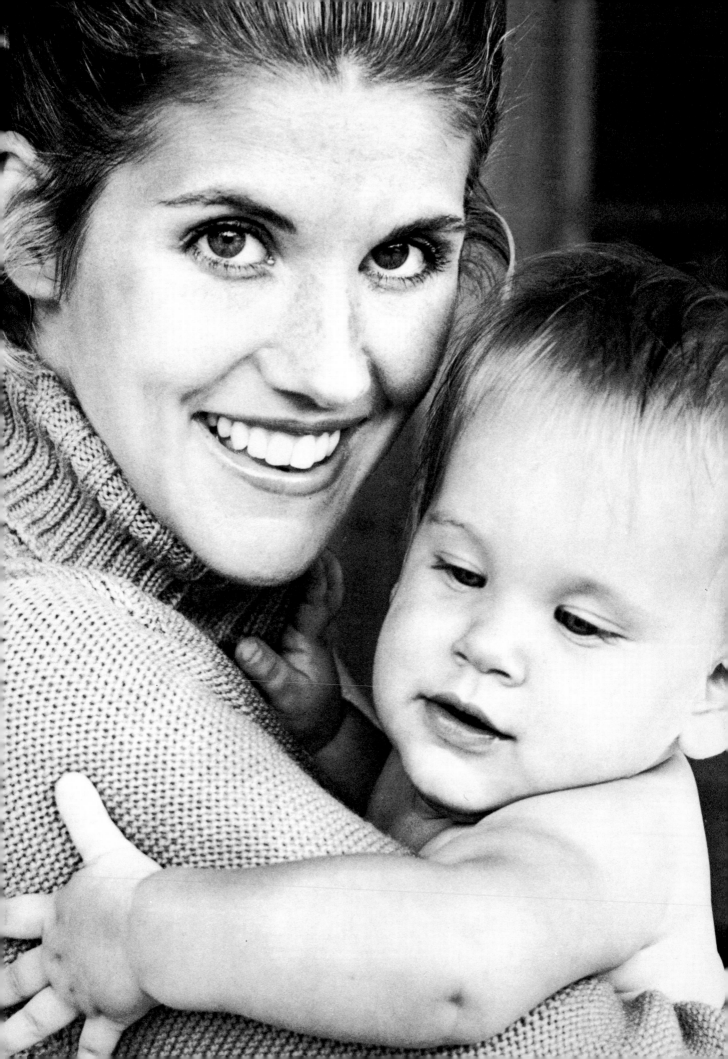

FROM
CAREER WIFE
TO MOTHER

Once Judy Conze and our editors had a good look at her daily routine, it seemed the soundest idea to divide her day into two parts. Morning was the most hectic—breakfast, shopping and so forth—so fussing with makeup and clothes had to be kept to a minimum. In the evening, when she wanted to look more appealing to pick up her husband for dinner with a few friends or for just the two of them, she needed a more finished hair style.

Beauty changes:

Since Judy has good healthy skin, she needs only a cleansing routine to start each morning, plus an occasional pick-up facial mask, and a thorough cleansing before bed. She had a professional facial at a salon, too, but actually you can do facials at home easily with any kind of mask you like; just follow the directions on the label. She also had her eyebrows shaped at the salon to learn how to lift them.

Morning time-saver routine:

The quick makeup routine we gave Judy requires nothing in the morning but a clean face braced with a light astringent to absorb any excess oil. Then a slick of moisturizer. Mascara, blusher and lipgloss; that's all.

Special occasion:

Judy's special occasion makeup: First, for circles or shadows under eyes, *right top*, she uses a faint blushed coverup, *right center*. Over that and her entire face and throat, a smoothing of beige foundation with moisturizer in it. She is careful to even the foundation out over a spray of freckles across

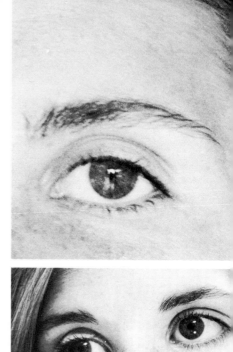

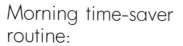

her nose. Then Judy smoothes a terra-cotta cream blusher across her cheeks—it makes you look as if you have just the faintest, most delicious sunny glow. With dark blue eyes like her's nothing is prettier than a mauve shadow over the entire lid. Instead of heavy eyeliner, which tends to close the eyes, she opens and brightens them with lots of black mascara on the upper and lower lashes. A tawny lipstick plus an overcoat of colorless gloss finishes the job.

Hand savers and time savers

Judy's hands showed the effects of the furniture refinishing she had been doing. Hand cream, cuticle cream and a good nail buffing changed the picture to the pretty one, *below*. In the future we suggested she wear rubber gloves with globs of cream under the nails.

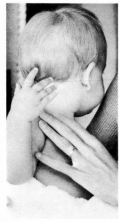

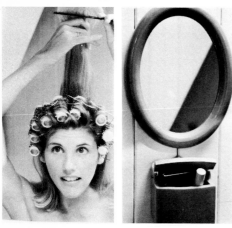

Judy now knows how to use electric rollers, *above left*, to give her hair body or curl enough for any style she wants in a few minutes. *Right*, She now keeps a small mirror and little makeup box in the kitchen, so she can put on her makeup—mascara, blusher, lipgloss—at the same time she is getting her family's breakfast.

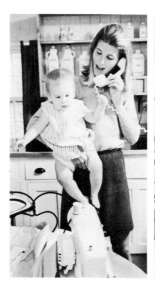

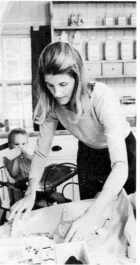

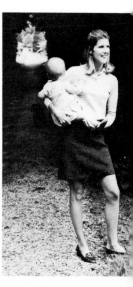

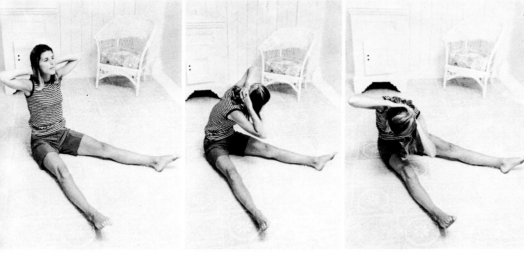

Bringing up
your figure
after baby

2-months-after-baby-comes, exercises for the waist

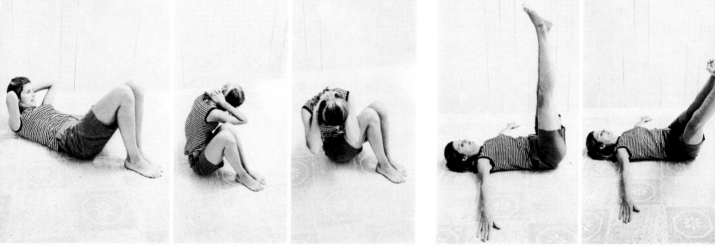

Exercises to get the stomach in shape: first three photographs; last two photographs show more waist trimmers

New mother exercises:

Judy needed daily exercise to bring her figure back to its pre-pregnancy firmness, so we suggested the ones above, subject to her doctor's approval. Waist: Sit with legs apart, fingers clasped behind neck. Reach left knee with right elbow, keeping left elbow as high as possible. Then switch. Do six times, each side, increase to twelve. Waist again: Lie with arms at side, legs in air. Slowly lower legs halfway, first to left, then to right. Do six times each side, increase to twelve. Stomach: Lie with knees bent, fingers clasped behind neck. Sit up bring arms to outside of left knee, then right. Do three times each. Bosom: This exercise can help support a flabby bosom by tightening up the muscles that surround it. Grasp wrists, as in photograph *right*, elbows bent and at shoulder level. Push elbows toward each other, wrists firm, for six seconds, relax and repeat six times. These body firming exercises can start about two months after the baby is born.

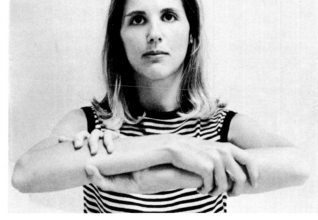

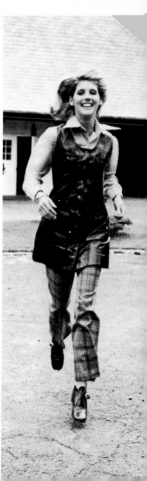

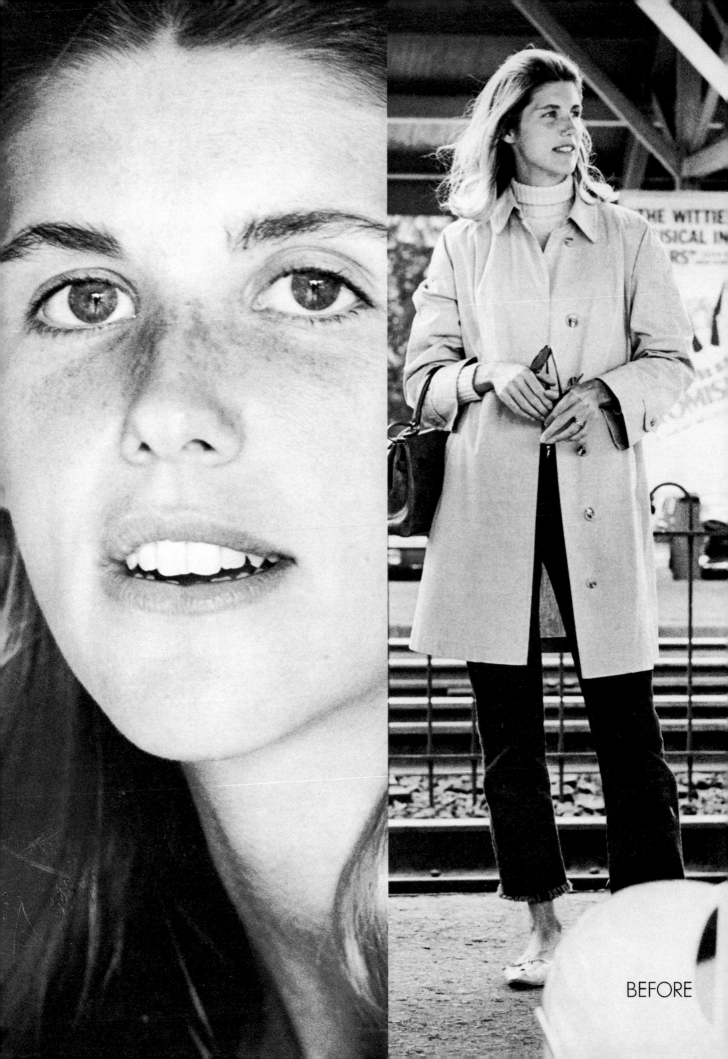

BEFORE

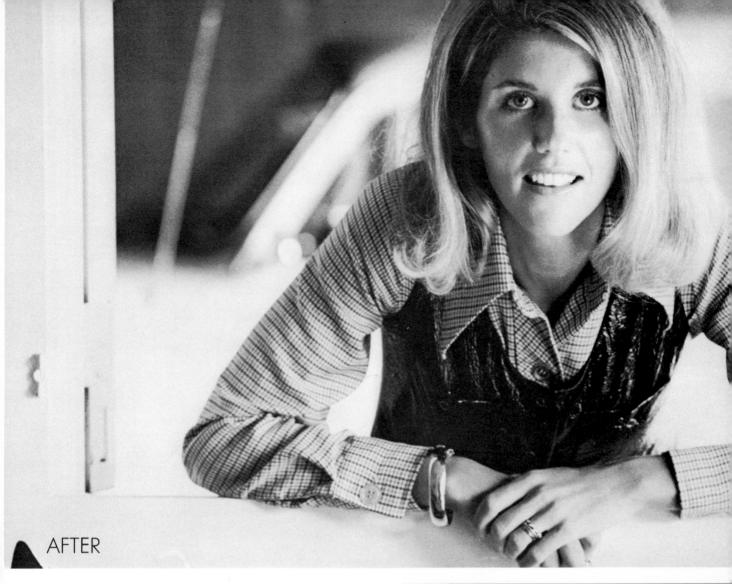

AFTER

FROM CAREER WIFE TO MOTHER

One of Judy Conze's predominant needs was a good basic hairstyling that she could adapt to different looks. On the *opposite page,* you see her at the station as she used to look when she took her husband to meet his train or picked him up —a girl without any makeup because she didn't have time, a girl with hair that had gone so long without a cut that the shape was limp and the ends beginning to split. Our beauty editors pointed out that a visit to a good beauty salon every six weeks or so for a trim would make the upkeep in between visits simpler. We took Judy to the Elizabeth Arden Salon where Adrienne brightened the color of her light brown hair by adding more pale blonde highlights, which would need little touching up, as little as two or three times a year. Then Alain Gervais gave her a good cut, showed her the soft casual style you see *above* and how to make the pony tail wrapped with tiny braids, *right*, for evening. A few minutes with electric rollers give Judy enough body and curl for both of these styles.

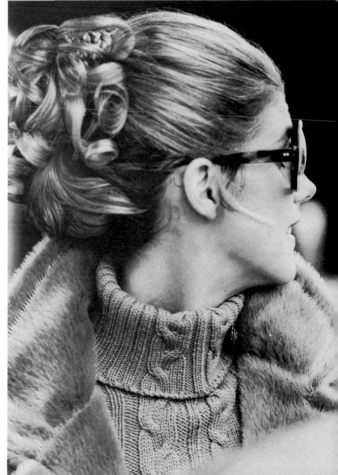

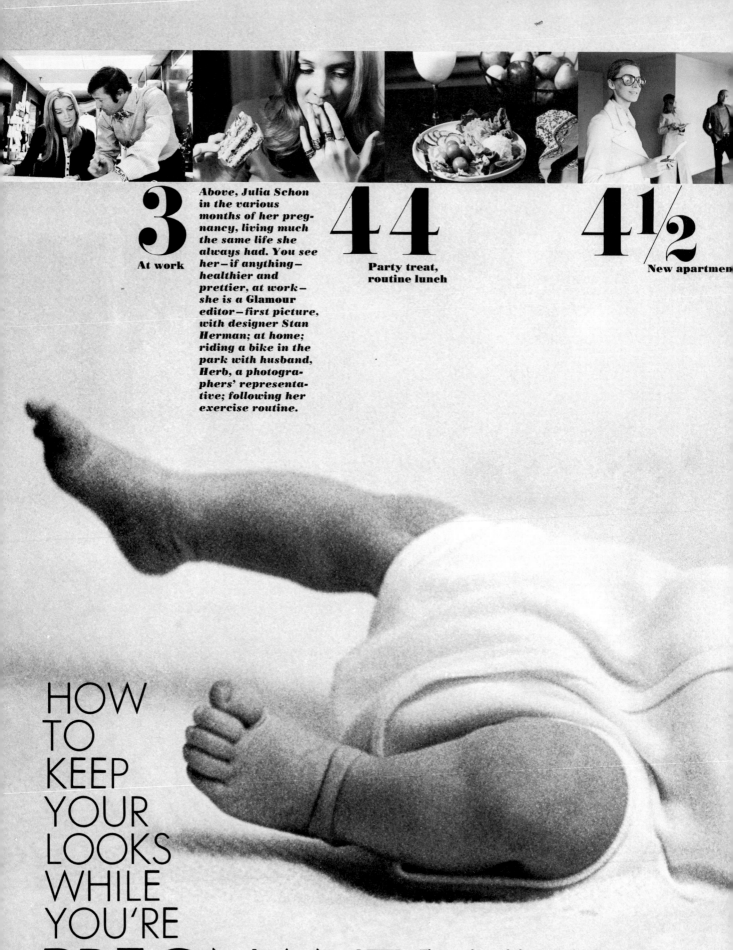

3 At work

Above, Julia Schon in the various months of her pregnancy, living much the same life she always had. You see her—if anything—healthier and prettier, at work— she is a Glamour editor—first picture, with designer Stan Herman; at home; riding a bike in the park with husband, Herb, a photographers' representative; following her exercise routine.

44 Party treat, routine lunch

4½ New apartment

HOW TO KEEP YOUR LOOKS WHILE YOU'RE PREGNANT

The mother of five-pound, eleven-ounce Peter Baird Schon, *above*, promised herself that she was going to look as good as she felt the day her doctor told her she was pregnant. She refused to slip into the drag of saying "I'm pregnant, I can't do any-

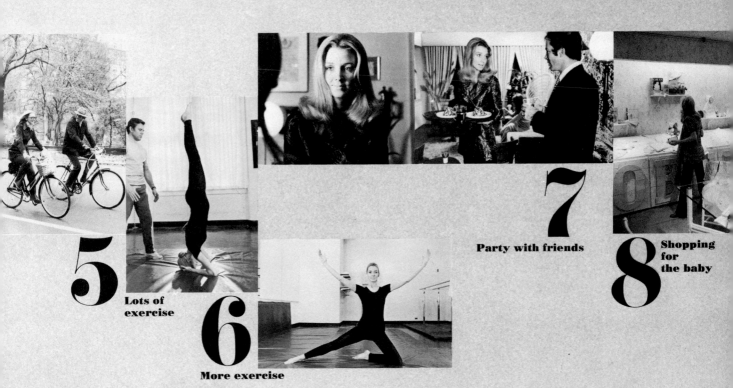

5 Lots of exercise

6 More exercise

7 Party with friends

8 Shopping for the baby

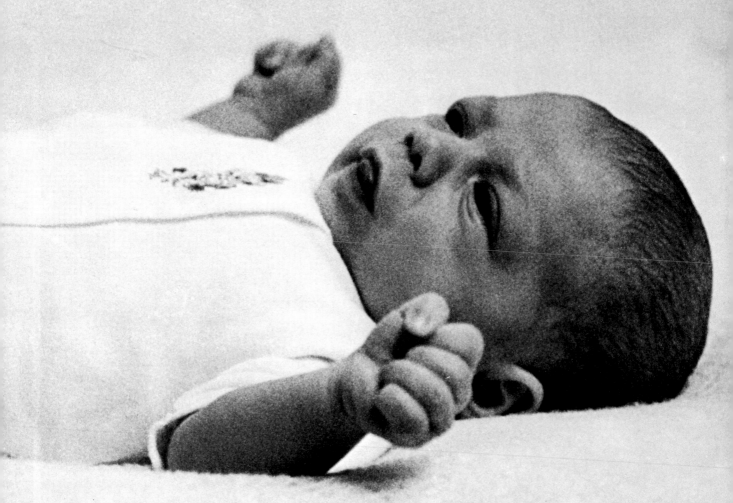

thing." In the course of keeping that promise, Julia Schon made sound discoveries about how to look and feel great right up to the minute the baby is born. The health and beauty routines she started during pregnancy can work as well for most ex- pectant mothers. Her attitude pays off not only during the months before the birth, but is also in- surance for a better figure and looks afterward. Here and on the next pages, follow Julia through the changes from her first to last month.

*Julia adapting her
regular lifestyle
to pregnancy.
Below, at work with
clothes designer
Stan Herman; office
lunch of salad
and milk substituted
for a sandwich.
Right, long jacket
with pants gives her
a neat slimming look.*

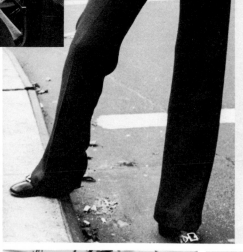

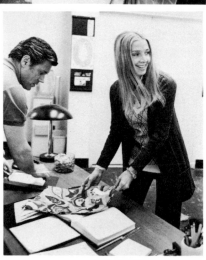

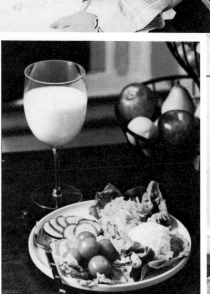

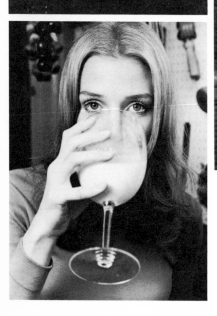

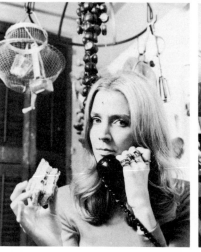

*Julia and husband,
Herb, going to
childbirth classes,
second row, right.
Directly above:
Julia signing in for
maternity exercises
with Larry at the
Gala Fitness Studios
in New York City.*

48

Behind any beautiful expectant mother is an enthusiastic beauty attitude, determination to keep looks and health polished and perfect. Julia Schon is proof of it. The single most important factor in her success was her decision *not* to consider herself any different from her unpregnant self. She insisted on making her regular lifestyle work while she was pregnant.

A lifestyle for pregnancy

Julia continued to work a full-time schedule, and doing it, she said, "was a morale booster." It gave her a psychological lift to be able to put in the effort. To counteract the tiredness she sometimes felt, Julia took an hour's nap every evening when she came home. The active physical life that she and her husband, Herb, like—skiing, bike riding, walking a lot—was something Julia would have felt sedentary without. Skiing was out of the question, but Julia substituted maternity exercise classes for it, and got more than her money's worth.

Maternity exercise classes

They were fun—with a half-dozen or so other expectant mothers. Julia's doctor approved of them, and she exercised twice a week for an hour each time. The exercises were not only assurance of firm muscle tone during pregnancy and after, but they helped take some of the stress off her back and stomach muscles. "It wasn't until the last two months that I really felt pregnant."

Most cities have maternity exercise classes and if this idea appeals to you, Julia suggests watching a session or two first to get the feeling of the thing. Then if you decide on the classes, be sure to check with your doctor.

Anxieties and beauty don't click

There isn't a woman in history who hasn't felt some fear at the thought of having her first child. Julia wasn't any different, but she discovered that after a few classes in natural childbirth, which both she

BEAUTY ROUTINE
For the first few months of pregnancy

and Herb signed up for, her anxieties began to relax. "Knowing what's going on in your body and what to expect helps even if you don't intend to have natural childbirth," Julia said. Besides, sharing this with your husband makes him feel a part of the whole venture; he doesn't get into the "left-out" syndrome. So many men really do begin to feel sacrificed, everything for the mother-to-be and baby, nothing for them.

No trick dieting

You have to face it—there aren't any substantial substitutes for the old high-protein, low-carbohydrate diet. Trick and fad dieting is less likely to work and less good for a pregnant woman, as Julia found out. In a rush of enthusiasm, the first day she found out she was pregnant she went to the supermarket and stocked up on all sorts of offbeat diet food, candies and sweets that she thought would satisfy her cravings. Most of them are still in her kitchen cabinet. In the first month she discovered that it was milk and eggs, lean meats and salads that satisfied her most, all parts of the high-protein, low-carbohydrate diet that most doctors prescribe. Really sticking to the diet in the first few months of pregnancy is a must, Julia thinks, and easier too. It was later, toward the end months, that she really started craving funny fattening things, like sodas at bedtime. If you're strict with yourself in the beginning, you can make a few exceptions later if the urges get harder to resist. Julia even found herself baking pies, which she never did before, but luckily a small slice was enough to satisfy her appetite.

How to turn some of your regular clothes looks into a maternity wardrobe

Practically everyone has at least one long cardigan sweater or long vest which are marvelous slimmers, plus a pair of jersey or other knitted pants. A few of Julia's pants fortunately had elastic waistbands which, of course, gave as she grew. At first she could wear her regular shirts, later she bought a few tops cut wider at the bottom, but not great full maternity smocks. She never really had to give up these put-togethers, and suggests that if your pants don't have elastic waistbands, you might invest in a pair or two that do. If you're not comfortable in pants, get the same slim look by wearing long cardigan sweaters or vests, shirts with skirts. A long scarf either tied like a man's tie or just looped softly at the neck with the ends trailing down the front is a perfect elongating accessory. More tips, next page.

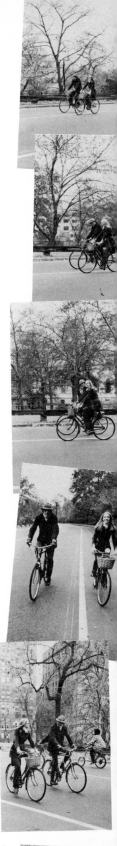

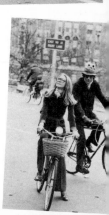

This is the time—those last draggy months—to pull out all the stops and find new beauty tricks and fashion ideas to lift your spirits. Going along with the fashion ideas started on the preceding pages—the non-maternity maternity look—now is the time to buy something new and fabulous. So many maternity dresses are so dull and unusable after the pregnancy. Julia solved that by substituting regular clothes that she was sure she could wear afterward. For instance, a wrap brocade jacket to wear with pants for evening; an A-shaped velvet dress. Anything that wraps, too, is a particularly good pregnancy look, especially if you have to buy a big-investment piece like a coat.

Exercises right up to the last day

The end is no time to let up on exercises, although on certain days Julia did find herself wondering if she had the strength. Once she got to her class, she said it was always a lift. She felt more supple physically and emotionally. In fact, the day Julia's labor began she was planning to go to her exercise class.

Skin and hair changes to make

Hormonal change can affect hair and skin, and pregnancy is a tremendous one. Julia found her normally-clear skin getting oilier and even had some breakout problems that were pretty depressing. She didn't let them run on, but went immediately to a dermatologist for something to help combat the changes. A trip to your skin doctor is really worth the fee because he can usually control the problems easily by giving you a new cleansing and treatment routine geared to cutting down the oil, or vice versa if your skin tends to dryness with pregnancy. He might prescribe a special shampoo and conditioner for hair which often takes on the same changes as skin, since the oil glands that feed the scalp feed skin as well. Julia's hair followed this pattern and became very oily. Besides more washings with a shampoo for oily hair, she used an instant dry shampoo and electric rollers for between-time pickups. Another super solution is streaking or sunbursting, which adds marvelous lights and body to hair, tends to make it somewhat drier.

Not the time to make big beauty changes on whim

Almost every girl has the temptation to change her looks completely in the last months of pregnancy—to cut long hair short, go to a completely different color, or whatever idea takes you. But don't do anything so drastic that you can't reverse it. The desire is often just a whim that you'll be sorry you gave in to. Julia had an urge to cut her long blond hair very short, but she compromised by going to Christiaan of Henri Bendel's salon and got a new styling, the top layer cut slightly shorter than the bottom to give her fine hair more bounce and make it easier to curl. That same day Gregory, the colorist, gave her a few light blond streaks just around the face. The new long cut also helped solve the problem of hair loss that is usually apparent shortly after childbirth. The loss is part of a natural process and eventually rights itself; there's nothing you can do to prevent it, but you can give the appearance of more hair by adopting a fuller styling for the time being.

Experiment with makeup

Makeup to Julia became the prettiest of pickups. Whenever she felt she looked tired, she experimented with colors—pale lime, mauve and blue shadows on the lids where she had never worn pastel shadow before. She learned to add tiny clusters of false lashes to her own. More color than usual seemed to work best for her and she added a sheer berry lipstain, lots of gloss, and blusher in a tawnier shade than usual. The more little attentions you can manage, the better. The psychological lift is worth every bit as much as the physical one.

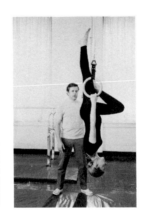

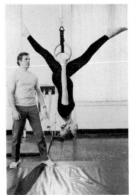

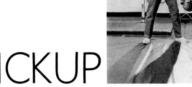

PICKUP IDEAS

For the last months of pregnancy

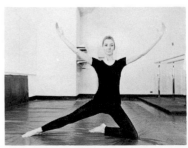

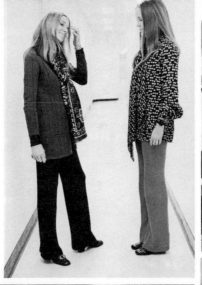

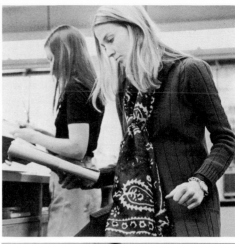

Right, Julia wears a long cardigan sweater, a shirt and Indian-printed scarf with pants. She found this one of her best pregnancy looks. Middle below, she experiments with more color in makeup and puts on little clusters of false eyelashes among her own.

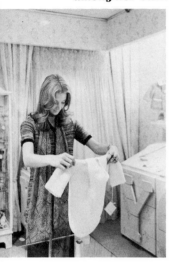

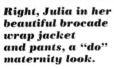

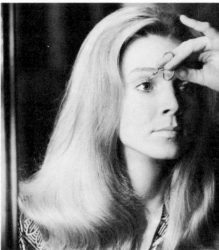

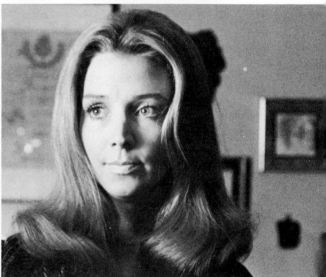

Right, Julia in her beautiful brocade wrap jacket and pants, a "do" maternity look.

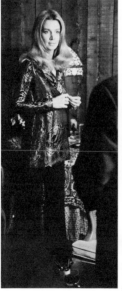

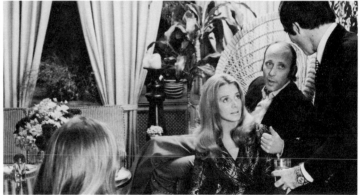

AFTER THE BABY

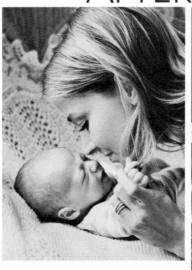

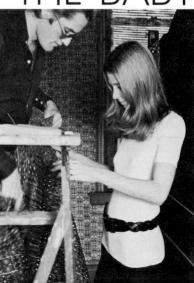

HELP FOR THE GIRL WHO'S PICKING UP THE PIECES
AFTER DIVORCE

"Going from marriage to a single lifestyle means developing a whole new attitude about yourself," says Yvonne Goodhue, a young divorcée who's learning that there are still new areas of her personality to explore. She is finding this new singleness completely different from her life before marriage. Besides having more responsibility for her son now, she feels that she's more mature, more concerned with making plans for a future. Sud- denly, she needs a new image that's more exciting and a wardrobe that's less casual and more job-date oriented. Her new lifestyle is not without problems and pressures, but on the whole she's found it a good challenge and actually more fun than she dared to hope. Following you can see how she changed her beauty image *below left* to the natural, fresh-spirited one *right*. Hair *right* by Paul Mitchell for The Crimpers.

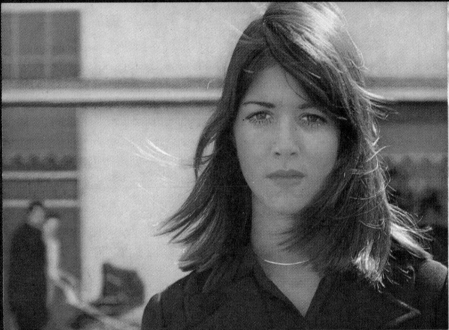

FRANCES McLAUGHLIN-GILL

BEFORE

AFTER

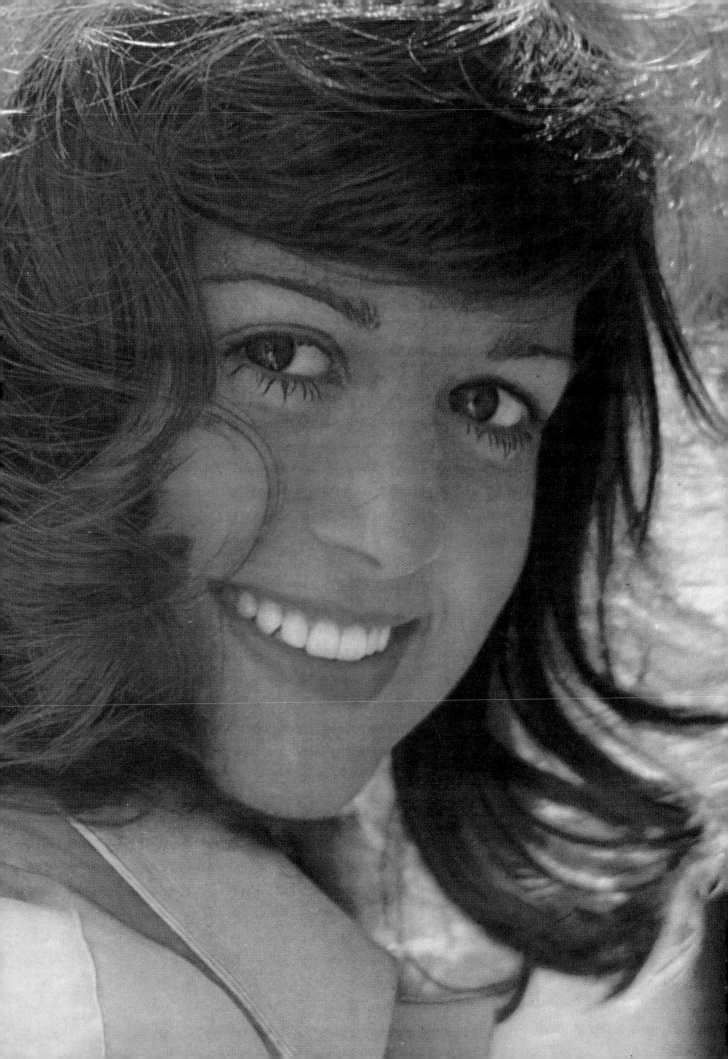

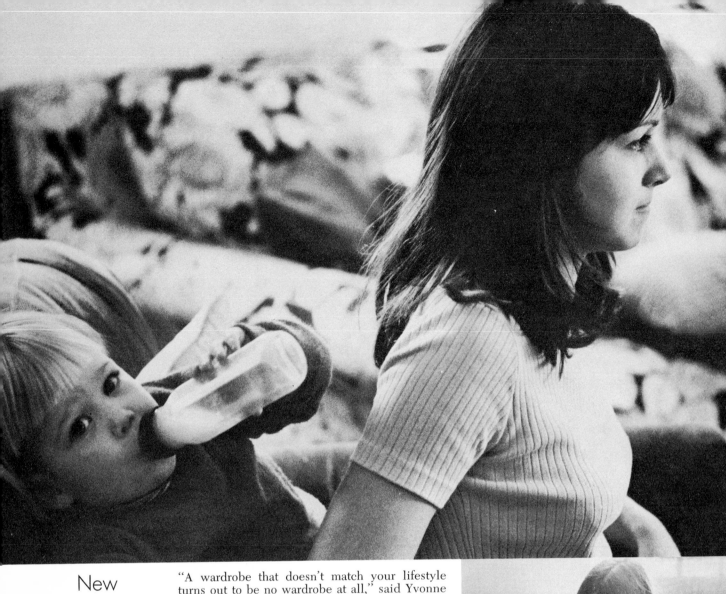

New problems need new solutions

"A wardrobe that doesn't match your lifestyle turns out to be no wardrobe at all," said Yvonne Goodhue. *Above* and *below* you see her with her two-year-old son, Jonathan, in the kind of casual clothes that used to work for her. But since her life now includes a job plus evening dates she needs looks that are a lot more polished. Making her dollars stretch far enough was another big problem. Yvonne's solution—since she continued to live in the same roomy apartment—was to take on a roommate. It not only eased the financial burden, it was a hedge against loneliness and gave her a new group of unmarried friends.

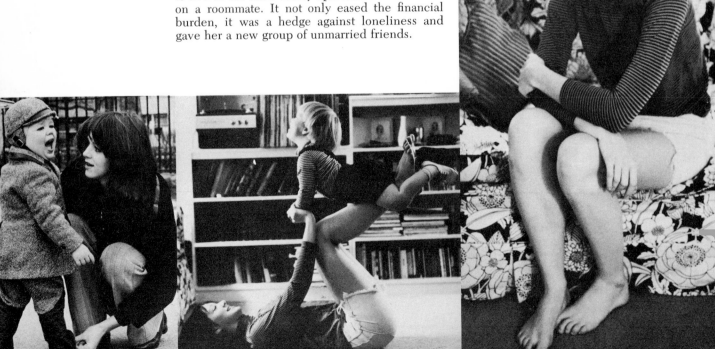

After the divorce, new ideas to help

Even though her new life means more responsibilities and less time for herself, Yvonne is determined to look prettier than ever before. She felt she'd gotten into a real beauty low just before her divorce, and her looks showed it. GLAMOUR's beauty editors suggested that she go for a full professional overhaul so that she could have the psychological satisfaction of seeing immediate results. We told her to have the works—a facial, leg wax, pedicure, manicure, arm-hair bleach, haircut.

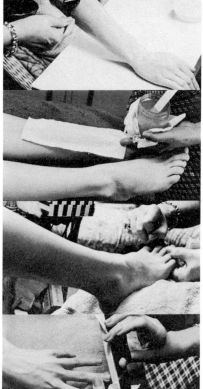

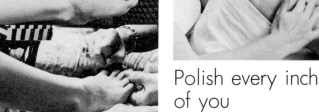

Polish every inch of you

An entire day of salon body-polishing from head to toe did wonders for Yvonne's morale. It also gave her a great chance to pick up some professional tips that made her at-home beauty life a lot more profitable. *Left above,* you see Yvonne at the Henri Bendel salon getting an arm-hair bleach for a smoother look in bare summer clothes, a leg wax, pedicure and a good manicure. She also had a tingling facial, *above.* When you go to a salon don't be afraid to ask for advice for continuing the routine at home.

New layers of hair

For a change of pace, Yvonne wanted to grow her hair longer. Her bangs had already reached the shaggy point. GLAMOUR sent her to Paul Mitchell, styling for The Crimpers, who gave her a fringed haircut that turned shaggy bangs into a big beauty asset. The bangs now blend into the short side fringe he cut to frame her face. He showed Yvonne how to blow her hair dry and get a super look at home with no set. "It's the best haircut I've ever had," she says. "It always looks good, and I've never had that feeling."

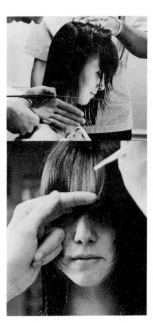

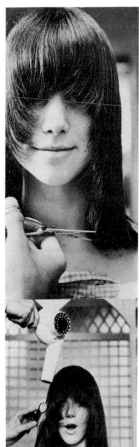

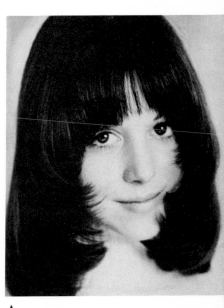

A new beauty image is a big morale booster

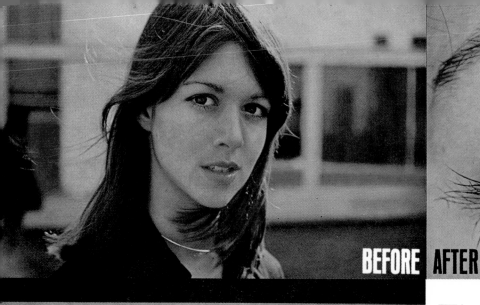

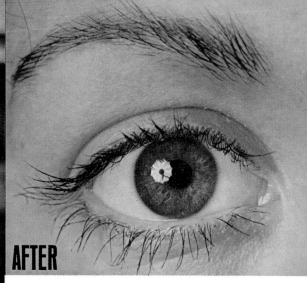

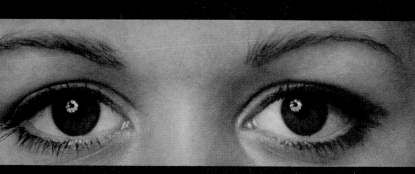

BEFORE AFTER

THREE NEW EYE LOOKS

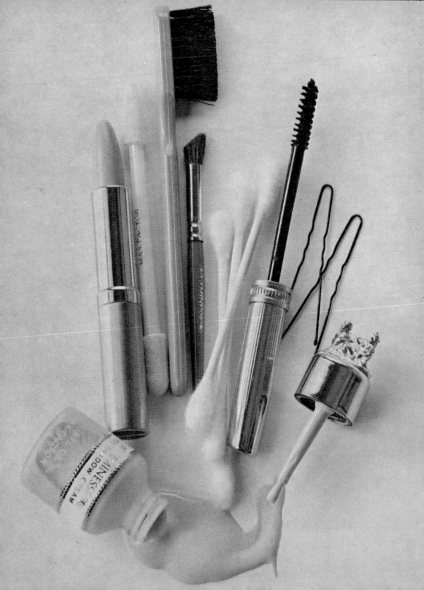

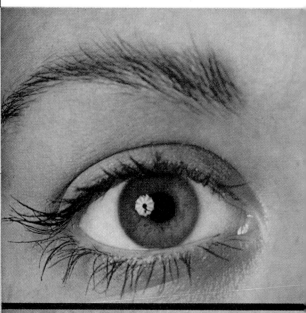

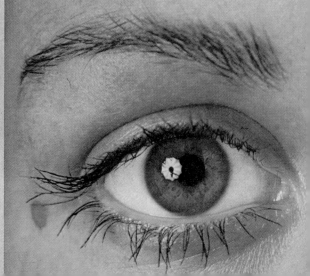

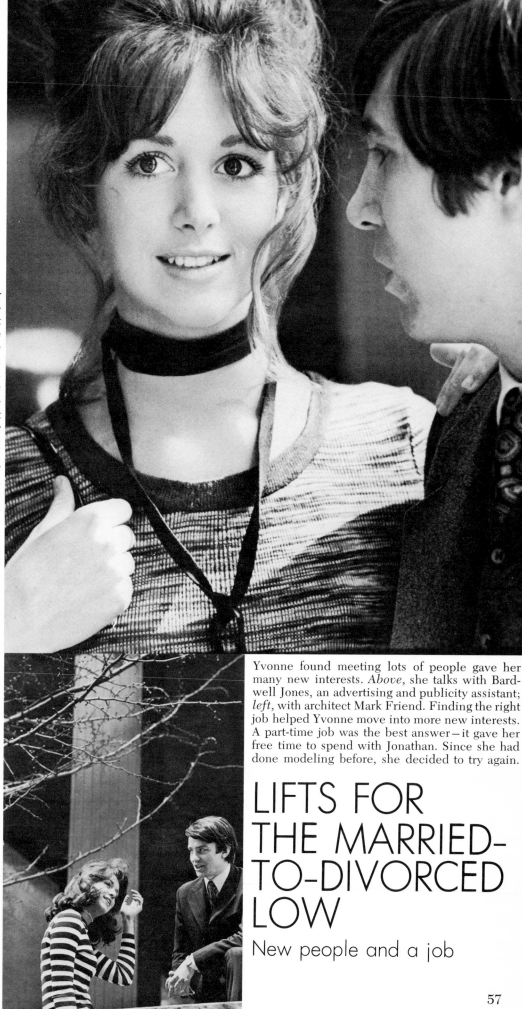

Yvonne has less time than ever to spend on makeup, so GLAMOUR's advice was to spend most of it on eyes. We gave her three different quick looks that she can choose from, depending on where she wants to wear them. They all use color instead of the black eyeliner she used to depend on to camouflage a slight droop at the outer corner of her eyes. *Opposite page top right:* The minimal makeup—it's done with blue green eyeliner drawn softly across the top lid and dotted on bottom lid close to lashes. Lots of black mascara is stroked on bottom and top lashes, which are very carefully separated with a rubber-tipped hairpin, and mascara smudges are wiped away with cotton tipped sticks. To tame brows, we suggested she brush them upward with a brush like the supersized mascara one in the photo *bottom left.* The eye *opposite center* is more festive —but takes just a few seconds longer. It's the same as the one directly above it, plus a dusting of turquoise shadow to intensify the color of her eyes. The bottom eye is a beautiful evening fantasy. It's shadowed with sunny yellow, lashes are mascaraed and curled. A small beauty mark is penciled in with blue liner just beyond the outer corner of one eye.

Yvonne found meeting lots of people gave her many new interests. *Above,* she talks with Bardwell Jones, an advertising and publicity assistant; *left,* with architect Mark Friend. Finding the right job helped Yvonne move into more new interests. A part-time job was the best answer—it gave her free time to spend with Jonathan. Since she had done modeling before, she decided to try again.

LIFTS FOR THE MARRIED-TO-DIVORCED LOW

New people and a job

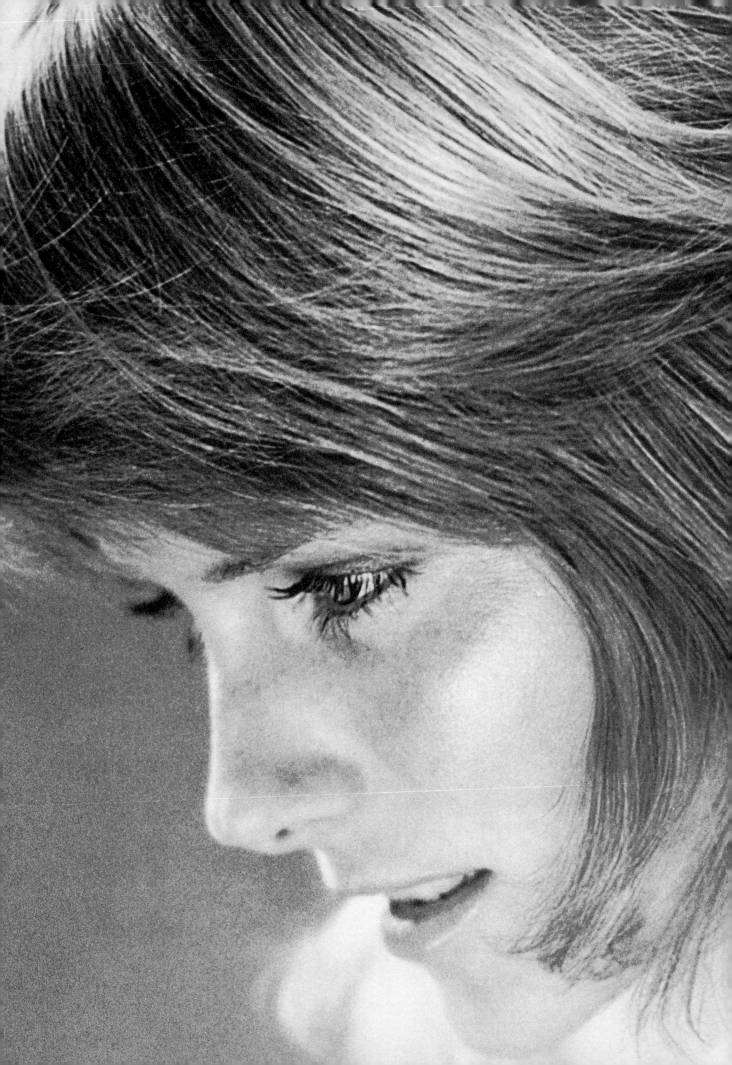

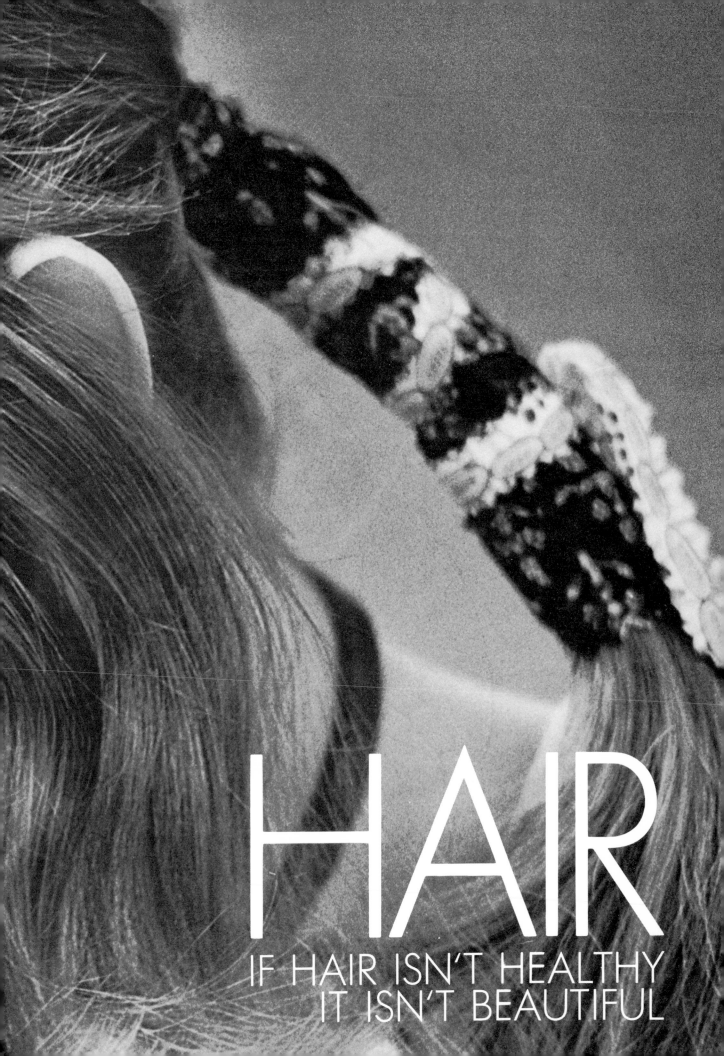

HAIR
IF HAIR ISN'T HEALTHY
IT ISN'T BEAUTIFUL

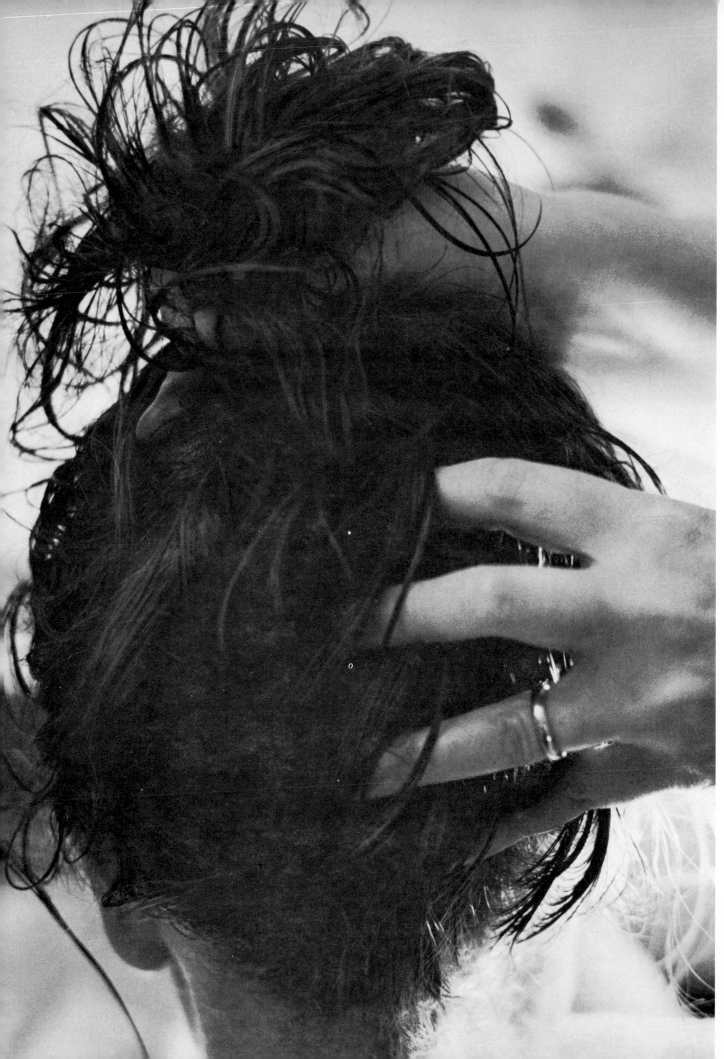

TREATING HAIR TO HEALTH AND BEAUTY

If hair isn't healthy, it isn't beautiful. That's why we start right off with this conditioning chart to get and keep hair in the best of health. Find your hair type and treat it to the care it needs. But first be sure you know the purpose of each treatment or conditioner called for—check them out on the briefing list below.

Hair type	Dry	Oily	Normal
For natural hair —hair that has not been tinted, lightened, permanented, straightened or overexposed to the sun.	1. Use shampoo for dry hair. 2. Creme rinse.° 3. Conditioning treatment once a month (fifteen- to thirty-minute application), no creme rinse. 4. Body-builder or setting lotion. 5. Hair creme between shampoos if needed.	1. Use shampoo for oily hair. 2. Conditioning treatment once a month (fifteen- to thirty-minute application). 3. Body-builder or setting lotion. 4. Dry shampoo between regular ones if needed.	1. Use a gentle shampoo. 2. Conditioning treatment once a month (fifteen- to thirty-minute application), no creme rinse. 3. Body-builder or setting lotion.
For tinted (any hair colored with a product except bleach), permanented or straightened hair, hair that has had prolonged exposure to sun, chlorine, teasing, or is broken in places.	1. Use shampoo for tinted hair, otherwise shampoo for dry hair. 2. Creme rinse.° 3. Instant conditioner once every two weeks (two- to five-minute application), no creme rinse. 4. Conditioning treatment once a month (fifteen- to thirty-minute application), no creme rinse. 5. Body-builder or setting lotion. 6. Hair creme between shampoos if needed.	1. Use shampoo for tinted hair, otherwise shampoo for oily hair. 2. Instant conditioner once every two weeks (two- to five-minute application). 3. Conditioning treatment once a month (fifteen- to thirty-minute application). 4. Body-builder or setting lotion. 5. Dry shampoo between regular ones if needed.	1. Use shampoo for tinted hair, otherwise a gentle shampoo. 2. Instant conditioner once every two weeks (two- to five-minute application), no creme rinse. 3. Conditioning treatment once a month (fifteen- to thirty-minute application), no creme rinse. 4. Body-builder or setting lotion.
For hair that has been bleached or bleached and toned with a pale blonde color.	1. Use shampoo for lightened hair. 2. Creme rinse.° 3. Instant conditioner once a week (two- to five-minute application), no creme rinse. 4. Conditioning treatment once a month (fifteen- to thirty-minute application), no creme rinse. 5. Body-builder or setting lotion. 6. Hair creme between shampoos if needed.	1. Use shampoo for lightened hair. 2. Instant conditioner once a week (two- to five-minute application). 3. Conditioning treatment once a month (fifteen- to thirty-minute application). 4. Body-builder or setting lotion. 5. Dry shampoo between regular ones if needed.	1. Use shampoo for lightened hair. 2. Instant conditioner once a week (two- to five-minute application), no creme rinse. 3. Conditioning treatment once a month (fifteen- to thirty-minute application), no creme rinse. 4. Body-builder or setting lotion.

Shampoo—pick the type made for your kind of hair—dry, oily, normal, tinted or lightened.

Dry shampoo—if necessary for control of oiliness between regular shampoos.

Creme rinse—will untangle hair after shampooing, softens it, helps control static electricity. Not a substitute for a conditioner and not to be used unless hair needs softening for control.

Conditioner—for strengthening and maintaining hair health. Improve feel and shine, help prevent breakage. There are two main types—instant conditioners left on the hair for two to five minutes before they're rinsed out, and the more penetrating ones that must be left on for fifteen to thirty minutes before they're rinsed out.

Setting lotions—help hair hold a set. Some, called body-builders, give extra body to fine- and medium-textured hair. For medium to coarse texture, a regular setting lotion will add enough body. There are setting lotions with built-in conditioners too, but their main job is setting the hair.

Hair treatments— what does what

° *To be used only if your hair is very coarse or fly-away because of its softening effects.*

SAVE YOUR HAIR FROM THE ENVIRONMENT

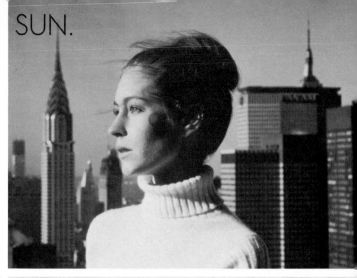

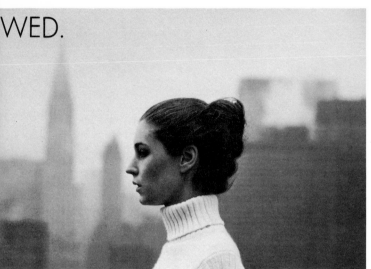

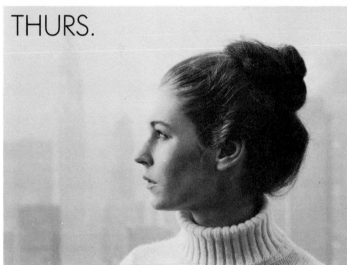

SUN

Sun is the worst enemy of hair. It can lighten the natural color, change the tone of colored hair, making it dull or brassy or bringing out reddish tints. The drying effect of sun causes breakage and split ends. To prevent sun damage, keep hair covered with scarves, sun hats, use an instant conditioner once a week, once a month give yourself a conditioning treatment that works deeper, takes longer—fifteen to thirty minutes.

HEAT

A hot environment heightens the natural condition of your hair. If it's dry, it will become drier; if oily, oiler. Hair gets dirty quicker in heat because of perspiration. Dry hair needs a shampoo designed for it, an instant conditioner once a week and a more penetrating conditioning treatment once a month, maybe a hair cream in between shampoos for extreme dryness. Oily hair requires more shampooing than usual with a shampoo geared to cut down on oil, a fifteen- to thirty-minute conditioning treatment once a month, maybe dry shampoos between washings. Normal hair will need more washings too than in cool weather, an instant conditioner every two weeks and a fifteen- to thirty-minute conditioning every month.

HUMIDITY

Hair is a barometer to humidity, said one dermatologist. It responds more quickly to it than skin. Since high humidity and heat often go together, you'll get the same effects as described under heat plus some. Curly hair becomes curlier, straight hair straighter when there is a lot of moisture in the air, and normal hair holds its set less easily. Use stronger setting lotions, wear simple styles that hold their shape without a lot of setting. Follow the above routines for both shampoo and for conditioning.

INDUSTRIAL POLLUTANTS

The most serious known thing pollutants do to hair that hasn't been colored or chemically changed by permanents or by straightening is to make it dirtier. Particles of soot, grime, smog, attach to hair, especially if it's oily, and stick to hair spray. One dermatologist believes that there is reason to support the theory that sulfur dioxide, *opposite page*, which acts as a bleaching agent in food, changes the color of hair, particularly tinted, bleached or treated hair. To protect hair, more washings, more coverings, especially for colored hair. More about special treatment of colored hair, *opposite page*.

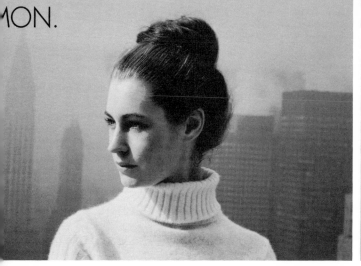

MON.

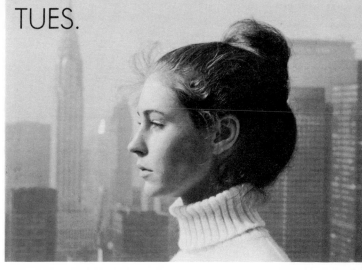

TUES.

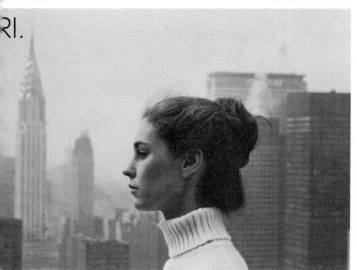

RI.

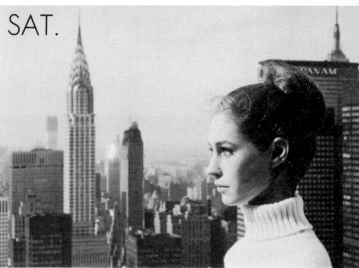

SAT.

What environment does to your hair is nothing short of drastic. We don't mean just what scientists are beginning to discover about the effects of air pollution on it, but all the other elements it is exposed to day after day, year after year, relentlessly — steam and natural heat, humidity, wind, air conditioning, sun, water, cold. To fight these elements consult the advice at *left*.

What the scientists say about environmental effects

Dr. Earle Brauer, the well known New York dermatologist, explained that "sulfur dioxide, one of the chemicals in soot, has been used in the food industry for many years as a bleach and preservative. For instance, the label on dried apricots tells you that sulfur dioxide has been added. This returns the dehydrated fruit, which becomes an ugly tannish-brown color, back to an appetizing orange. I can't believe that sulfur dioxide is so discriminating that it will alter fruit and other colored matter but not hair, particularly tinted or bleached hair. We know

the sun does it, and I'm sure the accumulation of soot on hair is doing it too. Hair in polluted cities can be protected by more frequent washings, wearing a scarf or cap when you go out."

You have to be more careful with it in every way, never even combing or brushing it as vigorously as you might do with untouched hair. It is more porous and fragile than regular hair. If it is colored, use shampoos, setting lotions, sprays and conditioners that are made especially for it, keep covered as much as possible when you're exposed to industrial pollution, always keep covered in the sun. The best conditioning routine is an instant conditioner once a week, a more penetrating one once a month. With permanented and straightened hair try to give some coverage when exposed to pollution and sun. High humidity will cause both straightened and permanented hair to crimp some.

HOW TO LIVE SUCCESSFULLY WITH YOUR OWN HAIR

What styles work
with what textures
and types of hair

The texture, the amount of hair on your head, its curliness or straightness, are facts you have to live with and face up to before your next hairdo can be a success. That's why the famous hairdresser Kenneth Battelle, who is the most insistent realist about hair, based all these next styles on those three facts before any others. Most girls know their hair type — fine, thin, curly; or coarse, thick, straight; or any of the other possible combinations. But many don't know the limitations of these types or won't accept them. They refuse to compromise between a style they want and what their hair can actually do. To help you recognize the best solutions to the different basic hair types is what these next five pages are really all about. Obviously, medium- to coarse-textured hair, in medium amounts on the head and straight, can take just about anything. This is lucky hair, and the styling possibilities are unlimited. It's the less malleable hair we're concerned with here, but even they don't have to be stuck with only one unchanging hairdo. According to the degree of thinness, curliness, etc., all sorts of things can be done in the way of styling and treatments: softening for thick, stubborn hair; straightening for curly; streaking or conditioning to give body. In fact, almost anything can be done with any kind of hair today. The trouble, Kenneth points out, is that sometimes what may have to be done to force a hairdo that is essentially unsuitable for the hair type isn't worth the difficulty of doing it. When you go to your hairdresser, bring up these matters. Ask what he would advise to give your hair more body, or to make it less wiry. Ask and ask some more. Insist on a cut that will almost give you the style without setting, that falls into line by itself. If it does not work, go back to the hairdresser, talk over the problems. A perfect hairdo rarely happens on the very first visit to a hairdresser.

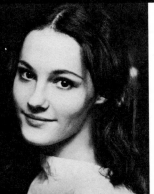

Hair type: fine, thin, curly. So fine that it just fell limp, left; so curly (see it damp and combed out, right, before it was set in rollers, far right) that any attempt to straighten it would have to be so severe the hair would probably lose body in the process.

Solution: Kenneth decided that the best thing for this very curly fine thin head of hair was to go along with the curl. He blunt cut the hair to control the shape, even all around except slightly shorter in the back. Then, because this type of hair has a tendency to split easily, he used a nonsoftening conditioner to give strength and body. This kind of body-giving conditioner coats the hair and acts like an invisible protective bandage. It must be applied after each shampoo. Actually, not all fine, curly hair is impossible to straighten. If it is thicker than this hair (that is, more of it on the head), straightening could have been quite successful. Straightening, however, always leaves hair with somewhat less body.

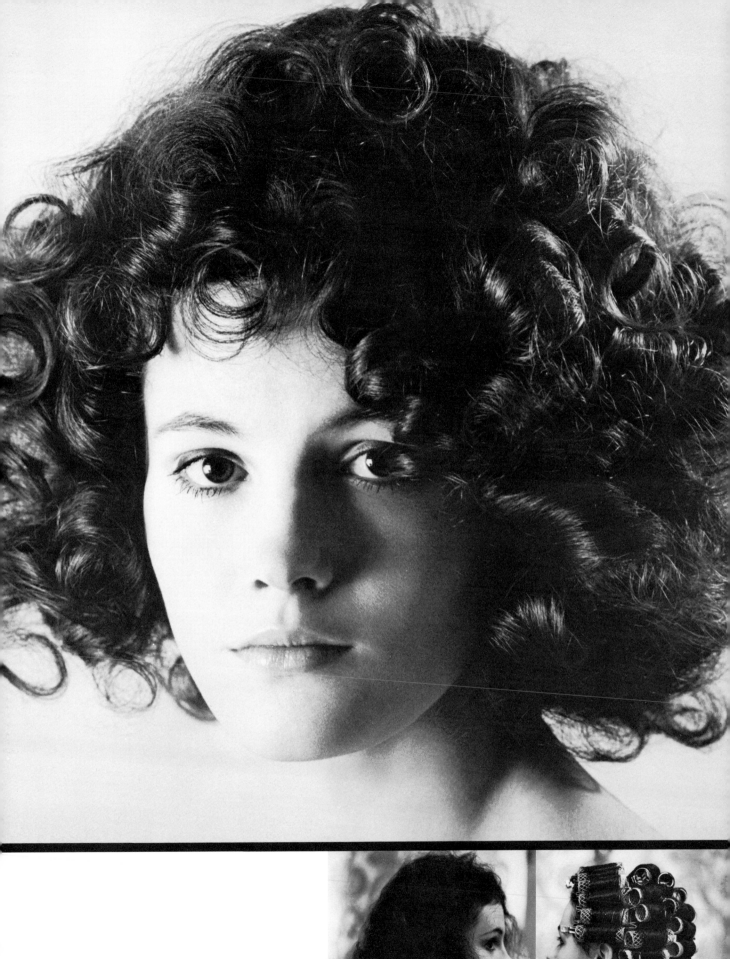
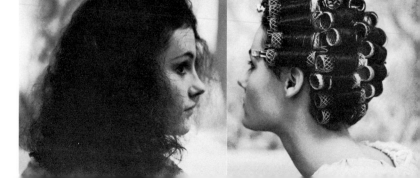

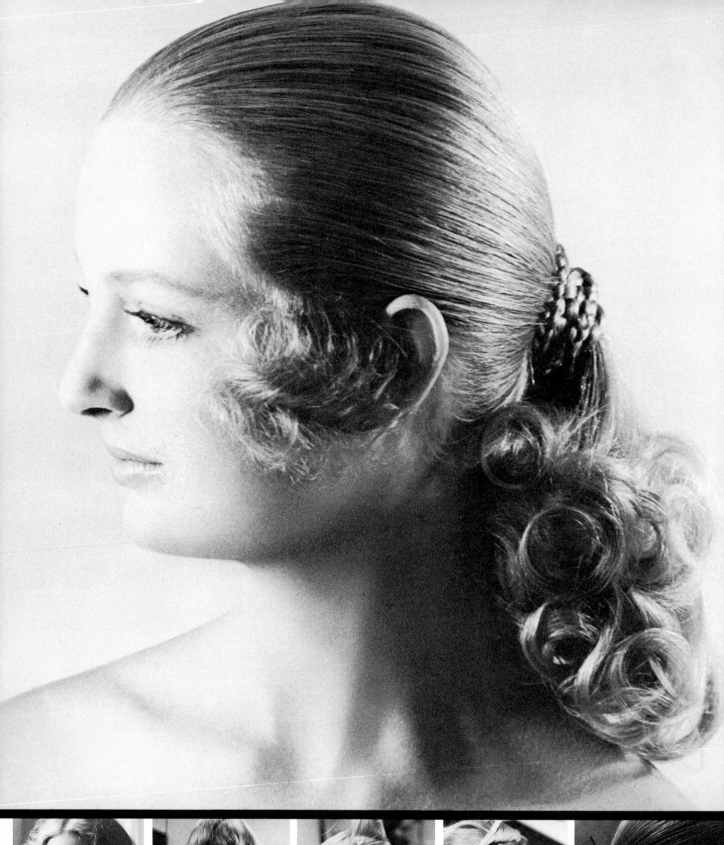

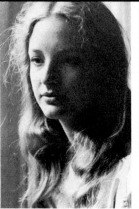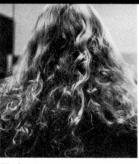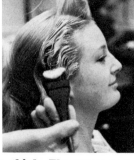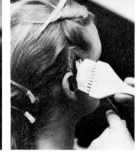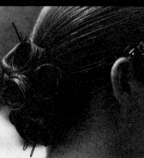

Hair type: wavy, coarse, thick. The wave pattern was strong except around the hairline, where it was excessively fuzzy—see left and directly above—not a smooth frame for such a well-defined profile.

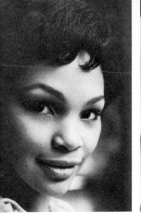
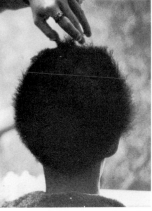

Solution: Curly, medium to fine hair is at its best natural, simply shaped around the head, particularly when the head and neck have the classic Nefertiti shape these do—see photographs *below*. Kenneth simply cut the hair close to the head, but not so close that falls and wiglets cannot be attached for a change of look. There are other solutions to curly, medium hair: It can be straightened and worn rather long with a blunt cut. Or you can go along with the curl, as Kenneth did with the fine, curly hair on page 65, setting it on small ¾″ rollers all over the head. (The smaller the roller, the more curl you'll get.) In either of the last two cases the cut has to be superb to really control the shape.

Hair type: curly, medium amount of hair, medium to fine texture. The straightened short style, above left, was undistinguished, neither here nor there.

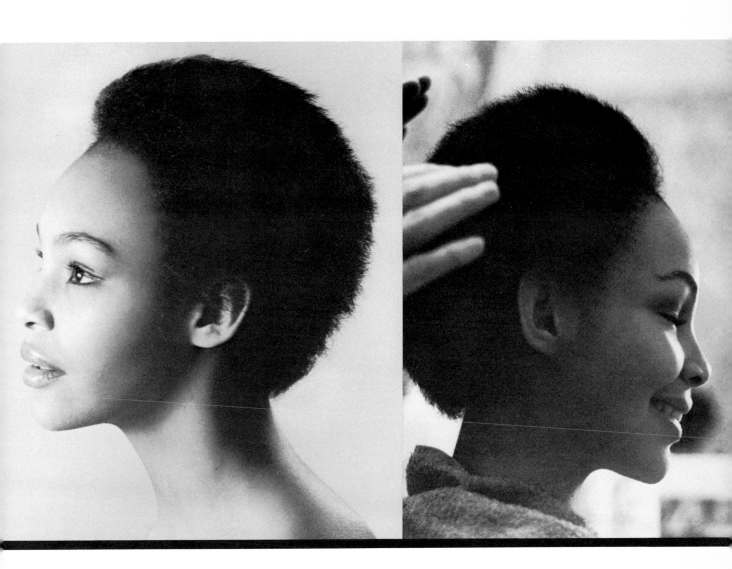

Solution: This wavy, coarse, thick hair, *opposite page*, could have been straightened throughout, but Kenneth felt straightening just two inches deep all around the front hairline would be sufficient, less expensive and less time-consuming. He chose the off-the-brow style, to expose the beautiful profile. You see two steps in the straightening process in the third and fourth small photographs, *opposite bottom*, and in the end photograph the easy, uncomplicated set for this style. The hair might alternately be set all over in very large rollers and worn down, too; the length would weight it so that there would be less wave.

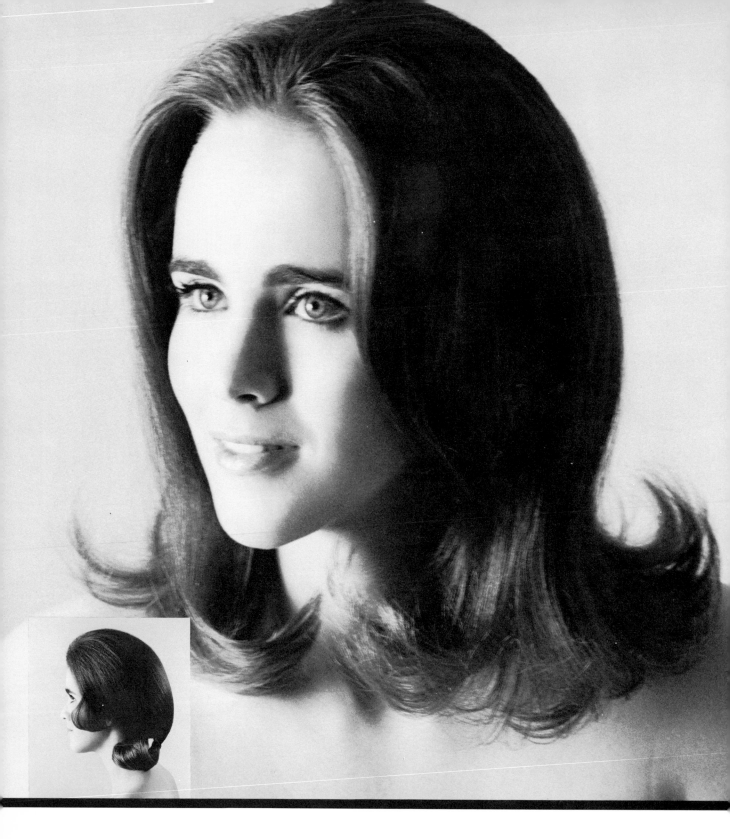

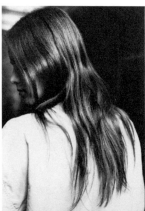

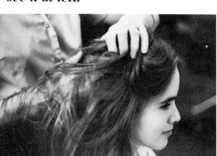

Hair type: fine, thin, straight. The hair has been allowed to grow in all different lengths without trimming— see it at left.

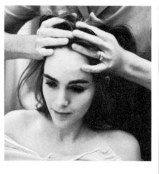

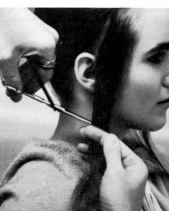

Hair type: coarse, thick, straight. This is really good hair but tends to be stubborn and is inclined to get very oily and lank.

Solution: Because this girl's coarse, thick, straight hair, *below*, inclines to oiliness and lankness a day or so after shampooing (see before picture *top left below*) Kenneth decided that streaking would help to reduce the oil. Streaking (see a step in the process *below center*) not only helps to reduce the oil but can give body to fine hair too; the more streaking, the more body. After the streaking, he shaped the hair with a blunt, even cut, then set one roller on the top, pin curls on each side and blew the rest of the hair dry with a hand blower. The hand-drying is really like brushing the hair into shape and gives stubborn hair a smoothness that full head of rollers would not. Kenneth does not feel that thinning is ever a solution to thick hair. The thinned strands, as they grow, push the others outward and compound the problem. Length is particularly good for this type of hair, since it weights the hair down in place. The blunt cut gives it the strong shape that allows it to fall right in line without setting.

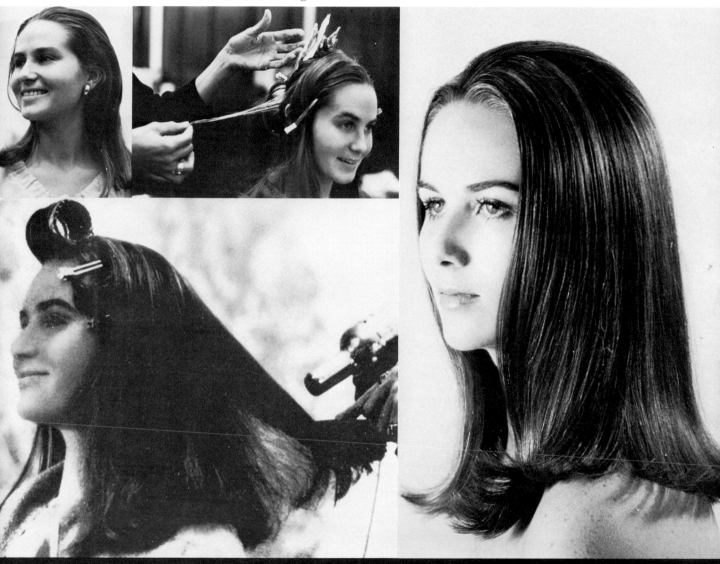

Solution: For fine, thin, straight hair like the girl's on the *opposite page*, the best solution is a blunt cut, even all around, a bit shorter in back than in front, but never any longer than shoulder length. This texture simply can't support more length. Kenneth cut two pieces on each side, framing the face from temple to cheek, shorter than the other hair because this is the weakest, thinnest area in anyone's hair. Shorter, it holds better and gives a sense of more fullness. The longer part is about as long (big picture, *opposite page*) as fine, thin hair should be, yet it is still long enough to be worn a second way (small picture, *opposite*), pulled back when the set begins to give out. To strengthen and feed the hair, Kenneth had one of his staff give a scalp-conditioning treatment, and after shampooing, he used a body-giving setting lotion.

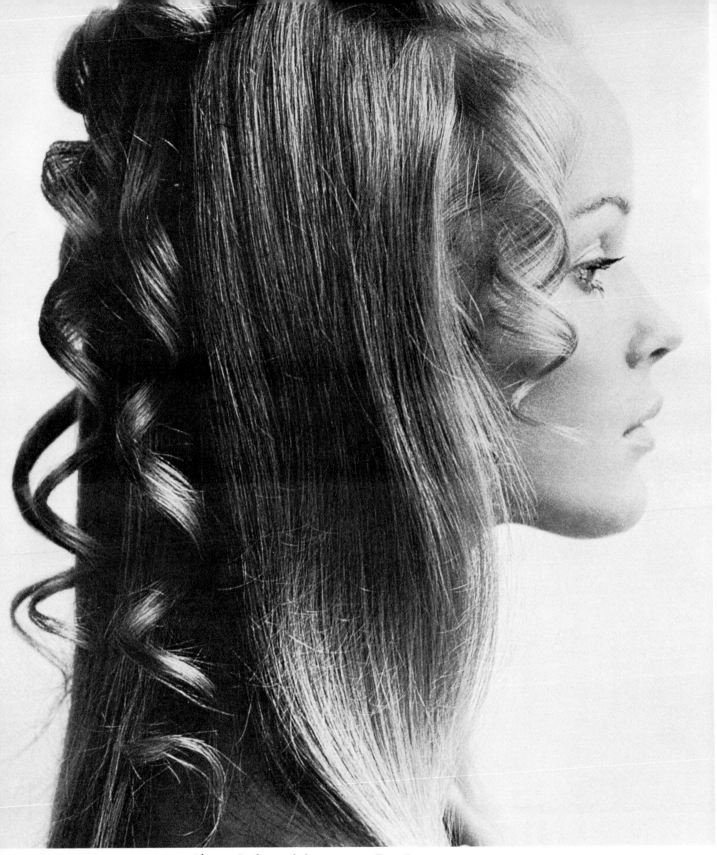

Above: Curly tendrils like these are made by setting wisps of hair in pin curls wrapped on a pencil or on your fingers, or on small electric rollers. *Right:* To set bangs see number 9 *opposite.*

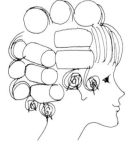
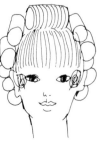
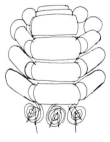

1. If you know nothing about hair setting discuss it with your hairdresser or a friend who does. Ask him or her to show you how to roll and attach rollers, ask them for advice on the size of rollers and be prepared to experiment with sizes.

2. The bigger the roller, the looser the set; the smaller the roller, the tighter. Most hairdressers use about six size ranges from ¾ of an inch to two inches in diameter.

3. The coarser or the curlier your hair is, the larger the roller you need—medium hair takes a medium roller; thin, straight fine hair a smaller roller.

4. Sets now are chiefly wound on rollers, although a few clips are usually used too. Clips make curls or waves that stay snug to the head; rollers are responsible for the pouffed wave or freer style.

5. To anchor the roller to your head use a clip at the base run horizontally through the curler and your hair. To keep the rollers in place on the crown of your head clip one to the other where they meet.

6. Work with thin sections, well combed out and not matted, of about one and one half to two inches wide. Never try to roll big matted hunks of hair.

7. Here are the two most basic setting patterns used by most hairdressers—from them you can take off on an endless variety of comb outs, short, long or medium.

8. Always use a setting lotion to make the hair more manageable and easy to handle, but be sure you read the label on the bottle or package. Some give body, some just make hair more docile, some add shine, others are for special kinds of hair, tinted, bleached, etc.

9. For flat bangs follow the setting pattern sketched *opposite page, below*. Comb wet bangs straight down and hold with setting lotion or clips at the tip ends, or with a piece of gauze or scarf tied over them. After they've dried and set, they can be made to look close or wispy just by separating with the fingers or a comb.

10. Don't take your hair down immediately after getting out from under a hot dryer. Either turn the dryer on cool or let the hair cool off at room temperature. Allowing hair to cool in the wave pattern while still on the rollers holds the pattern longer.

11. Touch-up sets. No one should have a hair style so incompatible with the type and texture of her hair that she has to wear rollers to bed. A good hair style doesn't need more than a half hour or so setting, preferably while you are bathing or showering and making up, before going out in the morning or evening. If your hair style needs more pick-up setting than this, it is wrong for your type of hair. Change to something easier and more suitable.

12. Rollers with brushes inside of them are rough on hair and can break it. End papers are great for setting. They hold the ends of the hair smoothly, help prevent them from crimping.

TIPS FOR AT-HOME SETTING

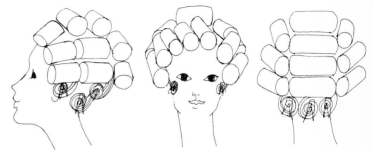

The set: Three diagonally placed rollers wind downward from side part across crown. Side hair rolls straight down; top back hair winds down. Small nape and temple strands go in clip curls at side and back.

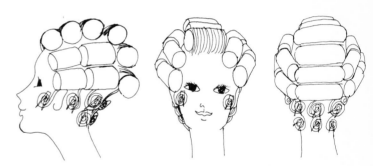

The set: Roll crown hair straight back from brow on largest rollers. Four rollers, all wound down, are placed in a double row on each side. Six flat clip curls at nape; two more, each wound forward, at ear level. Leave a long "stem" on the one nearest cheek.

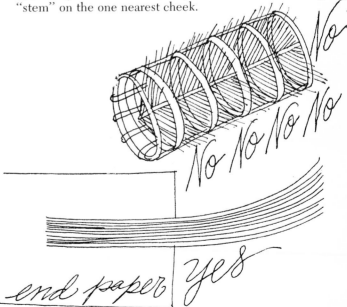

No No No No No

end paper yes

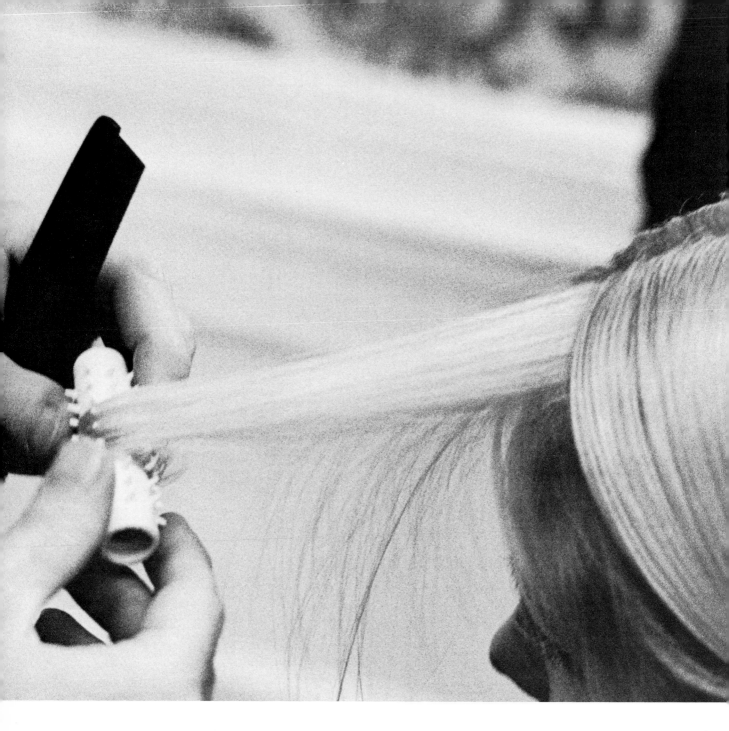

ELECTRIC ROLLERS

Almost everyone has tried electric rollers, but almost nobody realizes that they must be used differently on different kinds of hair if you want to get prime results. That's why we asked the famous hairdresser Kenneth to show how they work best on four basic hair types most women fit into—fine, wavy, unruly and colored hair. Follow his rules and electric rollers can start your hair working for you for a change, instead of the other way around.

HOW THEY CAN FREE YOU FROM BEING A SLAVE TO YOUR OWN HAIR

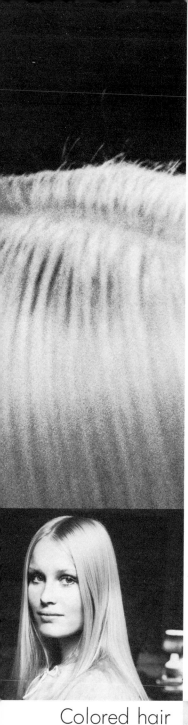

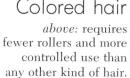

Colored hair

above: requires fewer rollers and more controlled use than any other kind of hair.

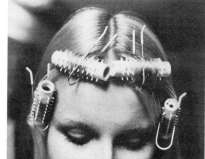

Color rules

Since colored hair is more fragile and usually drier than uncolored hair, you have to go easy and not use too many rollers too often—the heat can make it even drier if used too frequently. Use a few rollers for softness just around the face—like the soft, loose spiral curls on the colored hair, *above.* (In fact, follow this rule of controlled use of electric rollers on any head of chemically treated hair—i.e. straightened or waved.) *Left,* Kenneth sets four curls on smallest rollers, two on top and one on each side. To get the most curl, be sure rollers are completely cool before removing them, then comb through hair just enough to arrange the curl. To keep color-treated hair in shining good health and to add a little extra body, try using a conditioning spray made especially for use with electric rollers.

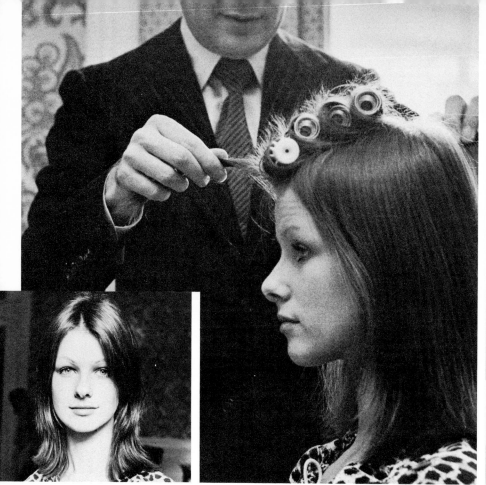

Fine, straight

hair, *above*, can get extra body from a good electric roller setting, *see right*.

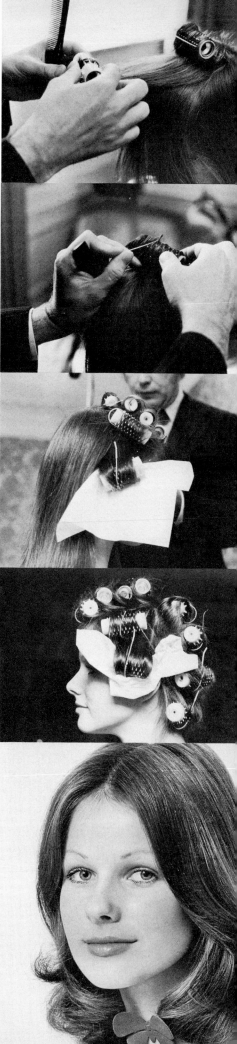

To give body to hair that's baby-fine and straight like the head *above*, Kenneth suggests using medium-sized rollers all over the head. Tips that help: Don't put too much hair on one roller, dampen hair slightly with a wet comb, *top right*, and leave rollers in hair until they are completely cool. Try a piece of tissue under a roller that's uncomfortably hot at the hairline. Don't overcomb your hair after the set or you'll take out some of the body.

Body rules

Stubborn hair

right, or coarse or flyaway hair, all can be tamed down by electric rollers.

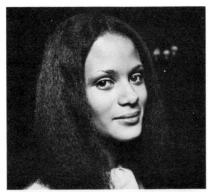

Electric rollers give unruly hair a smoother look. The setting here provides a smooth crown with control at the ends. Kenneth pulled the hair out smooth and straight before winding on each roller, then he wound it only halfway, leaving the hair at the crown straight. Use large rollers on top, and medium ones at the hairline. Always start rolling hair at the top, from the part as you see here. Unwind from bottom up. Curlers come out easier and hair won't tangle. Another way to help control this kind of hair is a special electric roller conditioner.

Stubborn rules

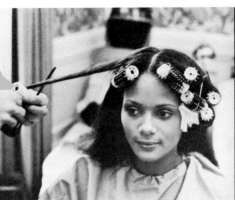

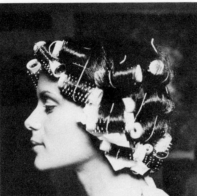

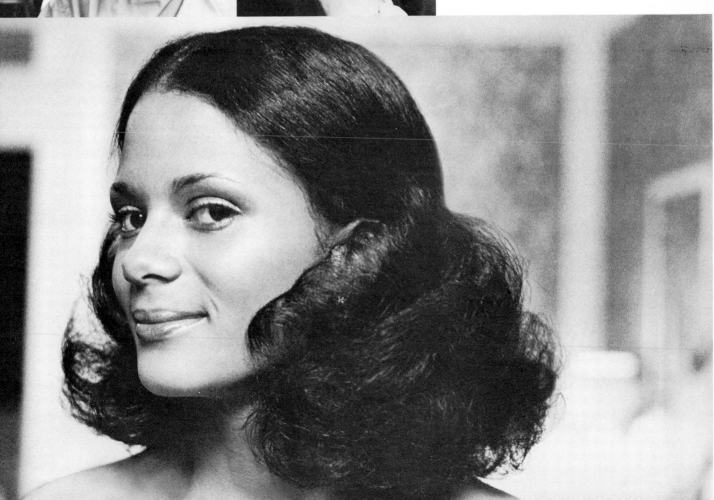

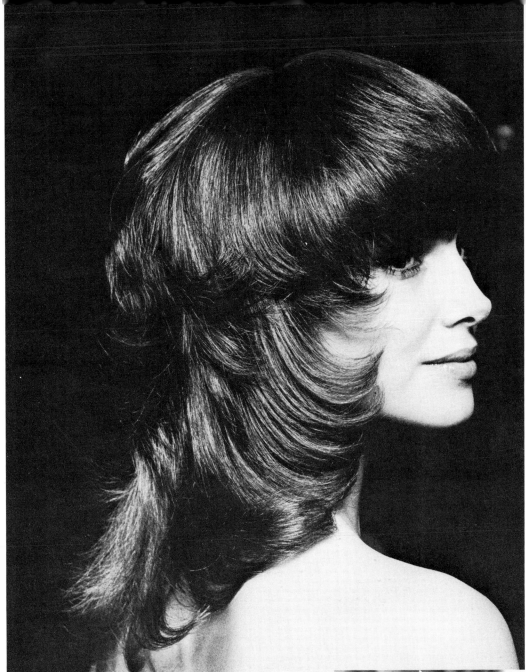

Naturally wavy

hair, *below*, gets beautiful control, *right*, from electric rollers strategically positioned in hair.

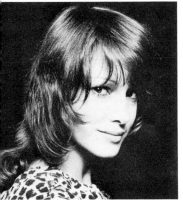

Control rules

If your hair is naturally wavy like the head here, what you can expect from electric rollers is control—not more curl. The hair here is layered short on top with longer sides and back. It can be blown dry, but to give the crown lift and smoothness, Kenneth used four rollers—one rolled forward, one backward and one to each side, *see bottom right*. Don't leave the rollers in too long—the first one should be ready to come out almost as soon as you've put in the last one. You can use electric rollers wherever you want a little extra control for wavy hair—around the face, through the crown—it depends on how you wear your hair. Large rollers will give the most control with the least amount of curl.

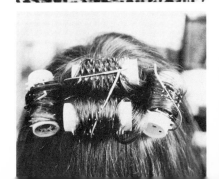

DON'T set hair every day with electric rollers. The heat can dry hair and cause ends to split or break. Three times a week is safe for normal hair, less for dry or color-treated hair.

DO use a special conditioner made for electric rollers if your hair is dry.

DO put rollers in first at the crown and then work down. Unwind bottom rollers first and work up. This keeps hair from tangling.

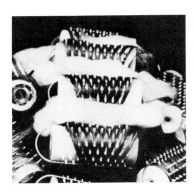

Cotton
pushed under rollers will keep them from resting uncomfortably on your scalp.

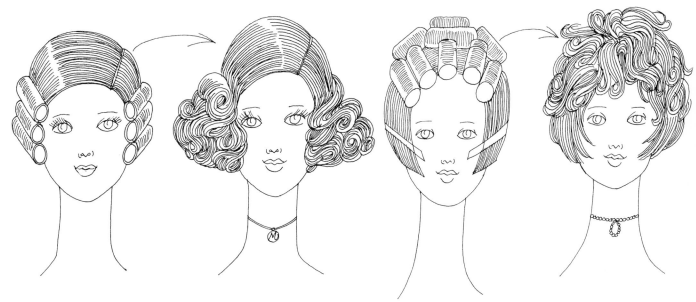

Here are two very basic sets for girls with medium to strong hair, preferably uncolored since they require a good number of rollers. You can set your hair by them and have a finished look in about ten minutes. Try using a conditioning spray especially for electric rollers. For the first set, which has a lot of curl at the sides but a smooth crown, you need chin length hair at least. You see the setting pattern in sketch one and the comb out in sketch two. For shorter hair with a curly top see the last two sketches. Set just the top of the hair, dampen sides and comb down smooth. Hold straight sides with tape.

Two speedy curly electric roller sets

A SUCCESS GUIDE TO WAVING, STRAIGHTENING, COLORING

WAVING

To change hair, which is mostly protein from straight to curly or curly to straight or anywhere in between, heat and chemicals are necessary. Something of the same thing that happens to an egg when it's boiled happens to your hair when it's waved. The dermatologist, Dr. Earle W. Brauer, in his fine book *Your Skin and Hair*, puts it this way: A hard-boiled egg is a typical example of protein altered by heat. Just as the egg put into boiling water hardens into a new firm position, your hair if you set it and apply heat—which alters (in this case softens) the hair's chemical structure—will take on the wave pattern of the set.

Electrically heated rollers, curling irons, hot combs and chemical waving all work on this principle. The more heat applied, the more changed the hair structure, which explains why too much heat can cause so big a change that you get fuzz instead of wave. Lesser amounts of heat used too frequently in the same places on hair can do the same thing. Excesses can cause not only frizz but hair breakage.

There are two kinds of waves given in most salons today—a body wave and a permanent.

Body wave

Given on larger rollers, body waves produce a wave pattern of one to two inches, whereas permanents require smaller rods, and they establish a curl pattern of a half inch to one and a half inches. Permanents give a tighter wave, body waves a looser one. Body waves don't change the overall shape of your hair any more than a lightweight little panty girdle changes your figure; they merely firm the line of the hair. They do not curl.

The decision to have a body wave should be made only after you have talked with your hair-dresser about your hair style in relation to the texture of your hair. Both style and texture determine whether a body wave is right or wrong for you.

Permanent

No one should ever get a permanent today with the idea that it will keep waves in the hair from one wash and set to the next. Any kind of wave needs some setting. Permanents are merely meant to hold the line of hair so that it springs back into shape after a set.

This wave pattern is necessary for certain textures of hair and better for certain styles, usually the short ones. Permanents give substance and adaptability to fine, layered hair, especially if you are trying to let this kind of hair grow out evenly to one length.

Anyone who has had trouble with permanents frizzing, or is afraid she will because of unhealthy or bleached hair, should talk over with her hairdresser the possibility of a test run—having one curl in each area (crown, sides, back, etc.) test-permanented before the whole head is done. This enables him to tell just how much heat is needed to ensure the right amount for each curl.

At-home waving

First inviolate rule: read the label and directions, then *reread*. Most of the disasters come from failures to follow directions, omitting steps and taking shortcuts. Each home wave has its own specific directions. Trust them, and follow these general rules so as to get the type of wave you want.

1. Waving rods follow the same rule as regular setting rollers: the bigger the rod in diameter, the looser the curl; the skinnier the rod, the tighter the curl.

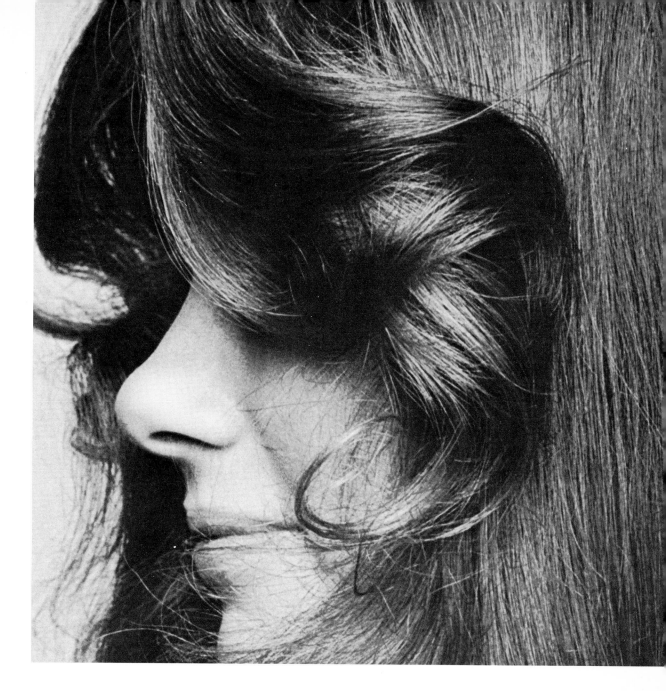

2. Consider the length of your hair—it takes one full wrapping of hair about the curler to make half a wave in the hair shaft. If you want very loose big waves, you'll have to use large rollers and have long enough hair to wind around them. If your hair is very short, say only two or three inches all over, you're forced to use small rods and get a tighter curl.

3. The hair farthest from the ends, that is closest to the scalp, will take the least wave because as the amount of hair rolled increases, less stress is exerted on that part of the hair.

4. The coarser your hair, the more curl it will take, the finer the least.

5. If your hair has been tinted, bleached or waved before, it is porous, i.e. has little breaks in the outer coating, or cuticle, of the shaft, and is more susceptible to the waving solution than hair with a perfect outer coating.

6. At-home waves usually come in three strengths—for fine, coarse or medium textured hair. Some are done in two steps: First, the waving solu-tion application and the second, a neutralizer which stops the wave solution's action and fixes the new shape. The one-step waves have in them a chemi-cal catalyst that allows the air itself to neutralize the waving solution; they work on a self-stop idea.

7. Be sure your hair is meticulously washed before waving—dirt or an excess of oil incom-pletely washed out can inhibit the action of the waving.

8. Always take a test curl before going the whole way. This requires a bit of time but it will allow you to know, before any irrevocable change is made, if you are using the right strength wave for your texture, the right timing. The same waving product that you used last time may not be right again because the chemicals in it, or in your hair coloring or bleach, may have changed your hair's structure.

9. Don't wave at all if your scalp or skin is irritated. Check in with your dermatologist.

10. Don't wave your hair more than twice a year, three times at the very most.

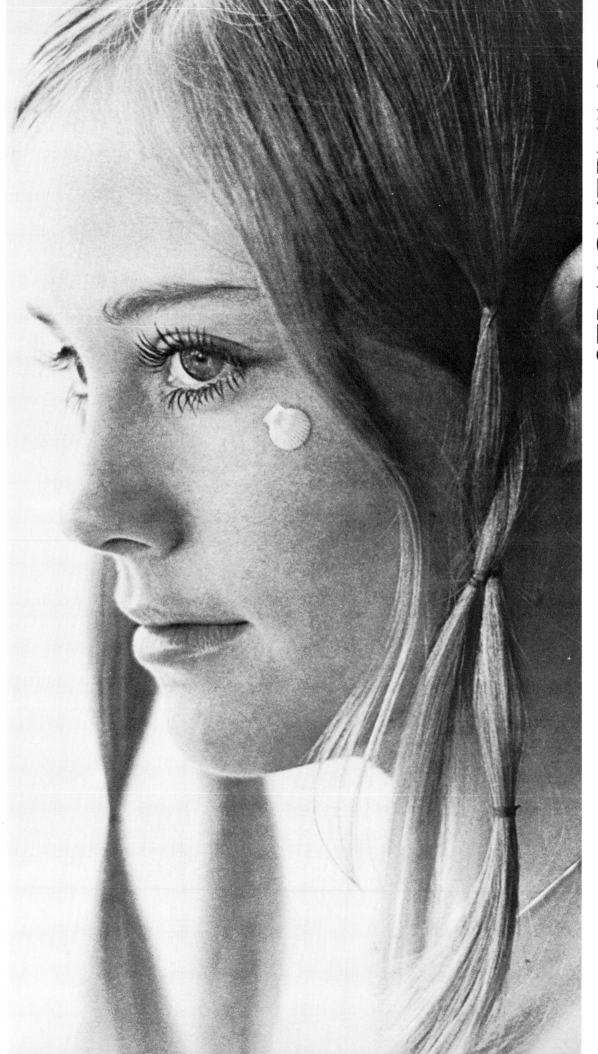

Straightening—as it is usually done today—is a permanent wave in reverse. Almost everything said about the reaction of hair to the waving solution in the preceding section applies to the straightening solution as well.

Other less effective and temporary straightening methods than the chemical one do not change the actual hair structure, such as waxes and gums that simply coat the strand and stiffen it. Heat is another common method—everyone has heard of girls who iron each other's long, straight hair even straighter with an electric iron on an ironing board; some cover the hair with wax paper and get the additional "fix" of the wax coating. This is dangerous, obviously—the hair could be singed and broken. In fact these are the dangers that any inexperienced person runs using electric heat to straighten hair, even the electrically heated combs designed especially for straightening. Besides, these methods are very temporary and lose effect in time and moisture.

Just as a wave chemically changes the arrangement of hair proteins to curl it, straightening alters the hair to relax the curl. Relaxing curl is really a more accurate description of what happens than straightening. Coarse hair is the easiest to straighten. The toughest section of hair of any texture to work with is around the crown and the hairline, particularly around the temples. Partial straightening can be done. That is, it is possible to straighten only the sections of hair that need attention and leave the others alone.

Most experts feel that overall straightening should be done no more than twice a year, preferably once—at the start of the summer when the hair gets loaded with humidity and becomes puffed. Straightening makes it less heavy. (In fact straightening has replaced extensive thinning as a remedy for unruly hair.) Hair that has been straightened and is spending the summer near the sea will react to humidity; it should be given the same attention as bleached or permanented hair, in other words it should be protected from the sun and salt water. Straightened hair might react a bit to chlorine in swimming pools, too.

At-home straightening

While it is possible to do chemical straightening yourself, it is more complex and difficult than home waving. Very few women can come near the quality of results that a real professional can.

No non-professional should attempt a straightening without first doing a strand test to see what happens to her individual kind of hair. If after doing to a few dozen strands exactly what the directions tell you to do to the whole head, the strands feel rubbery or sticky when wet, brittle when dry, if they become discolored or evidence a lot of breakage, *don't* go on.

To give you an idea of the complexities involved in straightening here is a brief description of how it is done. The hair is shampooed to remove any dirt or oil that could interfere with the straightening chemicals; the excess water soaked up with a towel; then the hair is combed free of tangles. The straightening lotion, which has been mixed and allowed to stand about fifteen minutes, is put on the hair with the fingers and worked upward until all the hair is covered, under as well as upper surfaces fully saturated. Next, the hair is combed carefully and gently, wrapped in a plastic turban for ten to twenty minutes to allow the solution to work. The next step is paramount. The hair has now been chemically softened. The turban is removed and the hair carefully combed straight to its full length all over—rearranging or relaxing the curl pattern. It takes about ten to twenty minutes of continuous combing—a difficult task for anyone to do herself particularly if her hair is long. After this the hair is rinsed, blotted and combed again. Then the entire saturating procedure is repeated but this time with a neutralizer instead of the straightening solution, all the time keeping the hair free of tangles. The neutralizer takes about five minutes and is then rinsed out. The hair is now ready for setting. The whole job takes roughly two hours, even a professional cannot do it in much less.

Anyone who attempts straightening, the professional or the do-it-yourselfer, must be meticulous in her workmanship. If the hair is inadequately saturated, if all the surfaces of each shaft are not covered, if the timing is off or the solution too weak or strong for the particular type of hair the results can be anywhere from just disappointing to disastrous in terms of the amount of breakage.

The health of the hair and scalp at the time of the straightening has to be good. Bleached, tinted, toned or previously straightened hair may not react as well to the same straightening process that they had in the past. If the condition of bleached, tinted, toned or previously straightened hair is in underpar condition, the real professional will refuse to attempt straightening. So you can see that you proceed on your own at some risk. On the other hand, virginal hair, that is hair that has never been chemically treated, may also be difficult to straighten. It may need a stronger solution left on longer. All these considerations, and more, are what make the Strand Test a step you can't dismiss.

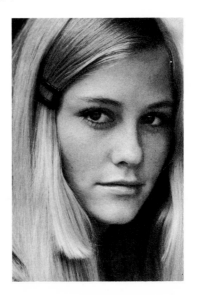

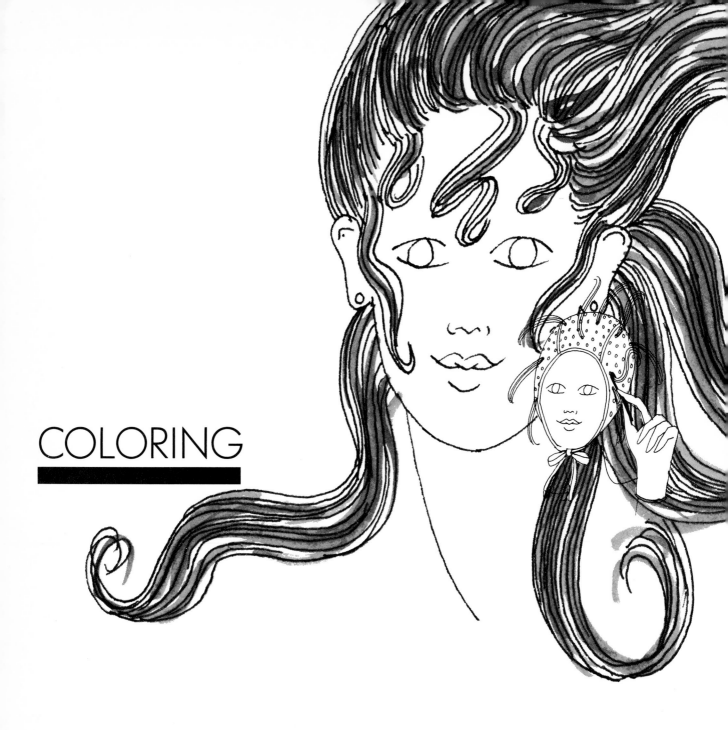

COLORING

Today, no cosmetic can achieve a greater illusion of naturalness than hair coloring. No one can tell, if it's done well and suits your skin tone.

Most skin shades are complimented by hair lightening, especially as the skin wears, and that can begin as early as twenty-five or thirty. The lightened frame of hair picks up skin, gives it a healthier, blushed tone. The darkening tints sometimes tend to muddy a complexion. That's why before taking the coloring step, it's worth trying on a few wigs or hair pieces in your local department store or beauty salon to see how the color change looks with your complexion.

With new hair color you may need anything from a change of foundation and blusher shade to a totally new makeup along with the dying or bleaching of your eyebrows. If hair, brows and makeup are off tone, no matter how superb the hair-coloring job, the look will ring artificial. "The

golden girl" with the long silky hair is one of the most glamourous images you can buy, but not if your complexion and eyebrows throw it off. To tone them costs money beyond the initial outlay for hair coloring, and, if you are trying to decide to make a major change from dark to light hair, realize what you are going to pay for it with both money and time. This coloring job has just as dramatic an effect on your wallet and schedule as it does on your looks, and its upkeep comes around regularly just like the rent.

Another consideration is whether to do the coloring yourself or have it done professionally. For instance, in lightening, some hair does not need a toner (a pale subtle tint) after the bleach has done its work, but the results can't always be predicted in advance because hidden tones "come up" during bleaching. Brown hair often proves to have a lot of red in it, and lightening will produce a strawberry

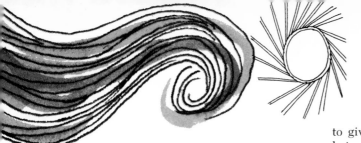

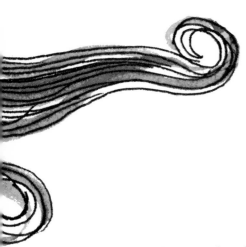

blonde. A "drabber" (often mixed with a toning tint) is then applied over the bleach to eliminate the brassy or reddish tones. Because of this bleaching is a job best left in the hands of a competent professional who knows how to cope with the perhaps unpleasant surprises revealed as the bleaching progresses.

The strand test

Bleaching or any other hair coloring change however can be made more predictable at home by the Strand Test. This is absolutely essential if you are doing the coloring yourself, especially if you've had coloring before and especially if you are using a permanent color that will not wash out. The chemicals in your previous coloring may not get along with those in the present one. The directions on the coloring package will tell you how to pretreat your hair to remedy this.

To take the test simply tie off two or three dozen strands of hair with a piece of thread and cut them off near the scalp. Do to the strands what the label describes for complete coloring. What happens to them is exactly what will happen to your whole head. Look at the results in strong light and if you are happy with them you can set to work confidently. If not, especially if you see that previously colored hair has reacted disappointingly, give up the self-coloring and take the problem to a hair colorist in a salon.

Once there, don't try to force the professional to give you changes he or she doesn't think your hair can take. For instance, going a shade lighter than he thinks you can go, or perhaps demanding a body wave that he thinks your hair can't sustain without breakage because of overcoloring. It is unusual these days to find a colorist who doesn't know his business better than you do. Hair coloring manufacturers make enormous efforts to ensure that colorists know how to use their products. There are exceptions to the rule, of course, and if you meet up with one, flee. The chances are, however, that you will be in the hands of a good colorist. So don't push him.

The patch test

Every bit as vital as the Strand Test is the Patch Test which should be done before it. A few substances involved in hair dying have a higher potential than most cosmetics to cause an allergic reaction to them.

In a salon, the Patch Test will probably be taken on a part of the skin just behind the ear but this isn't practical for home testing. An easier and just as reliable test area is the soft thin skin just in the crease of the arm. Twenty-four hours before you are planning to color your hair prepare a small amount of the coloring according to the directions (enough so that you can use it for the Strand Test, too). Wash a section of the skin about the size of a half dollar with soap and water, then dry. With a cotton tipped stick, swab the coloring product on the skin and leave it uncovered for 24 hours. Don't rub or wash off before this time is up or your test will not be valid. At the end of the time wash with warm water and if the skin is smooth, un-irritated and not itchy or in any way abnormal you are in the clear. If it is *not,* you mustn't use the product.

What kind of coloring do you want? Here are some guidelines to the marvelous range of hair coloring possibilities open to women today.

Lightening

To lighten your hair more than a few shades, bleaching is necessary. Streaking or sunbursting, which mean lightening only a few strands here and there instead of every strand, is a form of bleaching that achieves especially beautiful light effects in your hair and does not have to be touched up as often as the complete bleach job. For either, the hair is "stripped" with hydrogen peroxide, with a catalytic powder or liquid added, down to a pale wheat color. Stripping takes about an hour depending on the amount of color, artificial or natural, in your hair, the amount of hair you have and its texture. After the stripping, the hair is rinsed and ready to be toned any light shade you have chosen, silvery, golden, fawn, whatever. This two-step lightening process can sometimes be reduced to simply stripping, but the results can't always be predicted in advance because the toner may be needed to adjust hidden tones in the hair that crop up during the bleaching.

If your hair has been completely lightened, you will need a touch-up every six or eight weeks to cover the ½ inch or so of new hair that grows out. Just the new growth has to be bleached and then it along with the rest of your hair is usually toned to uniform the color. Since bleached hair has undergone chemical changes in structure it has been somewhat weakened, and, if the process is repeated too frequently, it can cause brittleness and breakage. You must take special care of lightened hair, using conditioners regularly (see chart on page 61), comb and brush it more gently than normal hair, apply shampoo, spray and setting lotion designed especially for it. If you are doing the touch-up stripping of the new growth at home be sure to protect the rest of your hair with a conditioner.

Streaking or sunbursting usually does not have to be touched up more than three or four times a year because the new growth blends in with the unstreaked strands. If the hair is worn prominently parted you will need to have streaking touch-ups more often since the new growth shows more readily on each side of the part than if the hair were partless. Streaking is, incidentally, a superb way to disguise hair that is beginning to get some gray in it.

Depending on the natural color of your hair and what you want to end up with it is possible to get a subtle lightening effect of just a shade or so without bleaching. This is done usually with a *permanent tint* in a one-step operation. The tint is mixed with a developer (peroxide) which takes some of the natural pigment out of the hair shaft and deposits new color in its place. Sometimes, especially with light brown hair, this slight change can be enough to create an illusion of blondeness. A permanent tint can be used on straightened or permanented hair. Although summer sun and a lot of perspiration may fade some of the darker tones in the color so that reddish lights begin to appear, the color will remain until new hair grows and until you cut off the old. As new growth shows you can have the permanent tint repeated all over the hair and it will keep a uniform color. (See too the section coming up on semi-permanent tints.)

Darkening

Darkening your hair is a much simpler matter than lightening it because prebleaching is not necessary. The caution here is choosing precisely the right shade for your complexion, one that will not dim and muddy it. Darkening is usually done with a permanent or semi-permanent tint. The description above of what you can expect of a permanent lightening tint applies to the darkening ones too.

Semi-permanent tints

These tints caused a minor revolution in hair coloring by eliminating the touch-up problem inherent in permanent tinting because they only last through several shampoos—two to four—and fade gradually away leaving no sharp line of demarcation between the tinted portion of the hair shaft and the growing-in virgin hair. But semi-permanent tints usually do not contain peroxide; hence, they will not lighten the color of your hair appreciably, if at all. Semi-permanent tints' greatest forte, is neither darkening nor lightening, but altering tones within the same shade range. Depending on the color used, a semi-permanent tint can subdue reddish glints in your hair . . . or it can supply them. It can add a rich sable glow to just plain brown hair, or turn a dirty blonde into a golden one. What these tints can't do is bring about a drastic change of color. The brunette who would become a blonde has no alternative to the bleaching-and-toning routine, with its attendant outlay of time and money. Some of the semi-permanent tints are not as good as others in helping to prevent with repeated use a kind of build up of color that imparts a dark heavy unnatural look to hair. For a non-professional to tell which kind of semi-permanent tint has less color build-up potential, she has to know that the product is a "non-peroxide, non-oxidation, metal complex organic dye," but this is hardly possible for her since the qualification does not appear on labels.

Temporary rinses

These are the most short lived of all forms of hair coloring; they last only until washed out. They contain no penetrating agent, simply coat the outside of the hair shaft with color. They have absolutely no lightening action at all; rather they brighten the hair by adding highlights within the same color family as your own—coppery, auburn, or golden. (They also are fine for toning down brassiness in overbleached hair.) They are generally hypoallergenic, and, unlike other types of hair coloring, require no skin Patch Test for a first-time user. Their extremely subtle effect is perfectly suited to the woman who wants to do a little experimenting without an irrevocable change. If she doesn't like it, she can wash it out and try a new shade.

Dos and don'ts for getting the best from a professional colorist: Do, if you go to one, know what you want. You should have some idea after reading this section on coloring. Don't just walk in and ask what he can do for you without giving him any clue to your likes and dislikes. He may think silky black hair is the most beautiful look in the world, but do you? On the other hand, if he tells you your hair won't take exactly the amber blonde shade you want, listen to him and don't insist on trying to get the impossible.

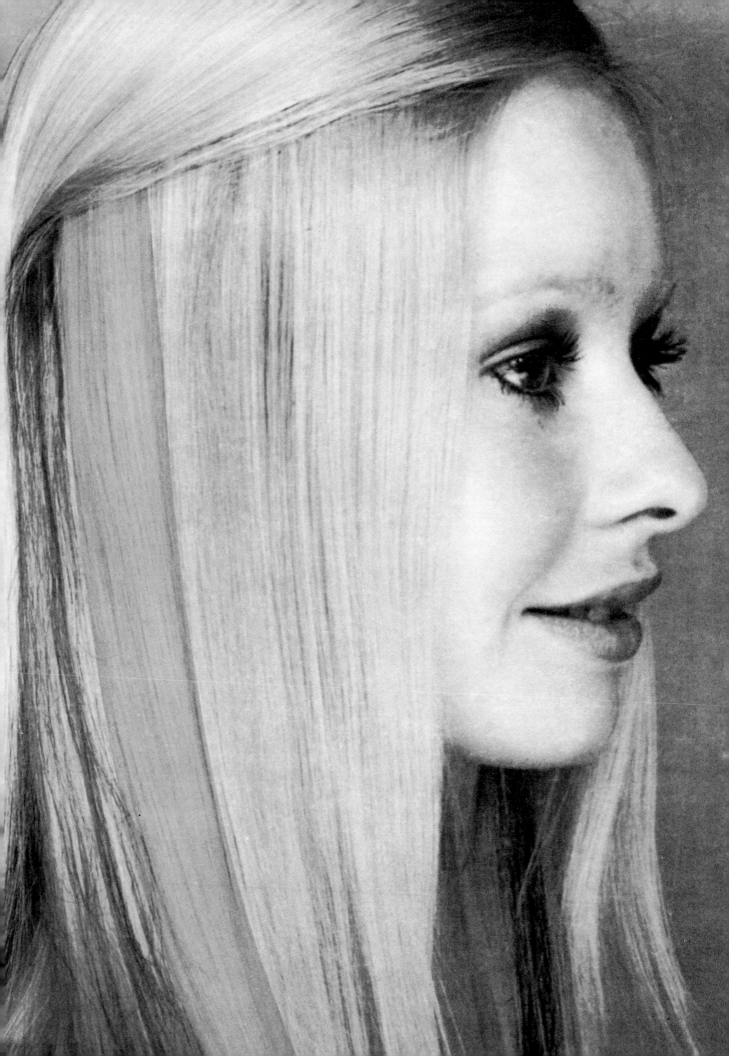

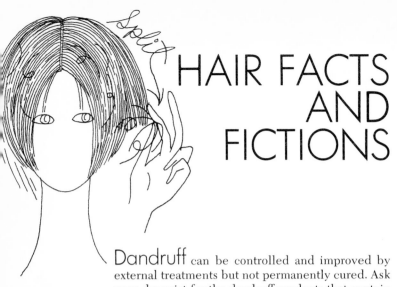

HAIR FACTS AND FICTIONS

Dandruff can be controlled and improved by external treatments but not permanently cured. Ask your druggist for the dandruff products that contain sulfur, salicylic acid, resorcinol, parachlorometaxylenol, or tars. There is a relatively new substance named zinc pyrithione that comes in a greaseless cream hairdressing or shampoo which helps even severe dandruff, particularly the hairdressing because it remains on the scalp between shampoos. If you do not find any of these things effective enough, go to your dermatologist. Dandruff incidentally is not contagious.

Brushing 100 strokes: This can, contrary to a long tradition of feminine belief, cause more trouble than benefit, especially to tinted, bleached or waved hair. One hundred strokes puts too much unnecessary wear and tear on chemically weakened hair, or any hair for that matter. Split ends and broken shafts of hair result, whereas the only probable advantage is a little extra shine. For very oily hair the result is a further distribution of oil all over the hair, down to the very ends of the strands. Brush your hair only enough to keep it in place and shapely.

Teasing ruffs up the hair shaft by raising minute sections of the outer coating so that they tangle with those of other shafts. This can achieve the illusion of more body but also hair breakage, particularly on hair that has been chemically

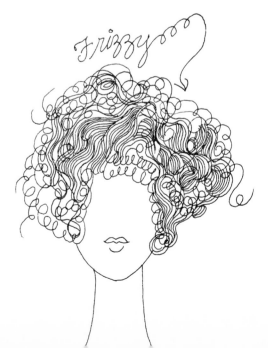

treated. Hair unaltered by chemical treatments, does not tease successfully. It is, ironically, the porous weakened cuticle that responds best to teasing and suffers most from it.

Split ends and shafts: The best solution is not to let them occur in the first place. Use preventive care: a shampoo designed for whatever type of hair you have, normal, dry, or oily. Brush gently and only for as long as you need to get the look right. Condition your hair once a month or so (see chart on page 61). Don't use rollers with bristles in them. Don't sleep on rollers. Don't roll too tightly. Don't use rubber bands to pull your hair so slick and tight that there is no give; this breaks the hair and pulls strands out from the scalp. If your hair is permanented, straightened, tinted or bleached, take even more gentle care of it, use only shampoos, conditioners, setting lotions, etc., made for chemically changed hair. Cover tinted or bleached hair in the sun.

If you already have split hairs, the only thing to do is have their ends cut off, or if the breakage is too high up to trim, wait till new healthy hair grows in. It will; these kinds of breakage are an external condition caused by external forces.

Dull, dry hair is hair which has had its outer cuticle or coating damaged or soiled. Normally the cuticle is hard and glossy, the hair shaft has a smooth silky but strong surface that reflects light and makes hair shimmer. If the cuticle is not smooth, it has been made porous by chemical change and it does not reflect light smoothly and evenly, any more than a cracked mirror does. The shine of hair is also influenced by the natural oils from the scalp glands. If there is a deficiency of oil hair can look dry and dull; on the other hand an over-accumulation of oil dulls it too, collecting dust and dirt to further tarnish the sheen. Washing will remove the oil; conditioners and scalp treatments will help to restore or supplement natural oils, conditioners will help strengthen porous hair shafts.

Hair loss: Not to be confused with breakage, hair loss means a decrease of scalp hairs. Every day a certain loss takes place, sometimes as many as a hundred hairs, and this is normal. The hair lost was in a resting state from growth, or rather the follicle that produced and bred it was. You may not even notice the loss because other hairs are constantly in a growing state to replace the lost ones.

If you are losing an abnormal amount of hair, see your dermatologist so that he can diagnose the situation correctly. Hair loss can be a result of certain systemic diseases such as thyroid, prolonged fevers. Only a doctor is qualified to decide.

Bald spots: Bald patches about the shape of coins that suddenly appear—disturbing as they are—are not usually serious unless you notice new patches appearing before the old ones have grown back or if the patches are spreading into each other to produce larger ones. The condition is known medically as alopeci aretata. Its cause is unknown,

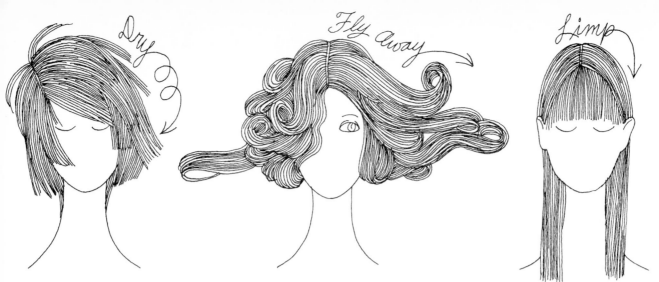

Dry   *Fly Away*   *Limp*

although emotional shock, among other things, is suspected. Usually the hair grows back without any treatment at all. If you find these patches you should nevertheless go to your dermatologist and have him start you on a routine to encourage hair growth.

After childbirth:
Many women after childbirth complain of a loss of hair. This is simply because during pregnancy alternating cycles of hair rest and growth do not happen. The rest is not experienced by the follicles, so that after birth, in order to re-establish the natural balance more follicles rest and more hairs fall out. It isn't necessary to do anything about this except not panic, just realize what is going on.

Towel drying your hair:
The "good, vigorous" rubbing of your hair dry with a towel is anything but good for it especially if you have hair loss problems. Rubbing increases tension on the hair shafts. Instead, wrap your hair in a towel and blot it gently.

Squeaky-clean hair,
i.e., just washed hair that squeaks when you rub it wet through your fingers, is to some girls a test of really clean hair. It is — so clean that a bit too much natural oil has been removed or else it wouldn't squeak. One or two shampooings at each washing are enough, don't overdo it.

Oily hair:
Use a shampoo especially made to facilitate the removal of oil. Wash as often as you need to, every few days if necessary. Brushing will not increase the oil but it will distribute it down to the very ends of the strands, so go easy on brushing. An oily scalp in teenagers usually comes along with acne, and they should use the special oil-regulating shampoos, too, to keep their hair as clean as possible. Many young girls think oily bangs cause their forehead skin to break out, but in the opinion of most dermatologists this is not so. One said, keep the hair and the forehead clean and the bangs can serve a useful purpose — to hide the acne, at least in that area.

Thinning
according to Kenneth merely compounds the problem it is trying to solve. Thick coarse or fly away hair, when cut so that certain strands are tapered shorter than others in an attempt to reduce the overall bulk, very shortly grow out and push the longer hair out even further than it was in the beginning. The solution can be straightening; or a good blunt cut and enough length to weight the hair down; or a creme rinse to soften and tame hair; or a combination of any or all of these.

Tangles:
A creme rinse is an almost automatic untangler but often leaves any but the coarsest, thickest hair too soft to manage. Never attempt to comb or brush through a head of wet tangled hair from the top down. Instead gently work in sections from the bottom up. In that way you remove the tangles towards the end first so that the ones from the top have some place to be combed down to and out. Starting at the top just causes a back-up of tangles like a traffic jam-up. Any kind of chemically treated hair is more susceptible to tangling because it has little breaks in it that snag with those of its neighbors. Be especially gentle and careful in untangling this kind of hair to prevent breakage.

Body:
You can brush it into your hair, wash it in, set it in, color it in, wave it in — in fact, arrive at it by just about any road you want to take. For the easiest body trick of brushing inside out; see page 108. All you do is bend your head downward, toss your hair forward over your face and brush it from the nape down. Then brush it back gently into the shape you want and you'll have the illusion of at least a fourth more hair than you started with. Of course, it won't last all evening but you can touch it up the way you do makeup.

There are body-builder shampoos and conditioners that actually do enlarge the hair shaft. There are setting lotions that do the same thing. Waving, streaking, bleaching, and many tints structurally enlarge the shaft, and this enlargement is as "permanent" as the processes themselves. No one has to worry today about getting body into hair.

Diet, vitamins, health food and hair:
If you eat a well-balanced diet, which by definition contains sufficient proteins, you are doing your best nutritionally for your hair. Dr. Cyril March, associate professor of clinical dermatology, New York University School of Medicine, said, "Medical science doesn't know of any food or special diet that will make hair healthier, fatter, thicker, sleeker, bigger or better in any way."

87

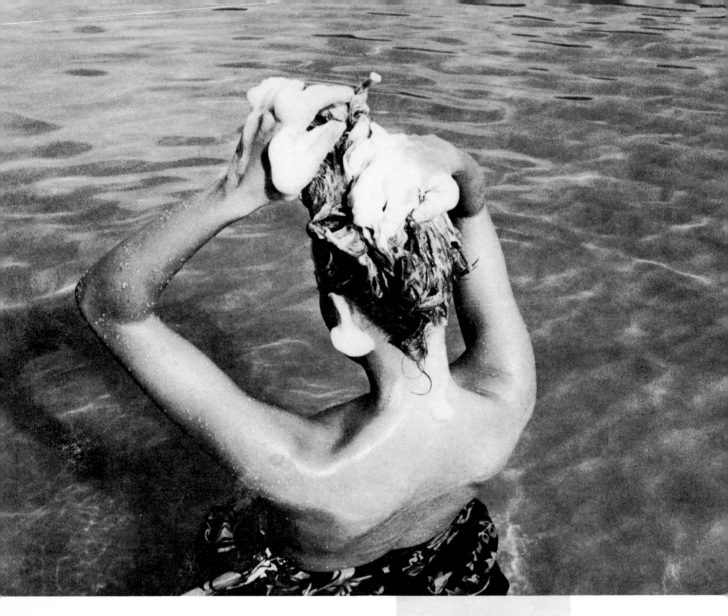

WEAR-IT-WET
SETS

Coming up may be your first problemless summer—
at least where your hair is concerned. You can look
pretty every minute whether you've come out of
the water at a nearby beach or club or just washed
your hair in an African or Mediterranean watering
hole because you just can't afford a room with a
shower everywhere you go. The trick is to master
the new wear-it-wet hair sets here and following.

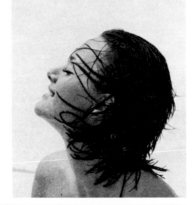

*The crescent tail set
corded, left below, and
on the courts is wet;
its dry version can be
either of the two big
heads you see on the
opposite page top and
bottom. The ribboned
top knot, opposite page,
on the girl in the striped
shirt on the golf course
is also wet; its later in
the day dry version
can also be either of
the heads in the large
photographs on the
opposite page.*

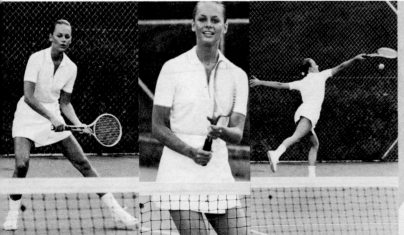

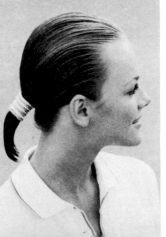

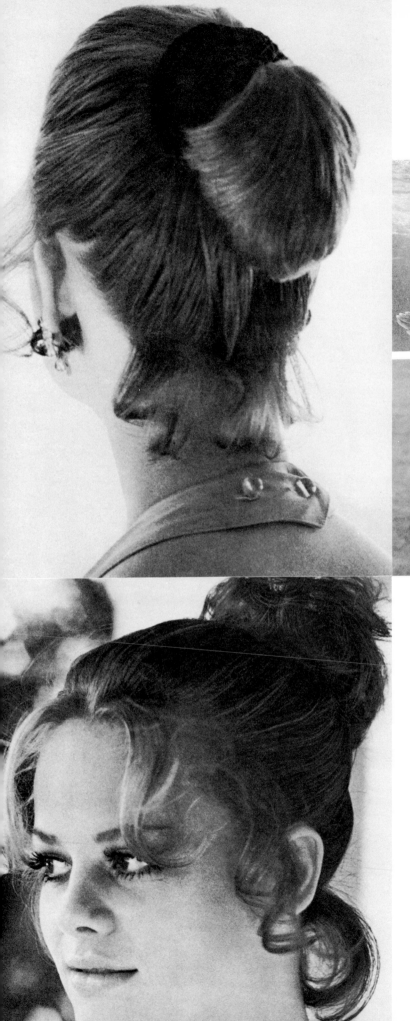

After you've checked through all the wet sets here and on the next pages to decide which one suits you best and matches up with your hair length, make sure you have a strong setting lotion and electric rollers on hand. (Of course if you have naturally curly hair you won't be able to get such straight lines with any of these sets, but you can still get very pretty wearable

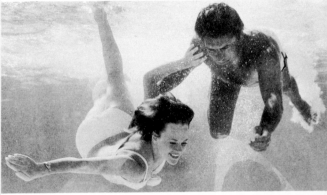

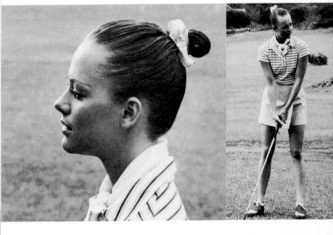

shapes.) The set for both the crescent tail and the top knot start the same way. Slick a strong setting gel through your wet hair—sleeking the hair back off the brow. For the crescent, bind it close to the head about two inches above the nape of the neck with a coated elastic band wound about with a flat ribbon or cord anchored with a tiny pin. Make sure the end of the tail is brushed under in a little crescent curl held in place by a generous dose of setting gel so that when it has dried and been combed out it will twist softly under. For the top knot sleek the hair up on the crown into a pony tail with a coated elastic band, comb the ends neatly under to make the little knot and anchor with bobby pins, then tie a ribbon about the knot. To do both comb-outs, part hair as in large photograph on this page, leaving enough at temples and nape for tendrils. Then brush hair up on the crown into a pony tail and anchor with a band. Curl tendrils with electric rollers. Brush the tail into a chignon like the ones in the large photographs. Smooth chignon can be held with bobby pins; curly topknot is finished by flipping out the wisps of hair with your fingers. 89

MORE WEAR-IT-WET SETS

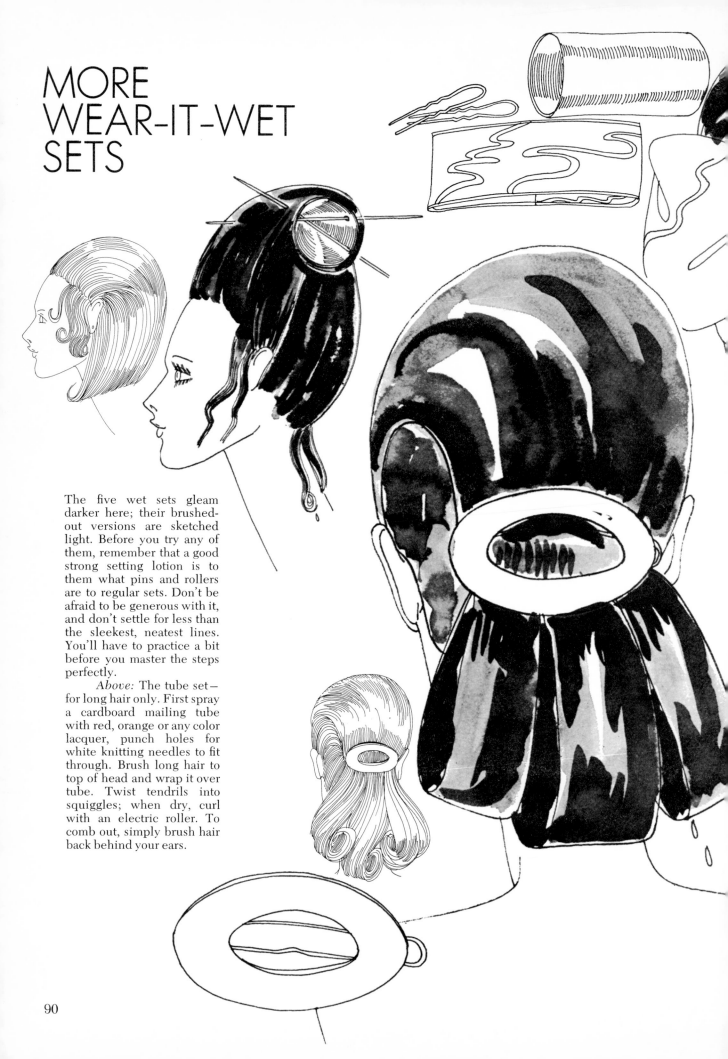

The five wet sets gleam darker here; their brushed-out versions are sketched light. Before you try any of them, remember that a good strong setting lotion is to them what pins and rollers are to regular sets. Don't be afraid to be generous with it, and don't settle for less than the sleekest, neatest lines. You'll have to practice a bit before you master the steps perfectly.

Above: The tube set— for long hair only. First spray a cardboard mailing tube with red, orange or any color lacquer, punch holes for white knitting needles to fit through. Brush long hair to top of head and wrap it over tube. Twist tendrils into squiggles; when dry, curl with an electric roller. To comb out, simply brush hair back behind your ears.

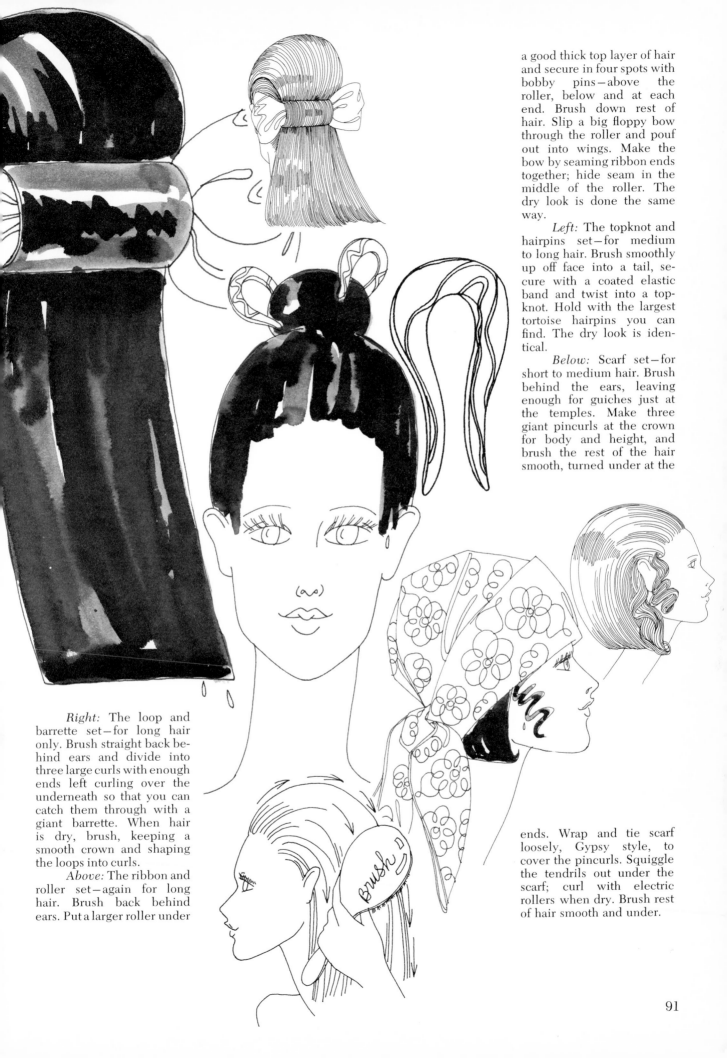

a good thick top layer of hair and secure in four spots with bobby pins—above the roller, below and at each end. Brush down rest of hair. Slip a big floppy bow through the roller and pouf out into wings. Make the bow by seaming ribbon ends together; hide seam in the middle of the roller. The dry look is done the same way.

Left: The topknot and hairpins set—for medium to long hair. Brush smoothly up off face into a tail, secure with a coated elastic band and twist into a topknot. Hold with the largest tortoise hairpins you can find. The dry look is identical.

Below: Scarf set—for short to medium hair. Brush behind the ears, leaving enough for guiches just at the temples. Make three giant pincurls at the crown for body and height, and brush the rest of the hair smooth, turned under at the

Right: The loop and barrette set—for long hair only. Brush straight back behind ears and divide into three large curls with enough ends left curling over the underneath so that you can catch them through with a giant barrette. When hair is dry, brush, keeping a smooth crown and shaping the loops into curls.

Above: The ribbon and roller set—again for long hair. Brush back behind ears. Put a larger roller under

ends. Wrap and tie scarf loosely, Gypsy style, to cover the pincurls. Squiggle the tendrils out under the scarf; curl with electric rollers when dry. Brush rest of hair smooth and under.

HOW TO CHOOSE A WIG

When you look at the wigs on the two following pages you will see what a difference the right and the wrong shape can make to the face. You can give the appearance of blotting out or diminishing the feature flaw by bringing some hair over it, not completely covering it, of course, but to slim down say round cheeks or a too broad forehead. Never leave the flaw totally exposed, but then don't be so self-conscious that you go overboard and start letting so much hair fall over it that everyone wonders what you are trying to hide.

Wig movement and color

Be sure the wig you buy has swing and motion. The one in the small picture below doesn't and that's partly why it looks "wiggy." It also needs thinning and trimming—more about that on the next pages. Don't pick a wig too far from your own hair color— your skin tone may not work with it. The long wig, *left,* is one pretty look to try. It has such freedom and movement that it can even be turned backwards—that's the way you see it in the large photograph, *opposite page,* with a few long hairs combed back. This doesn't work with every wig, but it's fun to experiment and it does give you an idea of movement to measure by.

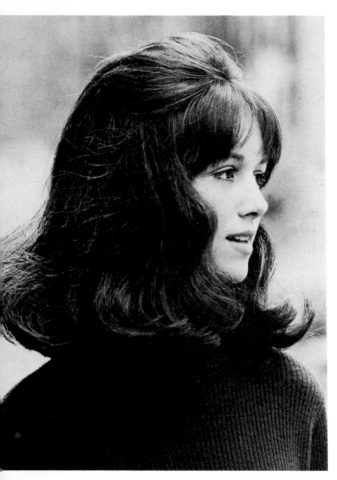

No motion

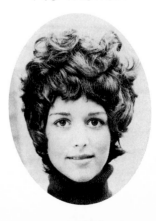

Not only the shape of the face is important in choosing a wig but the proportions of your whole body have to be considered. The girl in the little picture has a long neck. The height of the crown of the wig plus its overall shortness emphasizes that and leaves the neck exposed. The longer wig in the big photograph moves into the neckline and has a lower crown. Another point: Don't buy a heavy long, long wig if you are small, and don't buy a tiny little short wig if you're a big girl.

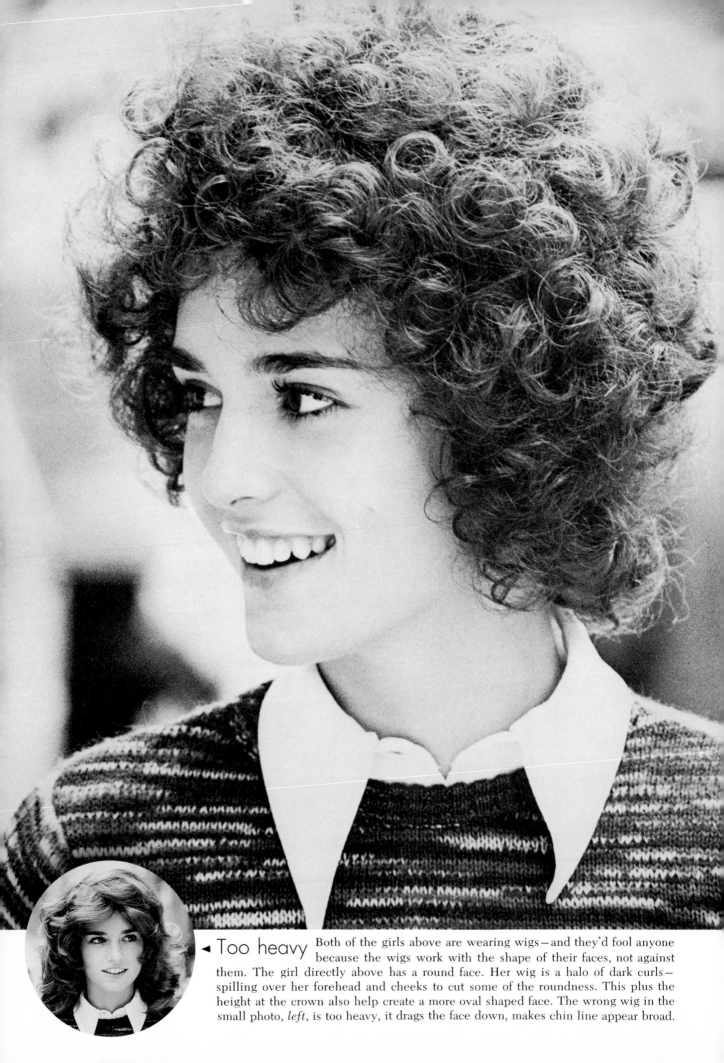

► **Too heavy** Both of the girls above are wearing wigs—and they'd fool anyone because the wigs work with the shape of their faces, not against them. The girl directly above has a round face. Her wig is a halo of dark curls—spilling over her forehead and cheeks to cut some of the roundness. This plus the height at the crown also help create a more oval shaped face. The wrong wig in the small photo, *left*, is too heavy, it drags the face down, makes chin line appear broad.

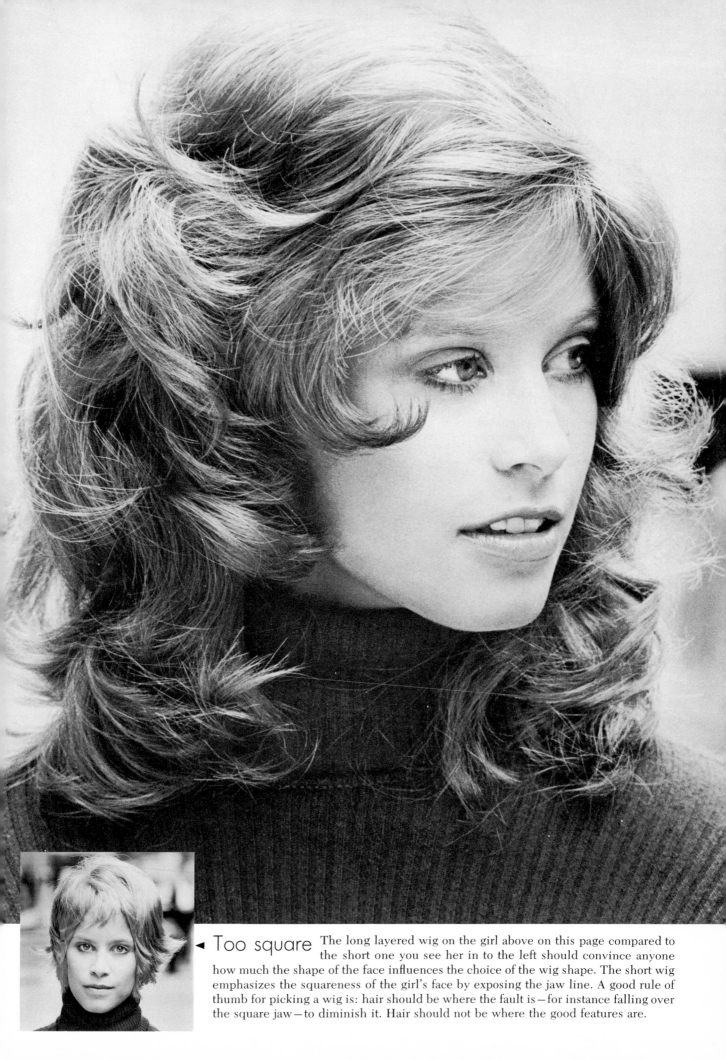

◄ Too square The long layered wig on the girl above on this page compared to the short one you see her in to the left should convince anyone how much the shape of the face influences the choice of the wig shape. The short wig emphasizes the squareness of the girl's face by exposing the jaw line. A good rule of thumb for picking a wig is: hair should be where the fault is—for instance falling over the square jaw—to diminish it. Hair should not be where the good features are.

HOW TO
CUT
AND THIN

Your wig will look more natural if it's thinned a bit and blunt-cut at the ends. Don't do this on a wig stand—because it doesn't stretch the wig base enough—and you can't do it on your own head. Have a friend who's good with hair or your hairdresser do it. Here's how it should be done—1. Put wig on. 2. Section it by center-parting and then parting again horizontally across the back earline so that you have four sections. Anchor three of the four sections with pins, leaving one bottom one free to start thinning. 3. Pick up a strand of hair at the very bottom of the wig—about one-half-inch deep

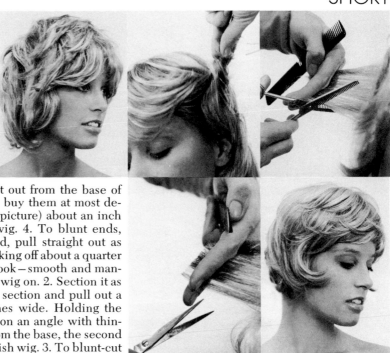

and three inches wide. Hold the strand straight out from the base of wig. With thinning scissors (scissors with teeth, buy them at most department stores) make one cut *at an angle* (see picture) about an inch from the wig base. Continue until you finish wig. 4. To blunt ends, re-section wig. Start at bottom, same size strand, pull straight out as before. Use regular scissors, cut straight across taking off about a quarter of an inch at ends. Finish wig. 5. The finished look—smooth and manageable. To thin and blunt-cut a long wig: 1. Put wig on. 2. Section it as you would for short wig. Start with one bottom section and pull out a strand about one-half-inch deep and three inches wide. Holding the strand perpendicular to the wig, make two cuts on an angle with thinning shears. The first should be about an inch from the base, the second about halfway down the length of the strand. Finish wig. 3. To blunt-cut ends, re-section wig, start at bottom with same size strand, holding it as before, and cut one quarter inch from the very ends of the hair. Cut straight across. Finish wig. 4. Compare wig here with picture 1 to see how big a difference there is.

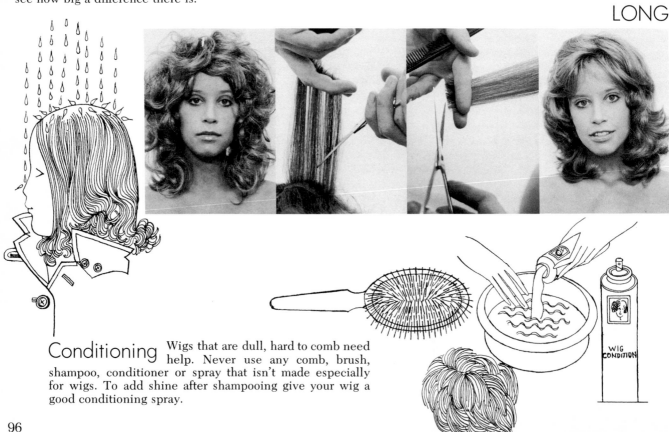

Conditioning

Wigs that are dull, hard to comb need help. Never use any comb, brush, shampoo, conditioner or spray that isn't made especially for wigs. To add shine after shampooing give your wig a good conditioning spray.

96

HOW TO
GET A
SMOOTH LOOK

MEDIUM

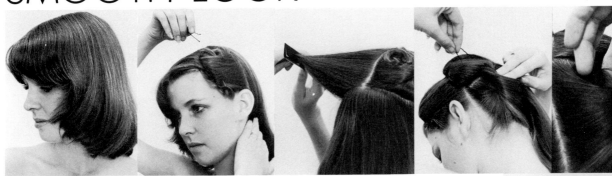

How carefully you prepare your own hair before you put your wig on can make a lot of difference in the way the wig looks. If your hair is lumpy underneath, the wig is going to look lumpy, too, and stand away from your head. Here's how to do a good flat hair wrap on medium-length hair so that your wig will hug the head and look smooth. 1. Comb hair free of tangles. 2 and 3. Make a center part, then a horizontal part at crown. Coil these two top sections into flat pincurls and anchor with short bobby pins — long ones may poke through the wig. 4. Make another horizontal part below the one at the crown about ear level. Divide this hair vertically so that you have four new sections. 5. Coil and pin them the same way. 6. This is the finished wrap (six pinned sections).

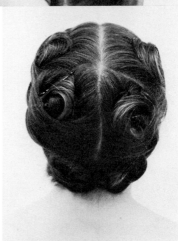

LONG

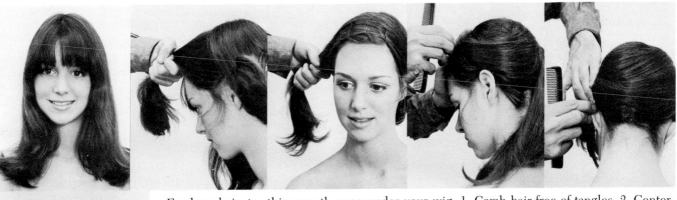

For long hair, try this smooth wrap under your wig. 1. Comb hair free of tangles. 2. Center-part hair extending the part all the way down the back of the head so the hair is completely divided. Now part it at the crown from ear to ear. You have four sections in all. (Use bobby pins to keep the hair from coming unparted temporarily if you want.) 3. Now take the front right quarter and wrap it into the left front quarter, smoothing with a comb and pinning as you work. Keep wrapping to the left so that the left side is wrapped toward the center back. Let the tail of all this hair hang loose at the center back. 4. Now pick up the back right quarter (the last section) and wrap into the front, smoothing and pinning. 5. Pick up the tail of hair you left hanging in back and wrap it in with the rest of the hair, pinning and smoothing. 6. Here's the finished wrap.

Some of the prettiest things you can do to hair are shown here — small fantasies that could be anything from a tiny "gold" butterfly to a long beaded braid. Pin them into your own hair or into a wig. 1. A long synthetic braid with tiny beads threaded through it. Wear it alone wrapped around your head Indian style, around a chignon, or as shown, as the third strand in a long braid made from your own hair. 2. A small postiche to pin on the back of your own hair or on a wig. 3. A spiraling "gold" chignon cap for your own or a false bun.

PARTY HAIR IDEAS:

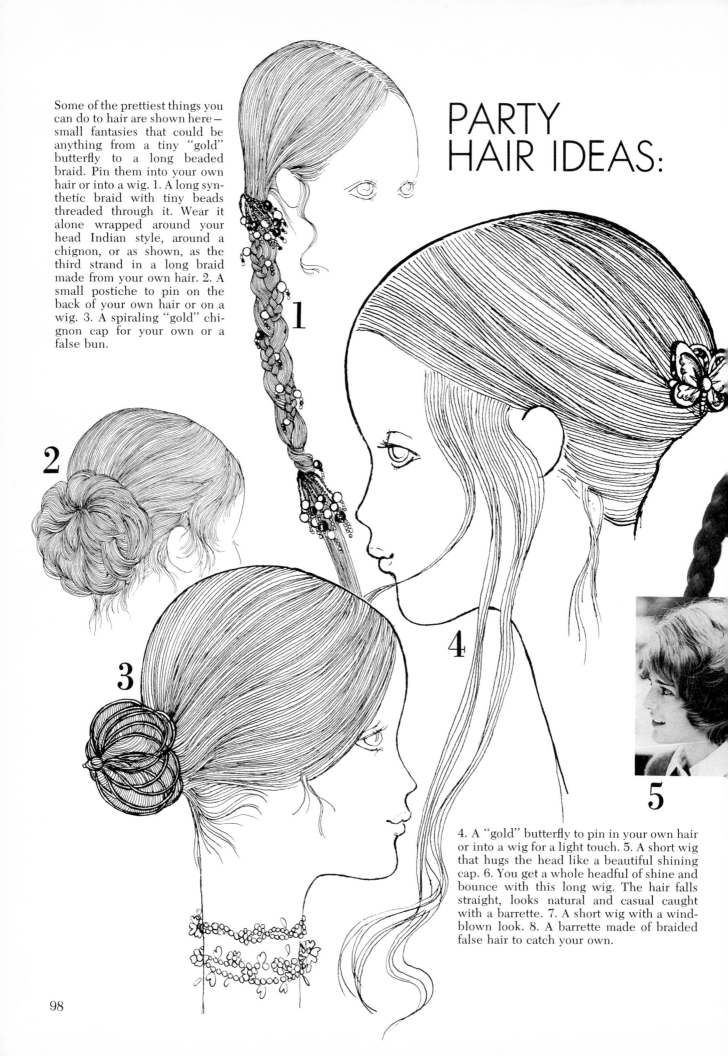

4. A "gold" butterfly to pin in your own hair or into a wig for a light touch. 5. A short wig that hugs the head like a beautiful shining cap. 6. You get a whole headful of shine and bounce with this long wig. The hair falls straight, looks natural and casual caught with a barrette. 7. A short wig with a wind-blown look. 8. A barrette made of braided false hair to catch your own.

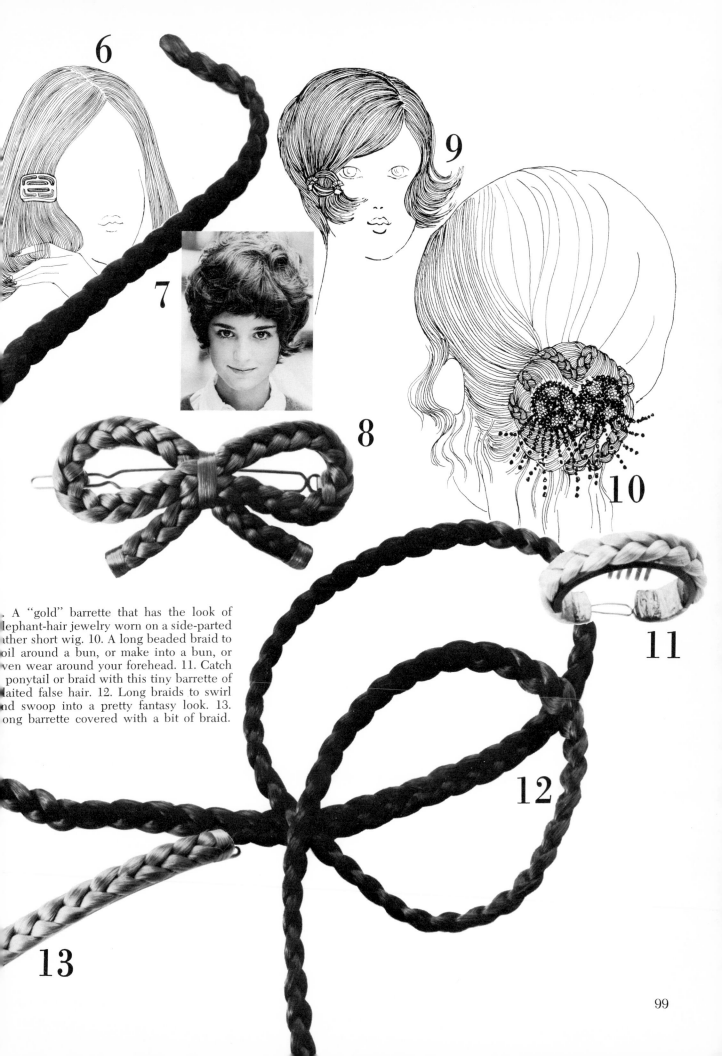

6

9

7

8

10

. A "gold" barrette that has the look of
lephant-hair jewelry worn on a side-parted
ather short wig. 10. A long beaded braid to
oil around a bun, or make into a bun, or
ven wear around your forehead. 11. Catch
ponytail or braid with this tiny barrette of
aited false hair. 12. Long braids to swirl
nd swoop into a pretty fantasy look. 13.
ong barrette covered with a bit of braid.

11

12

13

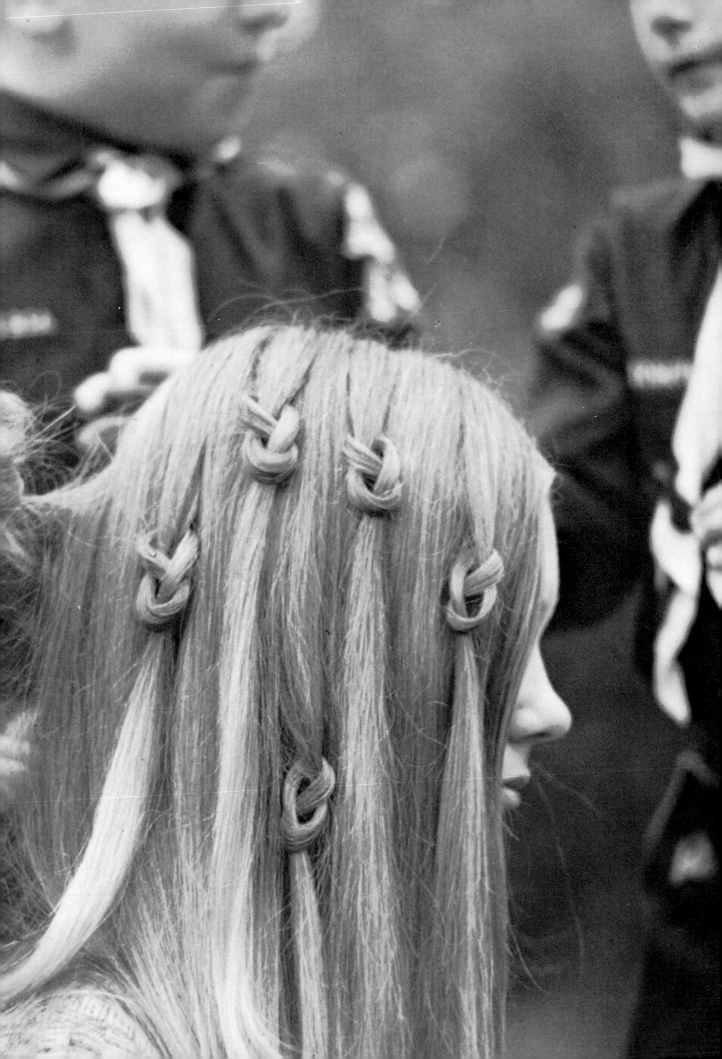

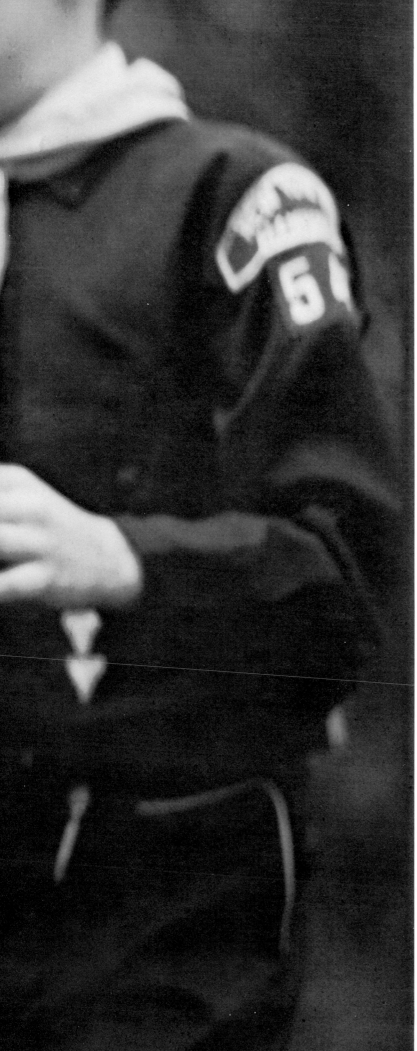

SCOUTS TO THE RESCUE— THE NEW HAIR KNOTS

Without cutting or growing your hair a fraction of an inch, you can find a dozen or so different ways to wear it on the following pages. All are based—Scout's honor— on authentic Scouting knots. Some are so simple even a Cub could do them; some may take a little help from your friends or hairdresser. All are meant to keep you from getting knotted up about what to do with your hair for fall. Have fun with it! Hair here by Alan Lewis.

LOVE KNOTS TO WEAR IN YOUR HAIR

Tying these little knots is almost as much fun as wearing them. They come straight from the Boy Scouts of America manual on knot-tying, but are tied with sleek, shining hair instead of the usual rope. When you try tying them, be sure to dampen the hair you're knotting so that it won't slip loose. *This page:* Pull one big piece of hair forward on each side of center part. Now pull a few small strands out at the very front and back and wrap them around the larger piece several times, see picture *far left*. Tie the ends of this small piece in a Half Hitch knot, see sketch *left*. *Opposite:* Hair can be center- or side-parted. Pull two pieces of hair out, the size in the picture, and tie a loose Sheet Bend—an old sailing knot. The diagram *below* shows you how to weave the hair. If your hair is center-parted, tie one on each side. Hair knots here and on the following pages were worked out by Maury Hopson and our beauty editor from the pamphlet *Knots and How to Tie Them*, published by the Boy Scouts of America.

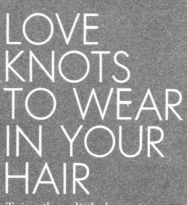

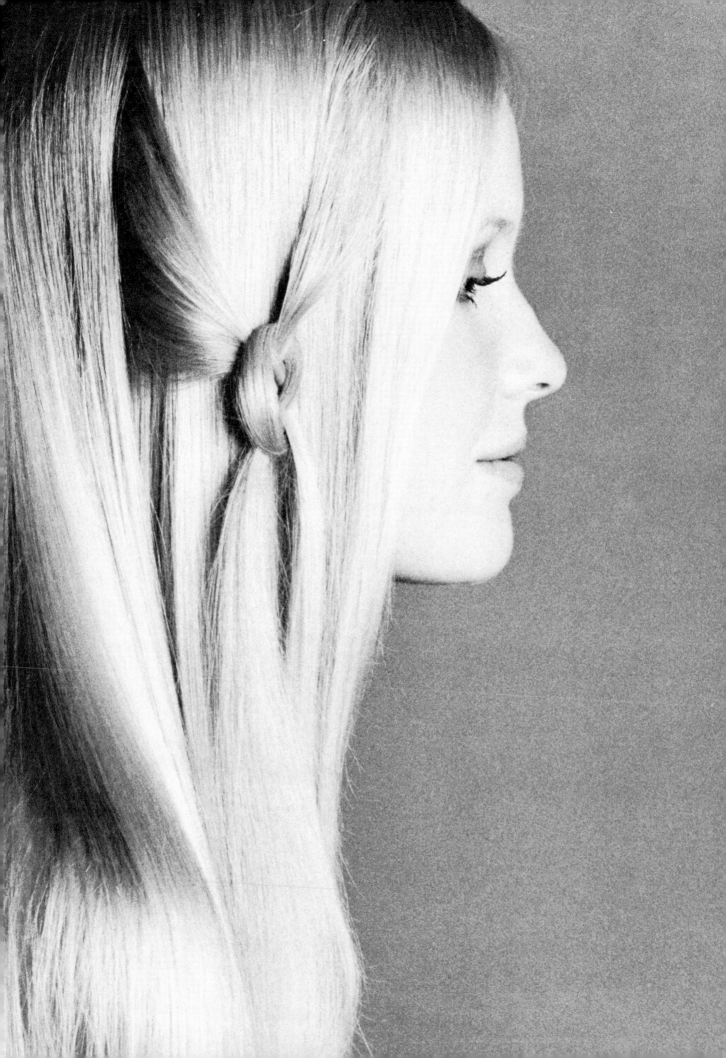

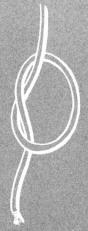

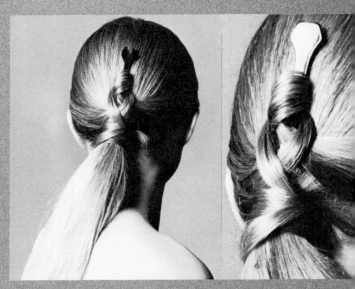

Here are more ways to tie your hair into shining little love knots. *Opposite page:* Pull out a fairly large piece of hair on each side of a center part, tie it into an Overhand knot. The diagram *left* shows you how. You can use very fine hairpins on the back side of any of these knots to keep them secure. *This page:* A ponytail caught with a Clove Hitch Over Bar knot and a pretty "tortoise-shell" ornament is one of the most romantic looks you could try. You'll need a friend's help for this one. Start by pulling hair back into a low ponytail—all but two small strands at the very front—and catch it in a coated elastic band. Stick the "tortoise" stickpin or hairpin into the elastic. Now bring the front strands to the back and loop them around the stickpin as you see in the diagram *right.* The knot on top in the diagram is the finished look pulled taut, but yours should be loose and plump like the one in the picture. *Right,* in the diagram you see the direction to loop the hair. You can tuck the remaining ends of the hair you tied underneath the ponytail and hold them with a fine hairpin. Hair by Maury Hopson.

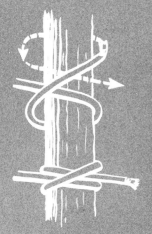

LOVE KNOTS TO WEAR IN YOUR HAIR

 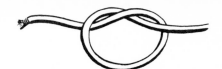

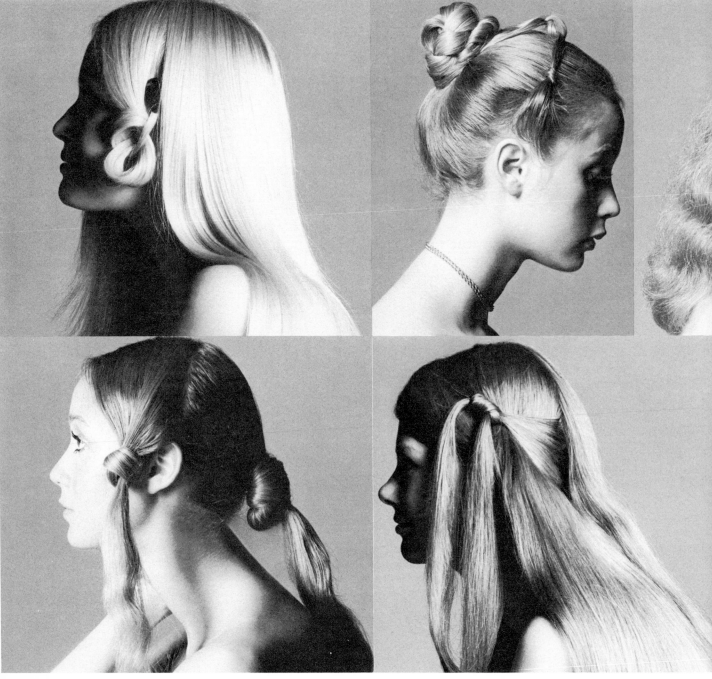

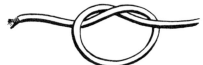 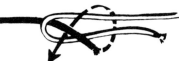

A Figure Eight knot, see diagram *at top left*, tied on one side of a center part is a fresh, pretty look. Pull out enough hair to make a nice plump knot, then clip end with a small barrette. Make three round, shining Overhand Knots for the look *at bottom left*. First, center-part hair; then make another part from ear to ear. Catch each of the three sections with coated elastic bands. Then make one Overhand Knot for each section, see diagram *at bottom left*. Be sure your knots hide the elastic bands. For the look at *top right* put hair up in a chignon at the back of the head, leaving out two small strands on each side above ears. Tie one Overhand Knot, diagram *at top right*, in each strand. Then tie strands together with an Overhand Knot and tuck the ends under the chignon with bobby pins. For the look *at below right* center-part hair, pull one thick strand out in front and another in back. Then tie them in a tight Sheet Bend knot. See diagram *at bottom right*. Fasten the knot to your hair with a small hairpin. Tie another knot on the other side of your head.

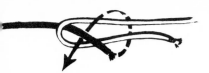 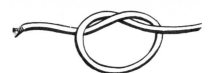

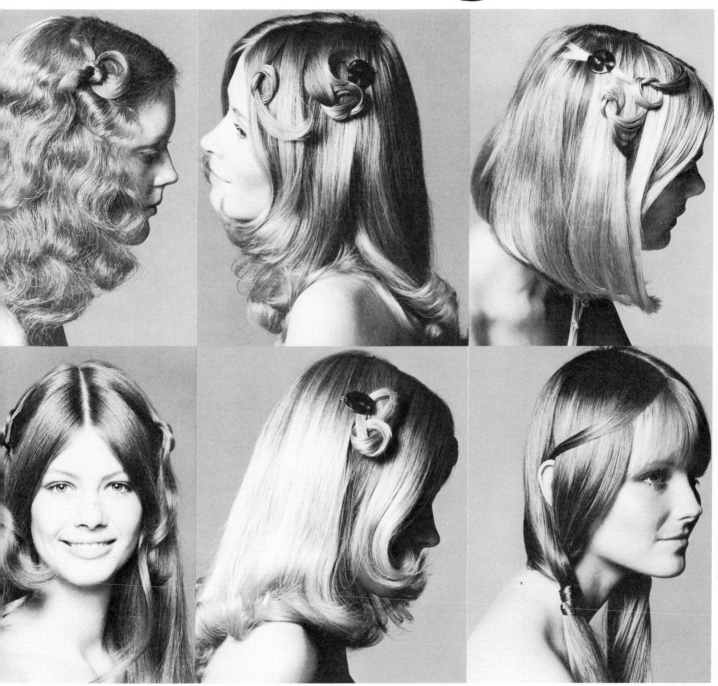

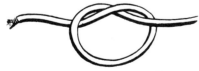 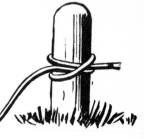

For top left, pull two small strands of hair out on each side of center part. Tie a loose Sheet Bend knot in each. If hair's curly, let ends curl; if straight, cover ends with a barrette. For *bottom left,* you can achieve this softly curled look by tying two Overhand Knots, see diagram *at bottom left,* on each side of a center part, and curling the long ends with electric rollers. The soft, lacy effect you see *at middle top* is done by tying several Overhand Knots in long hair. The diagram *at top right* shows you how to tie the knots. Clip the ends together with a pretty barrette. A "tortoise" barrette holds the ends of the loosely-tied Overhand Knots, at *bottom middle.* The look *at top right* is the same as the one next to it, but the hair is shorter. The knots are exactly the same, though. For the look *at bottom right,* split hair in half down the center. Pull out a small front strand on each side of part, tuck ends behind ears with bobby pins. Pull out two more small strands on teach side at nape of neck. tie them in Clove Hitch knots, diagram *right,* around each half section of hair.

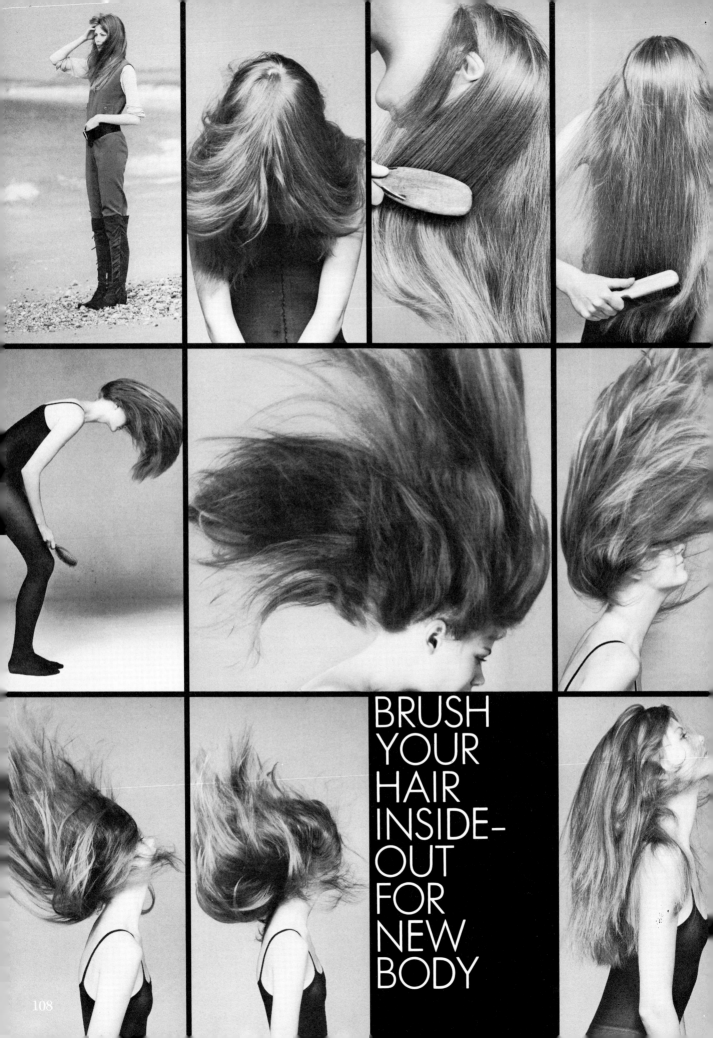

BRUSH
YOUR
HAIR
INSIDE-
OUT
FOR
NEW
BODY

108

you've often felt your hair ⟨liv⟩es its life in willful dis⟨ob⟩edience to you—it droops ⟨wh⟩en you want it sleek, ⟨str⟩aggles when you want it ⟨smo⟩ooth—try brushing it in⟨sid⟩e out like the model's do⟨in⟩g here. This reverse ⟨bru⟩shing helps give hair ⟨ne⟩w body and fullness with⟨ou⟩t any old-fashioned, hard ⟨on⟩ your hair back-combing. ⟨He⟩re's how to do it. Stand ⟨an⟩d bend your head forward ⟨so⟩ that all your hair hangs ⟨do⟩wn. Then begin brushing ⟨fro⟩m the nape of the neck ⟨for⟩ward as you see the ⟨mo⟩del doing in the top pic⟨tur⟩es. Give it a good brush⟨in⟩g, always *away* from the ⟨dir⟩ection of hair growth. ⟨Th⟩en stand up and throw ⟨yo⟩ur head back as the model ⟨is⟩ doing, *center* pictures and ⟨bo⟩*ttom left*. When all your ⟨ha⟩ir has settled back and ⟨do⟩wn, use your brush to give ⟨it⟩ a *light* smoothing, *di*⟨rec⟩*tly below*. The results— ⟨ha⟩ir that has a new lift, looks ⟨fre⟩e, uncontrived and natu⟨ral⟩, with all sorts of extra ⟨be⟩nefits like the polish and ⟨sh⟩ine a good brushing can ⟨giv⟩e it, maybe even a rosy ⟨glo⟩w in your cheeks from the ⟨inc⟩reased circulation of ⟨bru⟩shing and bending over.

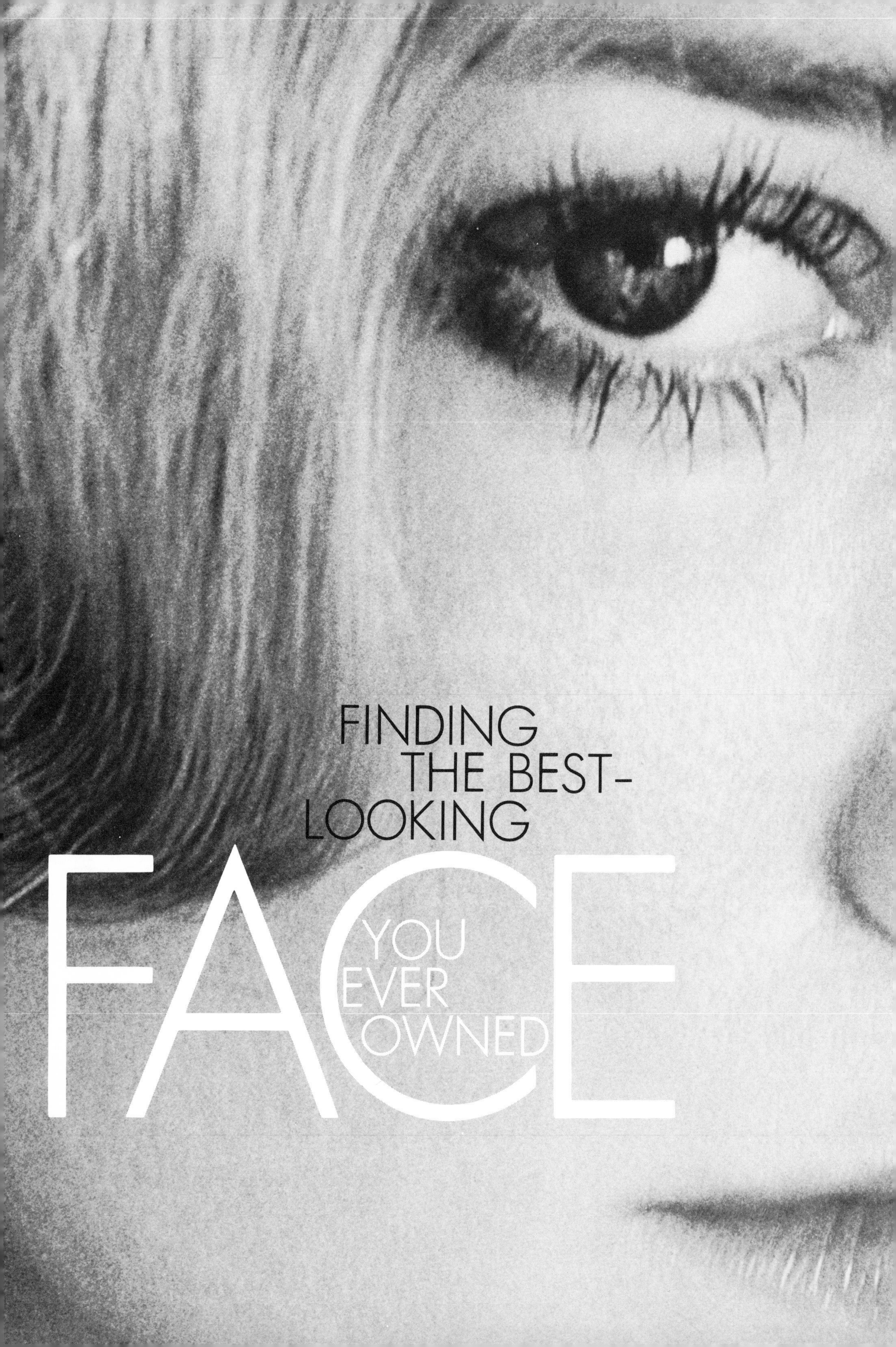

FINDING
THE BEST-
LOOKING

FACE YOU EVER OWNED

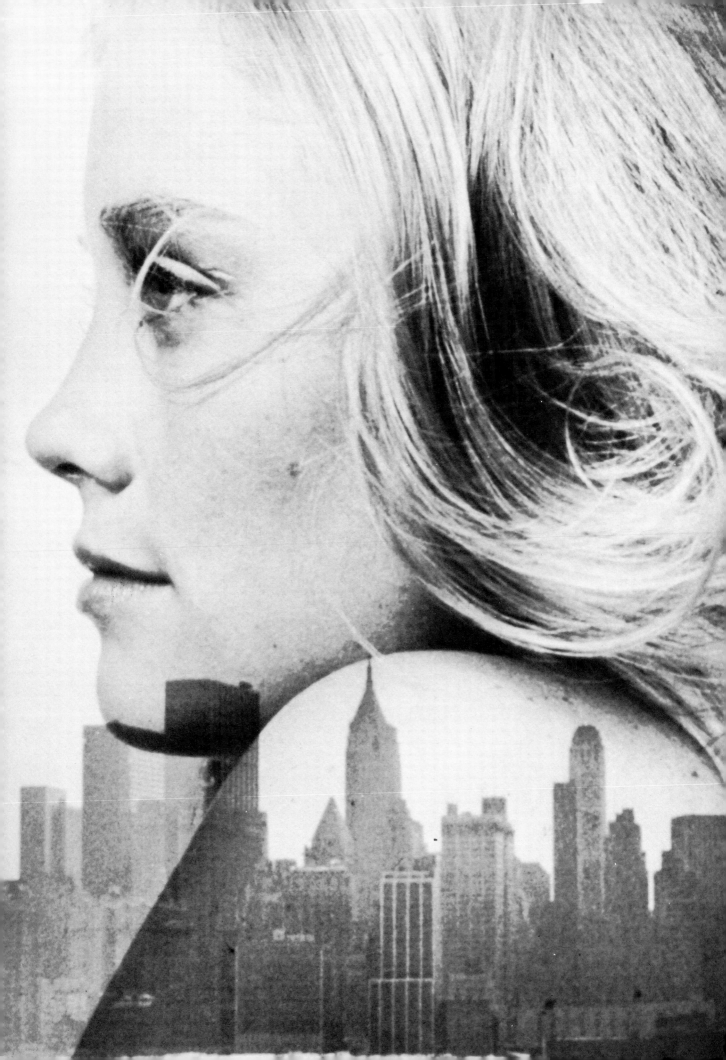

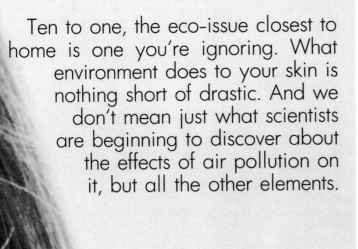

Ten to one, the eco-issue closest to home is one you're ignoring. What environment does to your skin is nothing short of drastic. And we don't mean just what scientists are beginning to discover about the effects of air pollution on it, but all the other elements.

SAVE YOUR SKIN FROM THE ENVIRONMENT

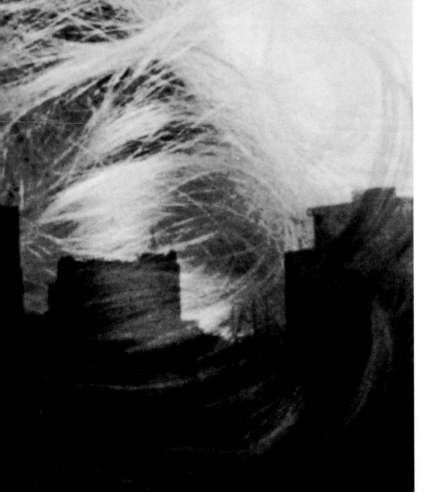

Environment is at work on your skin twenty-four hours a day every day. Nothing outside of heredity affects its look more than it does. To prove it to yourself, just take this simple test which Dr. Earle Brauer describes in his book, *Your Skin and Hair.* Compare the skin on your hands or face, which is exposed constantly to the environment, with the skin on your bosom or tummy, which is usually covered. The difference in softness, smoothness and color—unless you've been sunning naked—is undeniable, and the older you get the more noticeable it becomes.

(*Continued on p. 115*)

SKIN SURVIVAL CHART

	Hot and dry	Hot and humid	*Industrially* Polluted air
Dry Skin	*Dry skin gets drier in hot climates where there's little moisture in the air. What to have in your survival kit: For face—Moisturizer under oil-based makeup. Superfatted soap or cleansing lotion especially for dry skin. Emollient cream for night. Moisturized lipgloss or lipstick.*	*When there is a lot of moisture in the air, water does not evaporate from the skin as easily and not as much oil escapes as does under dry conditions. Humidity makes a better environment for dry skin, but it can't change the fact that your skin is dry. In hot, humid weather you're trying to perspire to keep cool, therefore some oil and water are lost, but not as much as in hot, dry climates. For face—Same treatment as in hot and dry, but use a lighter moisturizer.*	*Experts hassle over the degree of influence air pollution has on skin but until they're sure, follow these preventive measures: For face—Actually the moisturizer and oil-based makeup you'd normally use discourage grime, smog and chemicals from working into the skin. They make a protective barrier that lets contaminated particles slide off more easily when you are cleansing your face. Be very thorough with your cleansing routine. Once a week, add a deep cleansing facial mask for dry skin or a facial sauna. Carry mini freshening towels for pickups during the day, but be sure they are not astringent. If your eyes bother you, eye drops and eye pads while you're napping.*
Oily Skin	*Heat increases the oil productivity of skin, also causes oil to flow more readily. To counteract the increase: For face—More cleansing and freshening. Use a soap or liquid cleanser for oily skin, perhaps a mild antibacterial soap, a light astringent. Water-based or gel makeup and lipgloss. Perhaps the new oil-absorbent makeups. Moisturizer around eyes, on throat and lips at night. Mild astringent freshening towels or pads during the day, plus blotting powder. Twice a week a light astringent or pore-tightening beauty mask.*	*Your perspiration mechanism is working harder in order to cool the body, but the already moist air, like an overloaded sponge, isn't absorbing as much perspiration as dry air would. Perspiration mixes with skin oils, causes them to run and spread more easily. The routine to cut down on this extra environmental-induced flow of oiliness: For face—Follow the same treatment as in a hot and dry climate, maybe add more pickups and freshening during the day and more beauty masks at night. In extreme cases, a dermatologist might advise drugs that could slow down the oil activity.*	*Oils on skin help protect it against pollutants by acting as a natural barrier. For face—If your skin is just mildly oily you might want to add a moisturizer under makeup; otherwise follow same routine as in hot and dry climates. If necessary, soothing eye drops, pads.*
Normal Skin	*In a hot, dry climate normal skin gets drier. Combination dry-oily isn't a basic skin type—all faces have some areas that are oilier or drier than others. In dry areas, add moisturizer; in oily ones, absorb the oil with freshening pads. For face—Mild soap or cleansing lotion, light moisturizer under makeup or combo moisturizer-makeup, and lip protector or gloss. A night cream before bed around eyes, throat, mouth. A light beauty mask weekly.*	*Normal skin, like any other kind, reacts to heat and humidity by trying to produce more perspiration to cool the body, but this is not absorbed as easily in moist air as in dry, so it remains on the skin, mixes with oils stimulated by the heat, and causes them to spread. For face—Do what's outlined in hot and dry, use more pickups and freshenings during the day with mini towels and blotting powder carried in your purse.*	*Moisturizer should protect the skin evenly against pollutants. For face—Use a moisturizer under makeup or built in to it to protect skin against pollutants, especially the less resistant drier parts. Follow the same routine as in hot and dry.*

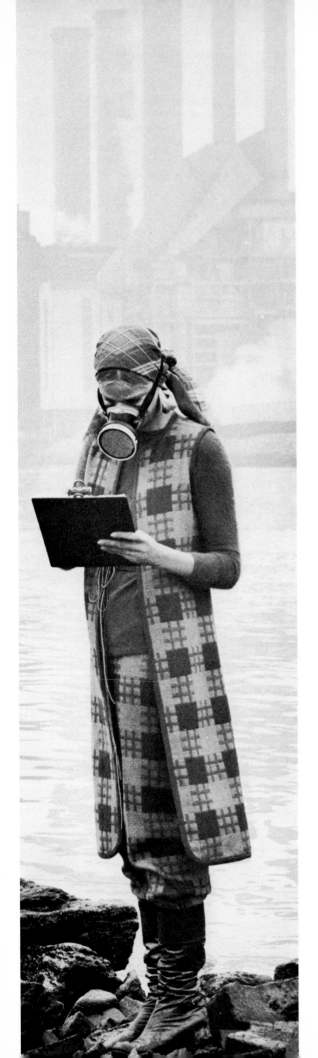

The better protection against environment you give yourself, the better your beauty chances. That's why we've made up these skin survival charts for every kind of condition most people live in. Pick out the elements you are exposed to and see how to save your skin from them. Start here with the brief chart on heat, humidity, sun and industrial pollution. There's more about their effects, along with those of wind, air-conditioning, steam heat, and cold further in the article.

Industrial city pollution

The smog, soot and grime that pollute the air in most of our big industrial cities land on your skin and don't just fly off. Exactly what happens is a matter of controversy among experts. Dr. Brauer, a dermatologist and medical director of the Revlon Research Center, said, "In industrial soot there are several chemicals. Sulfur dioxide is the most suspect one as far as skin is concerned. I first became concerned with this when I read a news item about the increased rate of disintegration of the statues and ruins in Rome and Athens since these cities have become industrialized enough to suffer from air pollution. The people trying to protect these works of art have discovered that the soot particles land on the surface, mix with water from the air, the sulfur dioxide goes into solution and turns into sulfuric acid. It is one of the strongest acids known. How much of this acid is deposited on the skin, how long it stays, what effect it has, we don't know yet. We do know that some sulfur compounds in quantity aren't good for the skin, they can cause undesirable irritation. It's difficult to find out what sulfuric acid in the environment does to the skin because we lack a control testing model. We can't just pour sulfuric acid on human skin—that would do damage. We have to get something that will reflect human skin as much as possible, plus creating chambers in which the actual environment can be simulated and controlled."

Until there is more exact information on skin contamination, there are a lot of practical things women can do to protect themselves from possible damage. The first is obviously to keep the exposed skin as immaculately cleansed as possible. Secondly, prepare your skin for going out into the environment with protective barriers such as moisturizers, foundations with oil bases, makeups that contain moisturizers and emollients. Dr. Brauer demonstrates what an effective barrier oil and oil-like substances provide by this quick test. He cleans two patches on the forearm with soap and water, then applies a test substance or protective barrier to one, but not the other. The next step is to drop a bit of soot on both to contaminate them. When the arm is put under a water faucet for cleansing, the soot on the protected area slides right off, while a residue remains on the other.

Set up an oil barrier like this on your arms and hands, as well as your face. Actually, it's a good idea to protect your entire body with a moisturizer or body lotion.

Industrial pollution is probably the least of the environmental threats to skin. Dr. Norman Orentreich, a well-known New York dermatologist, places much more importance on the effects of climate and sun: "After all, skin is always replacing itself, it is not a static thing. What was the bottom of the skin becomes the top about every thirty days, so pollutants or anything like that are constantly being removed." He doesn't believe there is enough scientific evidence that the normal pollutants in industrial city areas are affecting the skin. "Of course," he added, "if you are going to sit on top of a smokestack and stick your head into sulfuric fumes coming out, that would create damage. But one has to be practical. At the moment in our society I think the effect of pollutants on the skin is insignificant. It's like dropping a bottle of ink into the Atlantic Ocean at New York and worrying about detecting it at the Cliffs of Dover. Theoretically you could, theoretically one molecule will get there."

Humidity & heat

Dr. Orentreich believes the humidity factor is far more significant, along with sunlight, radiation and the thermal changes we introduce into life—steam heat, air-conditioning. This is why: Skin is a protective covering through which the body temperature is regulated to keep us in a state of equilibrium with our environment. As skin cells change and are shed they lose water. The body also loses water through perspiration. We lose this water to the environment, depending on the amounts of heat and humidity present.

If you live in Colorado, where the air is very dry and hot, you're going to lose more moisture from the skin to the environment than in a moderate climate or a humid one. The air is like a sponge. When it is dry it absorbs moisture from the exposed body surfaces. Heat also stimulates perspiration, which, as it evaporates, cools the body. In addition, heat increases the body's oil productivity. So you are losing both water and oil and need to return both by the use of moisturizers and creams. Even if you live in a hot humid place— Florida, Louisiana, the tropics—there is still some water and oil loss but not as much as in dry heat. That's because the heat is causing the body to perspire to keep cool, producing water that is not easily evaporated into the already moisture-laden air. The less evaporation, the more you feel the heat, and the more the body perspires trying to cool you off. The heat also makes the body oils more fluid, just as it does to butter. They mix with the perspiration and flow out of the body more readily. Hot, humid climates can be particularly difficult for very oily skin, since the already natu-

rally active oil glands are stepped up further. You need to get rid of the excess oil with frequent washings, mild astringents, pickups during the day with pads or mini towels designed for oily skin and usually containing some kind of astringent. If your skin is oily, but not excessively so, it will probably require a lighter moisturizer because it is, after all, losing some moisture and oil. A heavy moisturizer would make it even more difficult to perspire in humidity.

All healthy skin types automatically develop a certain equilibrium with their environments and can be helped further by cosmetics to replace moisture and oil loss or to absorb excesses. When you travel, say from Colorado to Florida, you'll probably need to give your skin, like the rest of your body, more attention because it does not adapt immediately. There are definite changes in a person's physiology from one area to another with lag periods involving sleep cycles and all sorts of factors. That is why a competent command will send soldiers who are to fight in tropical climates first to a hot, humid training camp in this country for a week or two. They have to be acclimatized or too many men would be lost to morbidity, they couldn't function properly and would become depressed.

Hard water

Much of the United States has hard water which contains mineral salts. In some places the content is higher than others. This means that ordinary soap doesn't lather well in it because the soap mixes with the mineral salts to form a precipitate of insoluble salts—the old familiar ring on the bath tub, plus an invisible coat of salts on your skin. If you rinse this coating off in clean water you are doing a reasonably good job of removing it. Anyone who has been on board a ship where evaporated water was used or in the Virgin Islands realizes the difference between water with and without these salts. In their absence, soap lathers profusely and you feel you'll never get it off.

The more you wash and bathe in any kind of water, the more you strip off the skin's oil barrier, especially if you use ordinary soap. This is not a denuding of the oils in the cells below the surface, but it is a denuding of the protective oil surface, which leaves the skin more susceptible to soot, wind and sun. A good solution to controlling this denudation in all seasons is to use a cleaning lotion that removes dirt effectively but is sparing in its removal of the natural skin oils.

Now that you know the effects of environment on skin and the possibilities of damage, join the ecology beauty crusade. It starts closer to you and home than any other part of the movement.

1 MINUTE SKIN TYPE TEST

The center strip down your face is the oiliest, in width from about mid-brow to mid-brow, in length from neckline to chinline. To find your skin type blot with a tissue just one side of your face within the oiliest area, blot in several spots, say forehead, nose and chin, each time with a clean part of the tissue. The results: Oily skin will show a considerable difference in gloss between the side blotted and the unblotted side. You'll also find a recognizable amount of oil on the tissue spots. Normal, or usual skin, will evidence only a slight difference in gloss and very little oil on the tissue. Dry skin signals no difference and just the barest trace of oil.

You'll read over and over again that some people have a combination skin type of oily and dry. Most dermatologists deny it. Outside of the oiliest area the skin may appear to be drier but it is actually still an oily type skin. Don't make the mistake of thinking a slight yellowish scaliness, even redness and a mild itchiness are signs of a dry skin. The scaliness is caked oil and skin refuse that would disappear if you used the right oily skin treatment. In most cases so would the redness and itchiness but if it doesn't, see a dermatologist.

BASIC CARE FOR THE THREE SKIN TYPES

Oily
Soap (especially for oily skin) and water washing every morning.

Take makeup off in the evening with a cleansing lotion, follow with soap and water washing or an astringent.

In extreme cases of caked oil, scaliness, redness, itchiness, follow the same morning and night care but use an extra strong cleansing lotion, astringent, soap designed for oily skin.

Dry
Cleansing lotion especially for dry skin morning and night.

Moisturizer under makeup and before bed, with special concentrations of oil and humectants for dry skin.

Normal
Soap and water washings morning and night.

If skin is very thin or fragile around eyes, ears, neck supplement or replace soap with cleansing lotion in these areas.

Before makeup use an astringent lotion.

Moisturizer under makeup and also before going to bed at night.

DOS & DON'TS

Do realize that if you have oily skin it is more prone to acne in the early years but you'll have less problems with dryness as you get older?

Dry skin types have more trouble in time—don't neglect increasing the oils and lubricants you put on your skin as it grows older.

All skin types will have to make some alterations in skin care as they grow older. Don't refuse to recognize the signs of changing dryness or oiliness, add or subtract what's needed.

Do for oily skin use water based makeup; for dry, oil based makeup; normal can use either.

COSMETIC
DO YOU KNOW EXACTLY WHAT DOES WHAT?

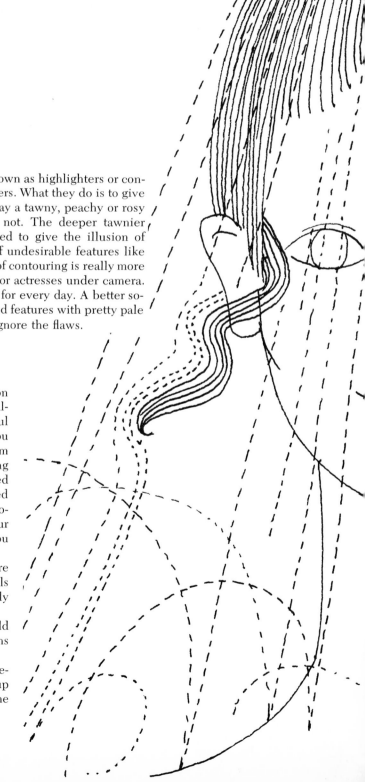

Astringents

These have a temporary pore-tightening effect, stimulate and often tingle the skin. They're bracing for oily skin. Take your pick between liquid, gel or saturated pad astringents. It's a good idea to read the label on the one you choose before buying it, just to be sure you know what you're getting, what the product is all about, and follow the instructions on use. In fact, read all labels on all cosmetics.

Blushers

These are sometimes known as highlighters or contourers, as well as blushers. What they do is to give added color to cheeks, say a tawny, peachy or rosy glow, either frosted or not. The deeper tawnier tones are sometimes used to give the illusion of fading out or "block" off undesirable features like fat cheeks but this kind of contouring is really more for professional models or actresses under camera. It is usually too obvious for every day. A better solution is to bring out good features with pretty pale highlight blushers and ignore the flaws.

Cleansers

There's a crowd of them so here's the rundown on what you should know about each one: *Soap:* Almost everyone uses it, but everyone is not as careful as she should be in choosing the right soap. If you have a dry- or oily-skin condition, or a problem complexion, be sure your soap is aimed at helping to correct the condition. There are super-fatted soaps for dry skin; drying ones for oily; medicated soaps for acne and other problem skins; hypoallergenic for sensitive skins. Check with your dermatologist if you have doubts about what you should use.

Liquid cleansers: Made for all types of skin, are more sparing in the removal of natural skin oils than most soaps, and are easy to remove by gently rubbing with a tissue.

Creams: A cleansing cream is often called cold cream and is generally better for dry or normal skins than oily.

Pad cleansers: Thick little wads of absorbent material saturated with a cleanser and good for touch-up cleaning during the day. Some are medicated, some astringent and are usually not for dry skin.

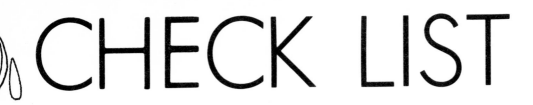

CHECK LIST

Cover-ups

These are matte makeups used to help camouflage minor blemishes, help cover shadows and redness. They range in color from flat white to the deepest skin tones. The white and paler ones can be used, too, to lighten or highlight certain areas of the face. There are sticks, creams, liquids.

Emollients

They are heavy-duty creams aimed at helping skin that needs oil. Under this heading come night creams to help lubricate the skin while you sleep, day ones to go under makeup, eye creams which are made especially rich because this is one of the first areas on the face to need oil to keep it from getting dry and crinkly.

Foundations

The purpose of a foundation is to help provide the look of better skin color and texture. They can give a matte or sheen to your skin, whichever look you prefer. Some have water bases and these are better for oily skin, others have oil bases and are for dry skins. Normal skins have a whole range to pick from. There are foundations that come with emollients and moisturizing ingredients to treat the skin all day under makeup. There are some foundations meant to be used without powder because they contain their own. Stick and cake foundations usually give heavier coverage than creams or liquid.

Moisturizers

They aid in keeping fluids in the skin by filming it over with the thinnest invisible layer of oil, plus preparing the surface of the skin to hold makeup longer. They come in different formulas for different skin types, oily, dry, normal. Some under makeup moisturizers have color to correct or heighten certain skin tones.

Powder

This sets the make-up finish with either a sheen or a matte look, and also provides for longer wear. Translucent loose powder is best for the final finish to your makeup—it doesn't affect the color—and translucent cake powder in its own little compact to carry in your purse provides for touch-ups. There are special blotting powders for oily skins.

Toners

They are milder skin bracers than astringents and have slightly clearing properties. (These are not to be confused with makeup that gives color tone to your skin.) Many normal or dry skins benefit from these. Another close, even milder relative, is a freshener, which cools and sometimes cleans the skin. Often astringents, toners and fresheners overlap; one product might be all three. Read the label.

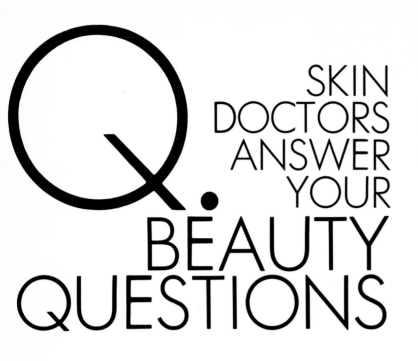

SKIN
DOCTORS
ANSWER
YOUR
BEAUTY
QUESTIONS

Keeping up with the newest medical findings in areas that affect your looks could drive you to a life of solitary confinement in the medical library. To side-step that poor prospect, GLAMOUR's beauty editors have stacked up some of the most often asked questions about recent developments in skin treatment—along with their answers from several distinguished specialists.

Q. *Short of seeing a dermatologist, what is the best thing to do for skin that's troubled with occasional or mild breakouts of pimples and blackheads?*
A. One of the most important things is keeping the skin immaculately clean. That's not so much to clear dirt from the surface but to clear it of the thin film of oil that's constantly being supplied and which can block the pores causing problems. Doctors recommend washing at least twice a day using hot water and a rich-lather soap. Massage the lather over the face from two to five minutes (the length of time depends on the oiliness of your skin and its sensitivity). Fingertips or a washcloth will do the job, but a soft-bristled brush (like a shaving brush) is the best. The friction and gentle massaging will strip the skin of the oily film and loosen blackheads. A cool-water aftersplash is optional. Finish off with an astringent made especially for oily skin. And if you use makeup, use medicated ones especially for oily skin. If this care doesn't clear the skin, the best thing to do is see a dermatologist. He can recommend special cleaning and prescribe lotions to dry up excess oil.

Q. *What can be done about acne?*
A. It is usually an affliction of the young. During the "acne decade," the years between thirteen and twenty-three, from puberty to the beginning of adulthood, most cases start and finish. Acne rarely continues after thirty.

The irony here is that this is an age when appearance can be desperately important, and a dreary, blemished complexion can seem unbearable at times. Being told you'll outgrow it is scant comfort. You probably will; but meanwhile, you have to live with it.

The only sensible beginning is to consult a doctor since acne is a disease, not just a beauty problem. There's no quick or miracle cure. It takes many weeks to get acne to improve but the more dedicated you are to your prescribed treatment, the sooner you'll see improvement.

Second, and equally important, is to try to keep the whole thing in perspective. Remember, you're by no means alone. From seventy to eighty percent of all young people suffer at one time or another from some degree of acne. Look around you. You'll find plenty of company for your misery.

Acne by definition, is a chronic inflammatory disease of the skin. There are several types of acne and much controversy over the treatment. The cure is different for different people. Acne may wax and wane with your general state of health or even with your moods (see question on emotional effects on skin). It may be blackheads; it may be more severe. But it persists.

One of the most important factors causing acne is a dysfunction of the endocrine glands which secrete hormones into the blood stream. Among those hormones are progesterone in girls, testosterone in boys. These hormones are chemical substances that travel through your blood stream from the sex glands to various parts of your body. In the case of your skin, the normal function of progesterone is to act on the oil glands, keeping the skin healthy and moist. When hormones get out of hand, however, the oil glands of the skin (face, chest and back are the target areas) are over stimulated, become clogged, then swollen and inflamed. You have acne.

Your doctor will probably put you on a skin cleansing and drying program. The cleansing program usually includes at least two soap and hot water washings a day with a complexion brush or cloth so that the gentle friction removes excess and caked oil and loosens blackheads. For in-between cleansing a medicated lotion and cotton pads might be prescribed. Skin drying is most often done with a lotion or cream usually containing sulfur, resorcinol, salicylic acid. It may be necessary to leave it on twenty-four hours a day or just at night depending on how severe the acne is. Some flaking or chapping follows but this widens the narrow skin openings in which oil collects and dislodges blackheads. The doctor will probably warn you that "face picking" is his business not yours.

To help disguise acne there are special lines of cosmetics with little or no oil in them. Ask your dermatologist about them. The majority of mild cases of acne clear up without a trace.

Q. *Is there anything really new to help acne?*
A. One of the most promising discoveries available now is tetracycline, a mild antibiotic that's particularly successful with most types of acne because it acts on the germs causing the infection. Doctors usually give a heavy dose of tetracycline pills initially, then taper off to a maintenance dose. This,

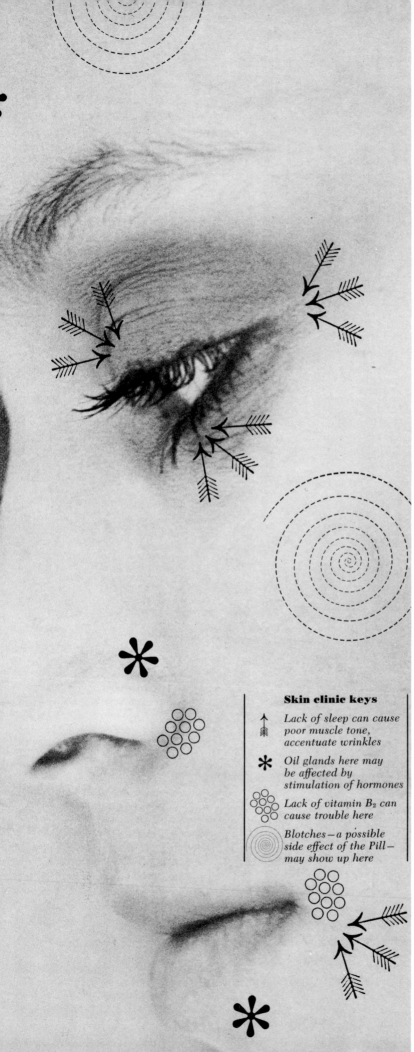

Skin clinic keys

↑ *Lack of sleep can cause poor muscle tone, accentuate wrinkles*

✳ *Oil glands here may be affected by stimulation of hormones*

Lack of vitamin B₂ can cause trouble here

Blotches—a possible side effect of the Pill—may show up here

along with scrupulous skin care, has proven very successful. But one of the times tetracycline is not recommended is during pregnancy since it is deposited in the teeth of the unborn child and discolors them. But skin usually improves during pregnancy because the increased output of estrogen hormone counteracts the oil-stimulating androgen hormone. This, in fact, is the basis of another new treatment. Estrogen is sometimes administered in straight doses for two weeks before the onset of each menstrual period. However, most doctors use this treatment only as a last resort because of the possibility of side effects similar to those sometimes encountered with the estrogen in birth control pills. Also, estrogen can only be used on girls because of the feminizing effects—like growth of breasts. (Note to girls who want to increase their breast size—don't jump to the conclusion that estrogen is the solution to your problem. It will only work in cases where estrogen deficiency is at the root of poor breast development. And even then, the side effects can be risky.) There is more research in the works. One new treatment still in experimental stages involves vitamin A acid. Applied to the skin, the acid has an irritating effect at first, but it unplugs pores to release the built-up oils.

Q. *What can be done for acne scars? How successful are chemabrasion and dermabrasion? What do they entail?*
A. Both of these procedures remove the top layers of skin so a new, finer one will heal over. Chemabrasion is done with an acid preparation which is painted on the skin. Dermabrasion—a mechanical rather than chemical process—planes down the top skin very much the way sandpaper smooths wood. But today these treatments are used only in selected types of acne scarring. There are too many drawbacks with chemabrasion. It's difficult to control the penetration of the acid and the results are often uneven. It can also produce an increase or decrease in pigmentation. Because of this, the line where treatment ended is often obvious, leaving a mask-like effect. Dark-skinned people are particularly vulnerable to this reaction. Dermabrasion has its drawbacks too. For one thing, it's not very effective on deeply-pocked skin since too many layers of skin would have to be destroyed to reach a satisfactory level.

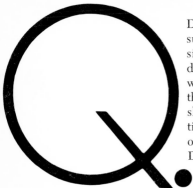

Doctors now are supplementing the surface abrasion with deep spot abrasion in the pock marks. They use a dental burr to break down the cell walls within the deep scar. When the skin heals over, the deep pits are shallower saucer-shaped indentations instead of deep cup-shaped ones, but may still be noticeable. Dermabrasion works best on shallow irregularities, but even then, many doctors hesitate to say how fine the results will be. About all they say is that skin will look better. But they won't promise how much better.

Q. *What is the latest opinion on oily foods like chocolate and peanuts in relation to skin? Do they cause breakouts or acne?*
A. According to Dr. Robert T. Binford, Jr. of New York Hospital-Cornell University Medical College, most doctors now agree that a diet rich in oily foods probably doesn't have anything to do with breakouts or blackheads. But hormones do. The onslaught of hormones at puberty or just before the menstrual period stimulates the oil glands to manufacture oil that with other skin cells blocks pores and forms blackheads. These act as plugs, causing the oil that's still coming full force to collect under the skin. Meanwhile, bacteria that is always present on and under the skin goes to work in the stagnant oil that's backed up in the oil glands and causes infection. Doctors are now reasonably convinced that an oil-rich diet has nothing to do with the whole process. In a way, it would be better if it did, because breakouts could be controlled simply by cutting out oily foods in the diet. But it doesn't work that way. Of course, a balanced diet is still necessary for overall good health which will show up in your general skin condition.

Q. *I'm in my mid-twenties and thought I was past the breakout stage. But my skin has flared up with pimples and blackheads worse than I had in my teens. Why?*
A. It's difficult to say. Some doctors say pimples at any age can be caused by emotions. But more than likely, the emotional factor is only secondary, if significant at all. In his book, *More Than Skin Deep*, Dr. Thomas H. Sternberg says that tensions and anxieties may lower the immunity of an individual to infection. And in that manner, emotions may be a factor. But skin breakouts are more complex than that, and possible causes should be explored by a dermatologist.

Q. *My skin started acting up a few months ago so I switched to hypo-allergenic makeup. But it hasn't helped. What's up?*
A. Lots of girls have this same problem, but very likely what's wrong isn't an allergy at all. Cosmetic allergies are not at all common. Most reputable manufacturers don't put known allergens, things that many people are sensitive to, in their products. So it's only a rare person who is truly allergic to regular makeup. But that's not to say that you couldn't be one who is. In fact, you could be allergic to regular and hypo-allergenic makeups. Hypo-allergenic just means you're *less likely* to have an allergic reaction—it's no guarantee you won't. If you suspect that makeup is your problem, see a dermatologist and have a skin Patch Test to tell if you register allergies. If not, maybe you've been using makeup that's too oily for your skin type and it's clogging pores. Maybe you're irritating your skin with a harsh soap. In either case, your skin is reacting in an unpleasant way, but it's not a true allergic reaction.

Q. *Recently I've noticed that the pores on my face have become quite large. what causes this and what can be done about it?*
A. Large pores are usually a matter of heredity. Pores can become enlarged because they've been overworked secreting excess skin oils over a period of time. Since the predisposition for oily skin is inherited, so is the predisposition for enlarged pores. There's not much that can be done about them. Chemabrasion is one treatment that can help, but few doctors use it, considering the drawbacks mentioned earlier. Other than that, cosmetics can cover pores to some extent, and astringents tighten them temporarily.

Q. *I've been taking sleeping pills lately. Can they do anything to my skin?*
A. Sleeping pills are among a list of drugs, including laxatives, headache mixes, antibiotics, tranquilizers and diuretics that can sometimes cause drug rashes.

Q. *Do birth control pills have any effect on the skin?*
A. A lot of girls have heard that their complexions will improve when they start taking the Pill. This isn't necessarily true. For still unexplained reasons, some girls *do* notice an improvement, but others say their skin got worse when they first started on the Pill although the condition leveled off a few months later. One New York dermatologist, Dr. Richard C. Gibbs, clinical associate professor at New York University Medical Center, thinks that a change is more likely to take place when girls go off the Pill— a change for the worse though. Once the body becomes accustomed to a certain level of estrogen, the backward adjustment can throw the skin off balance. But even this is not the most significant effect the Pill has on skin. According to Dr. Binford, the most important reaction to the Pill (in terms of the number of times it shows up—one survey reported it in about 29 percent of the cases studied) is a pigment change on the forehead and cheeks. The faint blotchy brown spots that appear are the same things our grandmothers probably called the "mask of pregnancy." Some doctors say an increase of estrogen in pregnant women and those on the Pill may cause an increase in melanin, a dark pigment, causing the uneven color spots. The only way to get rid of them is to stop taking the Pill. And many women have decided they'd rather have the slight spots than an unwanted child. Of those who do go off the Pill, some notice that the marks

fade gradually; but for others, they're there for good. In those cases, bleaching isn't much help. But since sunlight makes the marks darker, sunscreens do help keep the situation from becoming more noticeable.

Q. *What about IUDs? Do they have any effect on the skin?*
A. As far as is known now, no.

Q. *What can emotions do to the skin?*
A. Lots. Just about anything from making you blush to making your skin break out in patches of hives or aggravating a tendency to pimples and blackheads. For example, in stress situations, skin conditions like psoriasis (red patches often covered with white scales) or eczema (itchy weeping blisters) may be aggravated, or breakouts of hives can appear from apparently nowhere. Dr. Binford says this is probably caused by an imbalance in the autonomic nervous system brought on by tension. And although emotions don't cause pimples, they make them worse. The more you worry, the weaker your resistance, the more open to infection you are. If the tension situation is predictable—like taking a big exam or giving a speech—some doctors recommend a mild tranquilizer. And even in cases where the situation can't be anticipated and symptoms do show up, many doctors prescribe a tranquilizer plus more specific treatment for the symptoms.

Q. *Does pot have any effect on the skin?*
A. So far as most doctors think now, it doesn't have any effect on the skin. However, one doctor has suggested that excessive use of marijuana could upset the sympathetic nervous system and stimulate the sebaceous glands. You may notice that your sense of touch is heightened—but that's not because of any skin change. It's more likely a mental change. Reports show that under the influence of marijuana your past and future memories are decreased and your concentration on present stimuli is increased. This probably accounts for heightened sensory perception.

Q. *Is drinking bad for the skin? What does it do?*
A. Alcohol may dehydrate the skin for a short time, but that effect isn't lasting and won't cause any permanent problems. It can make an itching skin condition worse since it causes an increased flow of blood to the skin. Also, in extreme cases, very heavy drinking can cause loss of appetite—to the point that poor nutrition could produce symptoms ranging from poor skin tone to cracks in the skin at the mouth sides, scaly oily patches around the nose.

Q. *Is there anything that will prevent wrinkles?*
A. Wrinkling is a natural process in aging. The dryer your skin the greater its tendency to wrinkle. There is no way to prevent this but emollient cosmetics soften the skin, help to eliminate dryness and cause a retention of moisture which eliminates some of the finer wrinkling. That's why emollients should be used regularly by most women from their early teens on.

Q. *Can you catch warts from someone who has them?*
A. Warts, most doctors claim, are caused by a virus and like colds they are infectious and transferable not only to others but to other parts of the body of the same person. Some doctors imply that warts are psychologically triggered and can be treated simply and successfully by suggestion and placebos. Others remove warts either with an electric needle, acid or surgery. Your dermatologist may advise you just to leave the wart alone. Fifty to sixty percent disappear with no treatment over a period of years.

Q. *Can emotional troubles cause hair to grow on the body and face?*
A. There is considerable evidence that emotional stress may trigger the growth of excess hair on the face and body. Other causes are heredity, hormonal changes as a women gets older, specific diseases such as Cushing's Syndrome which can be produced by the prolonged use of cortisones. Anyone with excessive hair growth should see a dermatologist to discover the cause which of course determines the treatment.

Q. *What is the best way to bleach face hair?*
A. Peroxide with ammonia does a good job, not ordinary peroxide but beautician's peroxide which is 20 volume, 6 percent. Ask for it at your drugstore. You'll need to mix about 20 drops of ammonia to 1 ounce of peroxide. Apply the mixture with a saturated cloth and leave it on for about 20 to 30 minutes. You can also use a bleach that's meant for head hair but you have to test a patch of skin about the size of a nickel first to find out whether your skin can take the bleach or not. (See Patch Test on page 83.) If it doesn't irritate your skin, prepare the bleach just as directed in the instructions for scalp hair, and let it stay on the skin only long enough to decolorize the hair. How long depends on the color and texture of your hair, usually 20 to 30 minutes. Wash it off if you begin to feel any skin irritation and don't use it again.

Q. *My freckles get darker in the summer. Is there any way to keep them from getting worse or any way of getting rid of them for good?*
A. Freckles are hereditary. They are brought out or intensified by the sun. Stay out of it as much as possible, and try one of the bleaches especially made for them. But the lightening effect is only temporary and sometimes not worth the effort. About the best thing you can do is to try liking your freckles—a lot of people find them very appealing. Also when you are out in the sun use a good screening lotion, cream, gel or whatever form you like.

A.

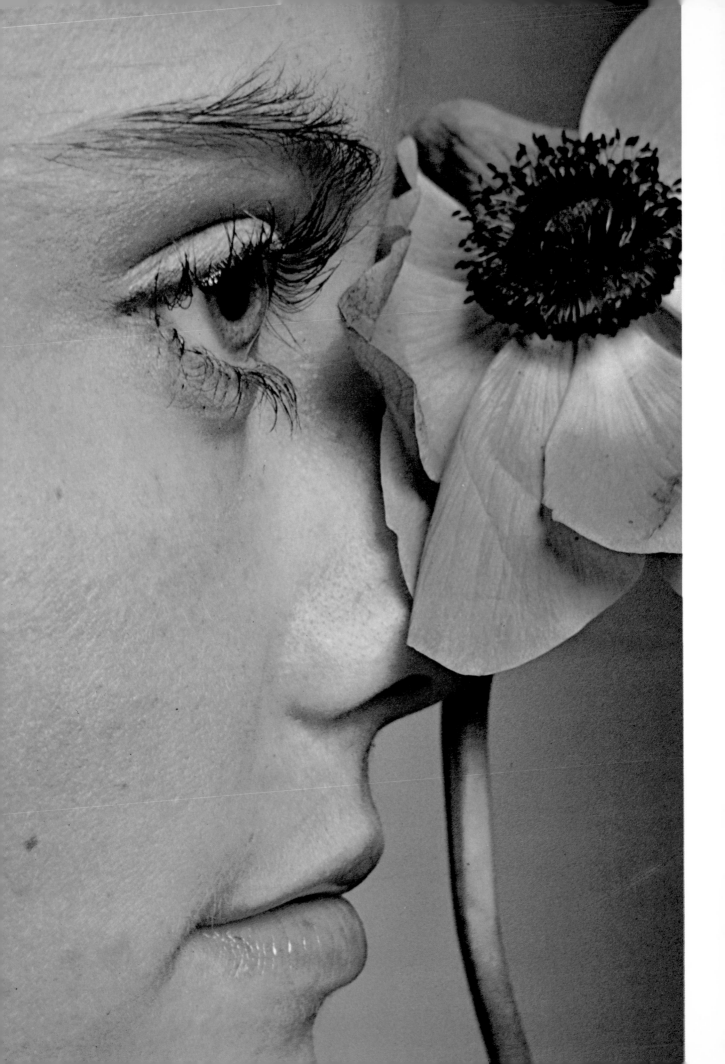

MAKE-UP

GLAMOUR believes in makeup that makes over but doesn't look too made-up, except for special-occasion dress-up times. Then there's a sense of play, an intended game of color and costume and magic. But for everyday, nobody wants to look like a put-on, which is the impression that unnatural obvious makeup or badly applied makeup gives. Actually today you have to look hard to find any kind of makeup that is heavy, opaque or cakey, it just isn't around. So the mistakes that do occur are usually in the use of the sheer new natural colors and consistencies. You won't slip into them if you follow the how-to section coming up—how to help correct feature flaws with makeup, how to do a perfect five minute face, how to play games for special parties, in fact everything you need to know about this fascinating subject.

FEATURE FLAWS

HOW TO HIDE NOTHING BUT STILL EXPOSE ONLY THE BEST

With sheer makeup—the next best thing to perfect, natural skin tone—the whole concept of contouring to put bad features in shadow with dark makeup and bring out good ones with light is exposed. That worked to some extent with matte makeup but not anymore. What replaces it is something beautiful, a new way of experiencing your face, hiding nothing but exposing the best. The new makeup honesty is the clearest thing to call it; to *do* it, all that's needed first is a fair assessment of your features. Then, put all your makeup power and technique on your good features, haunting eyes, unbeatable cheekbones, sexy lips, flawless skin, whatever, and the rest just naturally fades away.

So that there is no confusing the old contour camouflage and the new makeup honesty, we show examples of both here. The old way to slim a thick nose, *below left*, was to shade the sides with dark foundation or blusher, to put white or highlight down the center and bring out the forehead and chin with highlight. The new way, *below right*, is to emphasize your best features. Great cheekbones

OLD

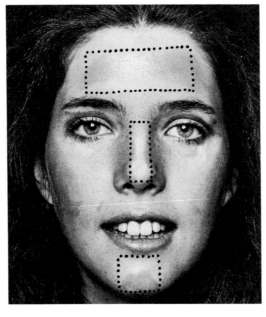

NEW

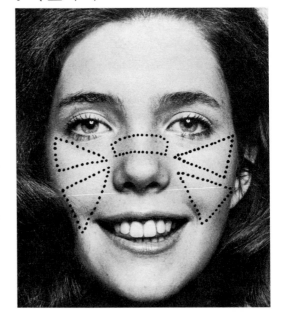

126

are emphasized with liquid gleamers in translucent, tawny or peach tones, and blushers. Over the bridge —follow outlines—goes blusher to give a healthy, fresh-air look; in the top triangles, gleamer; in the bottom, blusher. Blend.

Below left: The old way to slimming a wide face was to darken tones where cheek hollows should have been and extend eye shadow and liner out to cover wide temples. *Right:* The new way concentrates on eyes and lips. On the eyes, the sheerest shadows, lots of lash-lengthening mascara. Make the mouth sexy with pale lipstick or stain blotted then buffed with gloss.

OLD

NEW

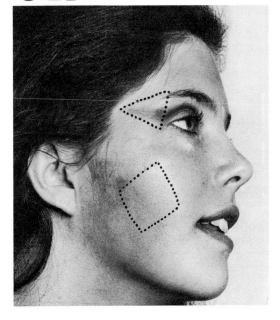

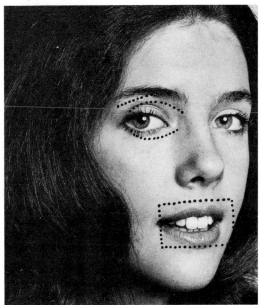

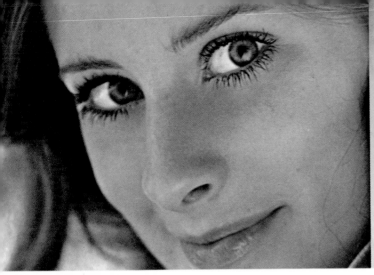

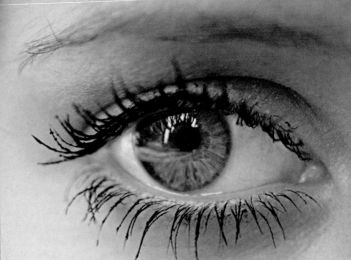

1 *Droopy corners lifted: 1,2.*

4

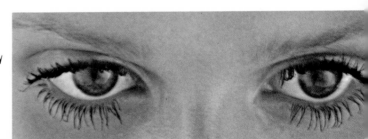

Round eyes ovaled out: 3,4,5.

7

Deep-set eyes brought forward: 7,8.

8

9

Small or narrow eyes enlarged: 9,10.

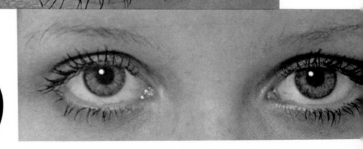

HOW TO MAKE YOUR EYES REAL WINNERS

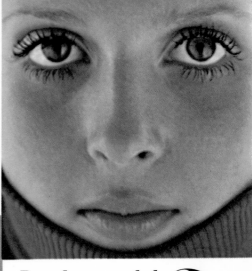

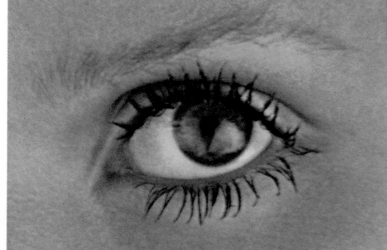

Round eyes ovaled out: 3,4,5.

3

5

6

Underbrow raised: 5,6.

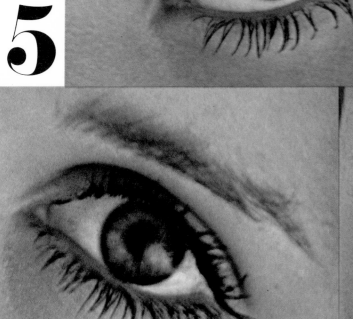

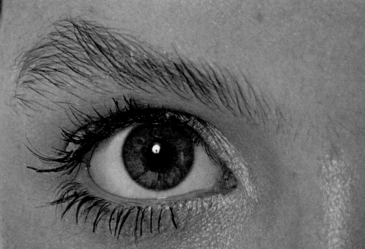

Overhanging underbrows raised: 5,6.

11

Protruding eyes set deeper: 11.

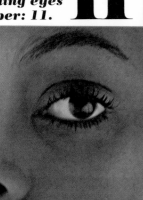

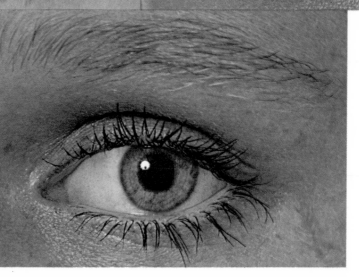

Small eyes enlarged: 9,10.

10

Details next page

TO CORRECT EYE SHAPES

It's a new kind of teamwork between lashes—false or your own—and makeup that turns eyes without too much going for them into real winners. This team work can either correct faulty eye shapes or make eyes that are already well-shaped into ideals.

BEFORE AFTER

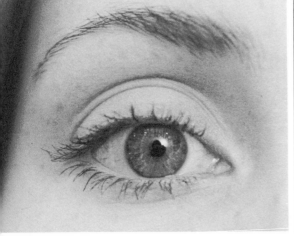 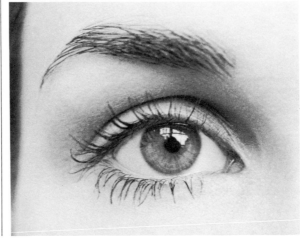

HOW TO MAKE YOUR EYES REAL WINNERS

Sketched opposite are the six basic eye shape faults. If you have one of them the captions to the right of each shape will tell you briefly how to correct them with makeup and lashes. You'll also see numbers by the sketches. Match these up with the corrected eyes in color on the preceding pages and you'll realize the real changes makeup can achieve. Check out too the basic rules for applying eye makeup and lashes on the following pages.

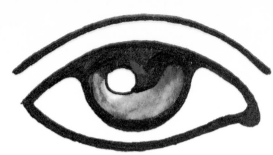

Droopy Corners

Tiny individual false lash clusters, top center only. Mascara top and bottom. Pale shadow on top lid.

1, 2

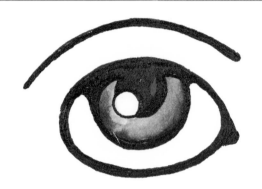

Round

Individual false lashes at outer corners, top and bottom. Mascara. Surround eye with medium-color shadow, extending slightly at outer corners.

3, 4, 5

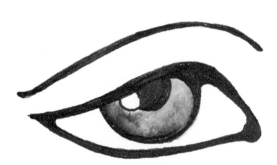

Overhanging Underbrow

Powder and mascara own lashes for more buildup. Medium-color shadow under bottom lashes, extending slightly beyond outer corners. This draws attention away from the brow.

5, 6

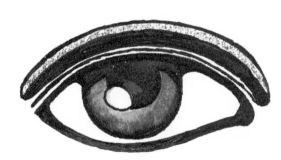

Deep-set

Trim false lash strip, keeping lashes very short. Apply on top only. Mascara. Use light shadow on the lid, under brow and just under the lower lashes.

7, 8

Protruding

Powder and mascara own lashes for extra buildup. Surround eye with medium- to deep-color shadow.

11

Small and/or Narrow

Powder and mascara own lashes for extra length. Use pale shadow all around the eye, buff to an almost-nothing finish.

9, 10

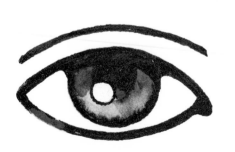

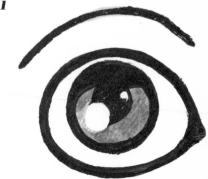

Although heavy shadowing and lining of any kind looks unnatural now, bear in mind the color-contour rule that deeper tones de-emphasize, and the brighter, paler ones bring out eye features. For instance, if you want to recess a protruding eye, use a deep blue or deep mauve shadow. To give more width to a narrow eye, surround it with a paler-color shadow like yellow or apricot.

Lash tricks: There are three ways to correct shape problems with lashes: use whole strips of the new invisible-base lashes; use tiny clusters of individual false lashes cut from strips; or powder and mascara your own (*see below*) to add thickness. The chart, *preceding page*, tells you which is best for your eye shape. If you use the invisible-base lashes, gently flex the base with fingers, *photo* 1. Even if lashes are "pretrimmed," *trim them again* for a natural look, 2. If you use individual clusters, cut two or three lashes as you see on this page, *top*

right. You see them being applied with tweezers on opposite page, *big photo.* The small numbered photos on opposite page show you exactly how to apply false lashes to bottom and top lids. In 3, lower lash has been dabbed lightly with surgical adhesive and is being pressed gently against lid, close to base of natural lashes. In 4, top lashes are positioned over lid. In 5, the lash coaxed into corners with the blunt end of an orangewood stick. Now that lashes are firmly in place, gently stretch eyelid with fingertip to keep lash from puckering on lid, 6. In 7, you see what the false lash looks like with no mascara—false and real lashes separate. In 8, both are mascaraed for a completely natural look.

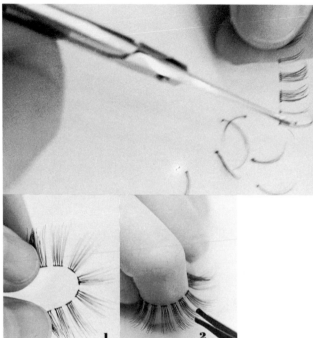

BASIC EYE MAKEUP AND LASHES RULES

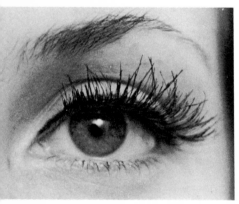

TIP: No matter how dark your own lashes are, use blond to medium-brown false lashes, and mascara them for the most natural look.

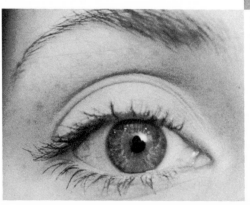

DON'T
No eye should ever appear looking this way —heavy liner, gooey mascara—generally overdone.

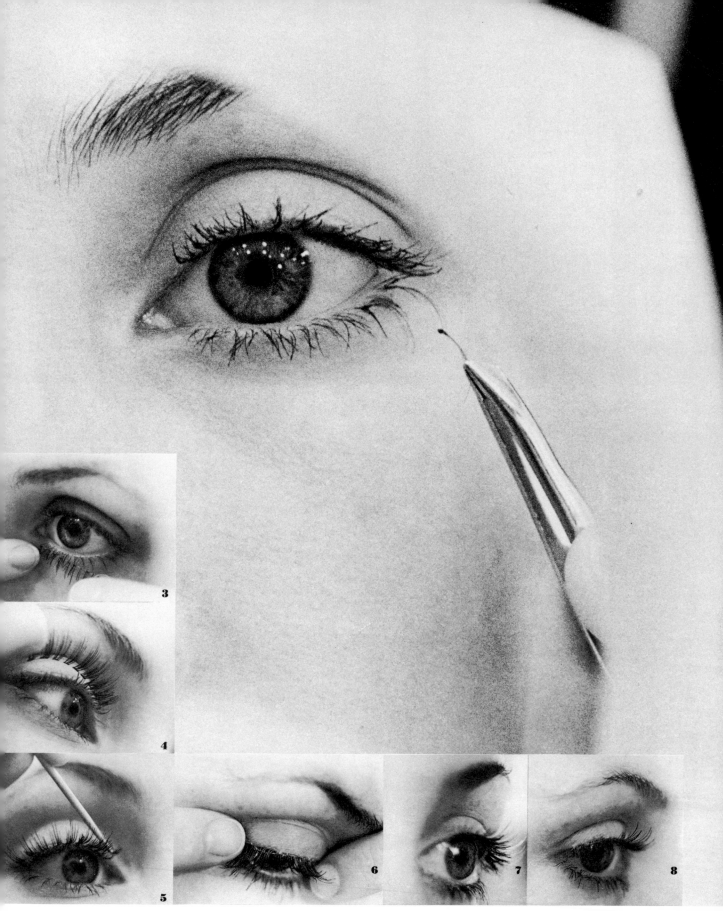

POWDER TRICK

To make your own lashes superbeautiful, powder them lightly with baby powder, then mascara them.

SHAPING IRREGULAR BROWS

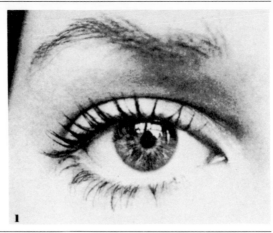

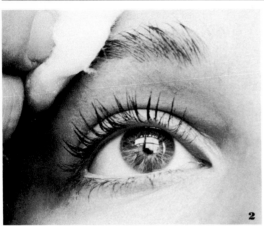

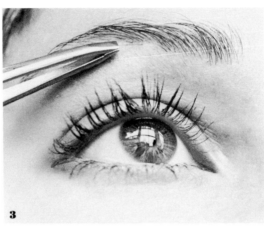

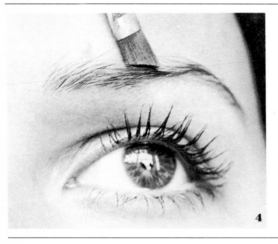

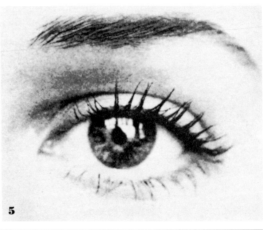

1. Basically, the brows here need filling in on top—the dip is too pronounced—and a little plucking underneath to clean up any straggly hairs.

2. Always cleanse the area that you're going to pluck with a bit of alcohol first.

3. Brush the hairs in the direction they grow so you can see the strays and misfits. Pluck any hairs that don't fall into the natural line. Go slowly so that you don't make any drastic mistakes. Keep brushing and rechecking.

4. To fill in dip on top, we used a powdered eyebrow makeup in the same shade as the brows, stroked on lightly with a moistened brush. Stroke makeup on in the opposite direction of hair growth to get the most natural look. Be careful not to get any on the skin underneath hairs, only on the skin in the dip, or brows will look too dark and heavy.

5. The finished brow. Dip is less obvious and the brow is even and cleaner-looking.

EYEBROW SHAPE-UPS

If your brows are carefully shaped and cared for, they can add as much to your eyes as the right shadow or long beautiful lashes. If they miss, the whole eye doesn't make it. That doesn't mean that every pair of brows has to look like every other pair of brows. Bushy ones, thin ones, irregular ones, all have their own individual charm and personality. The idea is to make the most of whatever you have. Here and following are a lot of ideas to help you do just that.

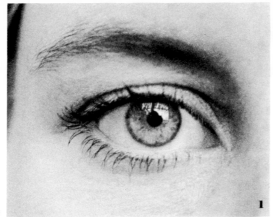

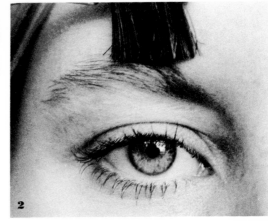

1

2

1. *These brows are bushy and most of the growth is below the bone structure so the eye area seems dark and heavy. The eyes are also very close-set. What's needed are thinner brows a bit farther apart.*
2. *Brows are cleaned with alcohol and brushed.*
3. *One row of hairs at a time is removed from below the brows (never pluck from above). A few hairs were removed from the inner corners to make more space between brows.*
4. *Eyebrow makeup is tested with a moistened brush to be sure the color is truly a natural for the actual brow's shade.*

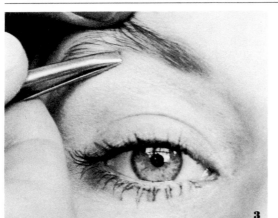

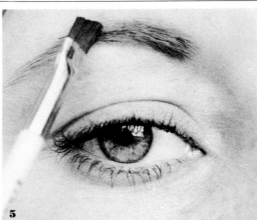

3

5

CONTROLLING BUSHY BROWS

4

6

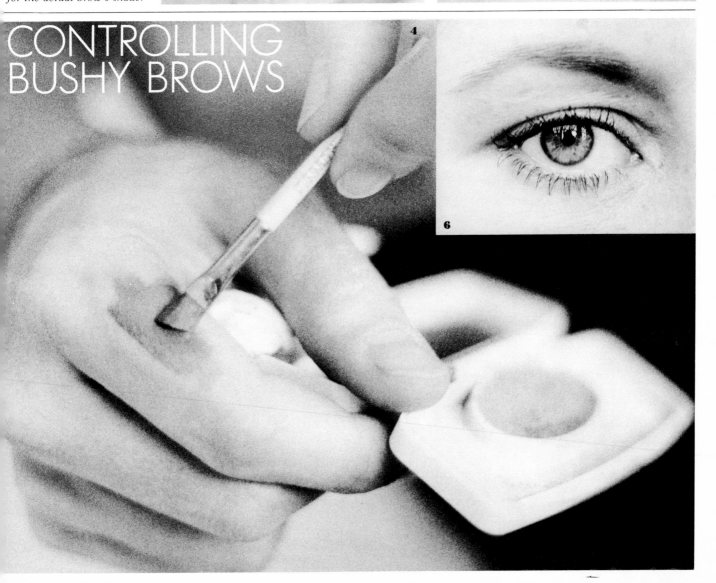

TAMING THICK DARK BROWS

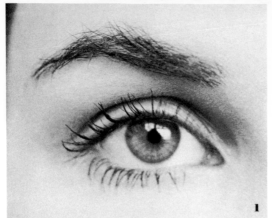

1

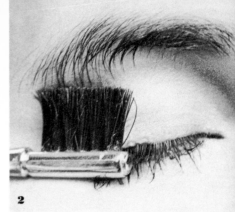

2

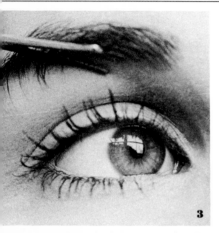

3

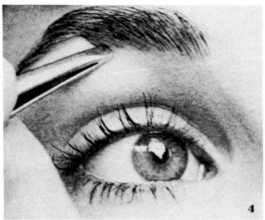

4

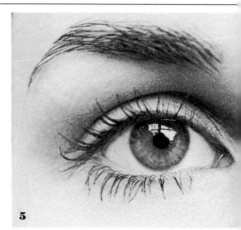

5

1. *These thick brows need to be thinned and lightened a little to open and soften the eye area.*
2. *The brows are brushed down to check their length.*
3. *Since the hair in these brows is long as well as thick, it's helpful to trim off the very tips of the hairs. This lets more skin show through so the brows look lighter. Use a snub-nosed scissors and trim the very tips. Brush hairs down and trim no shorter than roots of bottom row of hairs. Follow the natural brow shape as you go. Trim just a bit at a time.*
4. *One or two bottom rows of hair are plucked—depending on thickness of brows.*
5. *The brow after thinning. Now they are ready for professional bleaching. Always go to the best salon in town for this. It's not an at-home job because a special bleach is needed to keep hair from turning orange.*
6. *Bleach is applied with a flat bristle brush and left on about five minutes.*
7. *Bleach is removed with dampened cotton.*
8. *Finished brow. It will need to be rebleached in about five weeks.*

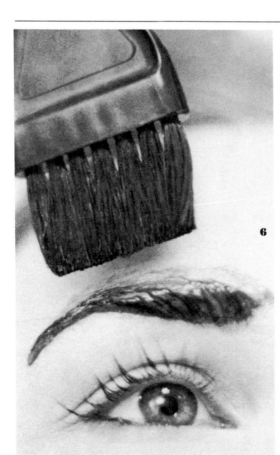

6

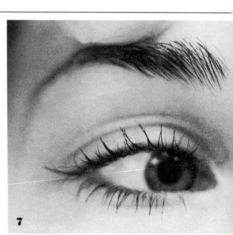

7

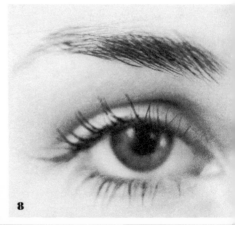

8

1. *These brows are too thin at outer corners and too sharply arched. It could be their natural shape or perhaps the result of overplucking.*

2. *Brush hairs so they fall into place.*

3. *To soften the severe points at the inner corners, push back hairs against direction of growth and remove one or two hairs. To soften the arch, pluck one row of hairs from under inner corners.*

4. *Remove any straggly hairs from outer corners.*

5. *To fill in outer brows, use a bit of powdered eyebrow makeup and a moistened brush. Match the color of makeup to your brows as closely as possible.*

6. *Clean excess makeup with cotton-tipped swab.*

7. *Finished brow.*

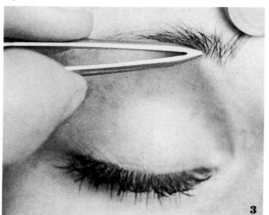

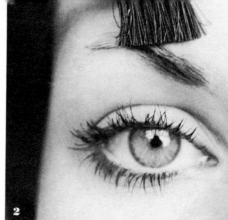

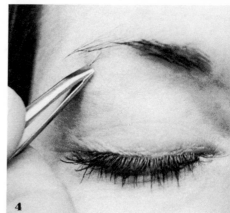

TIPS

• *Never pluck brows without first cleansing area by dabbing with alcohol.*

• *Pluck one or two hairs at a time to be sure you don't do anything too drastic.*

• *Use a magnifying mirror to help see what you're doing but keep checking total look in a regular mirror.*

• *Never make any definite points at the inner brow corners or at the center of natural arch.*

• *Check for new hair growth every two days and pluck. It's much easier to maintain the new shape if you pluck before hairs grow back completely.*

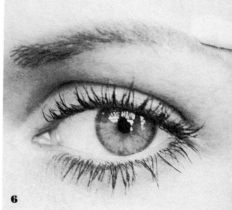

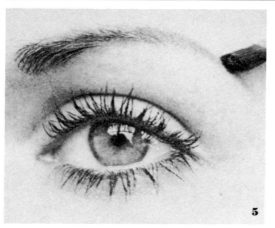

HELP FOR THIN OR OVERPLUCKED BROWS

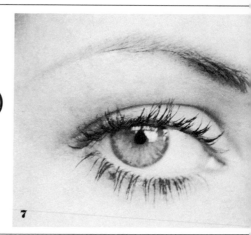

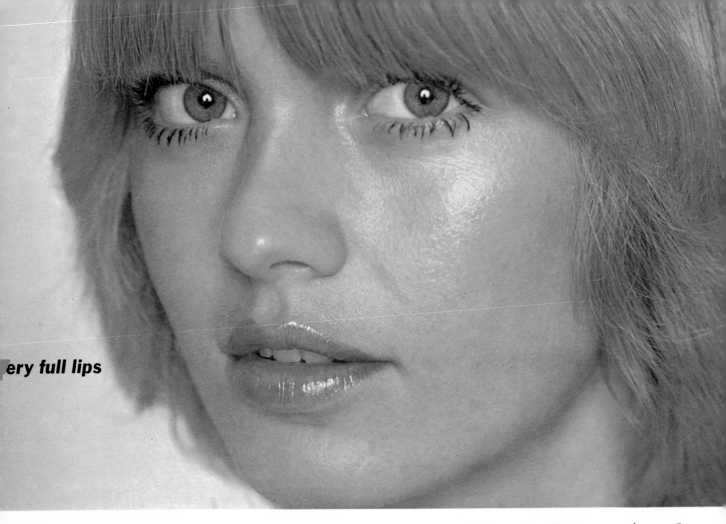

ery full lips

NEW SHAPE-UPS FOR LIPS

Clear deep see-through color is a more dramatic idea for lips than pale tones, and the lips that wear it are going to get a lot more attention than they've been used to. What's needed for this look is the softest, prettiest, lip shapes. All the lips here originally had problems. On the next pages, find out how we solved these problems—here the pretty results—and how you can solve yours.

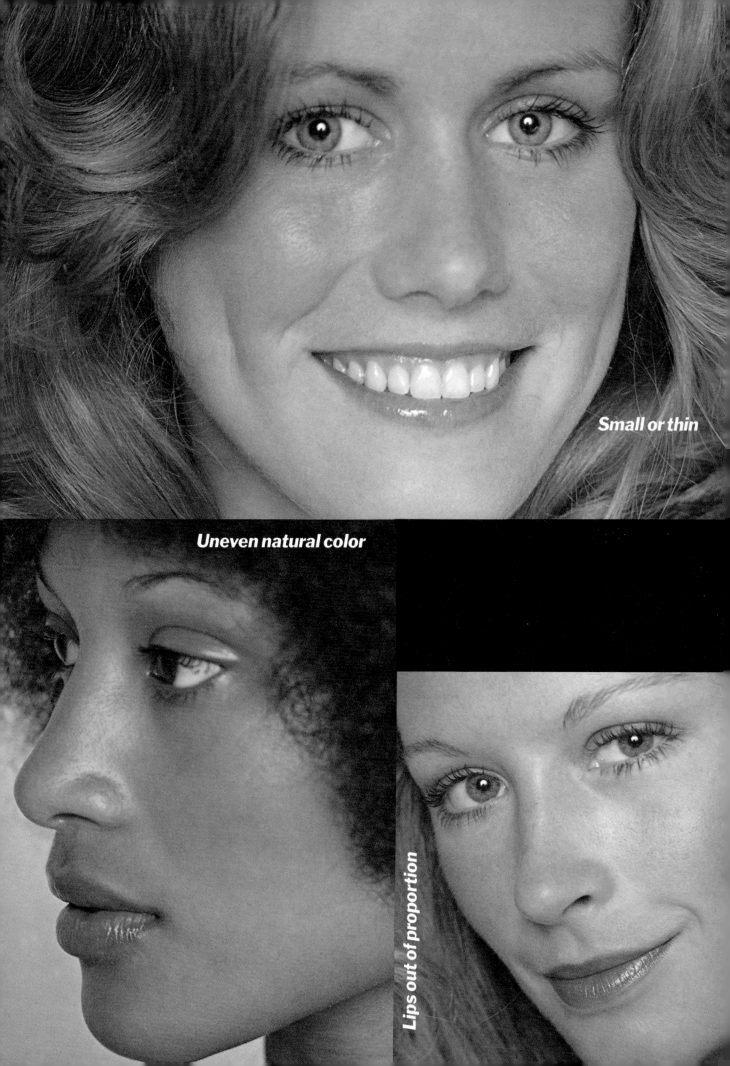

Small or thin

Uneven natural color

Lips out of proportion

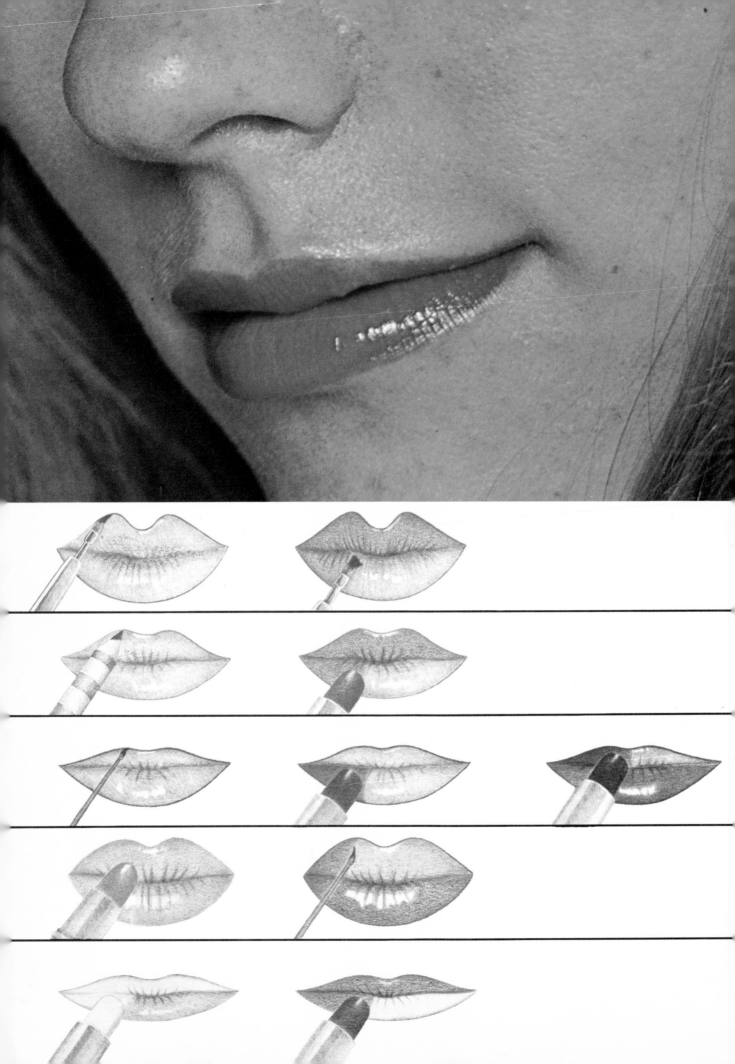

The deep-toned lipsticks bring lips in for a lot more attention than they get wearing paler, no-color lipsticks. That's why we take the five most common lip shapes and the problems that go with them and show you how to turn them into the softly sensual mouths you see on the preceding page and opposite. To make the chart below work for you, find your lip shape or problem and read across to find the solution.

Very full lips

There are two important things to remember for this lip shape. First, don't pick the deepest colors. The sheer bright cherry red here is about as deep as you should go. Next, apply lipgloss *before* you apply the color. Lipstick applied over a gloss doesn't appear as dark and has a sheerer texture. Another tip: always outline your mouth with a lip brush for a cleaner line, a more finished look.

Just right

You're the lucky girl who can wear most any color from the clear medium tones to the rich, deep mahoganies. Here are some ideas to help you shape the prettiest lips. Outline with a lip pencil first; using one a shade deeper than the lipcolor gives lips a nice definition. Here we used a soft, rich tangerine with a deeper russet outline, and finished with a no-color gloss.

Lips out of proportion

The lips here don't match each other in size. The top lip is thinner and smaller than the bottom. To correct this, try using two different lip colors, both in the same color family but one slightly deeper than the other. Here we used a browny burgundy on the bottom lip and a slightly deeper one on the top to bring it out and give the illusion of fullness.

Uneven natural color

Girls with brunette coloring often find the skin closest to the inside of the mouth a brighter pink than skin at the outer edges of the lips. This makes lipstick color look uneven. To correct this we've applied a pale green undercolor lipstick, then outlined and filled in with a brown-toned lipstick wand that has a brush attached.

Small or thin lips

Thin or small lips should never wear the deepest colors. The tawny earth colors look smashing on you, so do most of the clear brights. Use a sheer white lip base underneath. It keeps color from turning dark on lips, adds an inner glow to give the illusion of more fullness. On top we used a pretty, pale coffee shade.

Very full lips

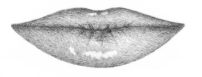

Just right

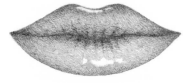

Lips out of proportion

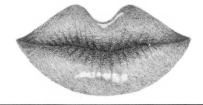

Uneven natural color

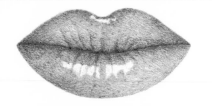

Small or thin lips

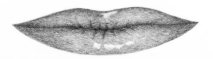

141

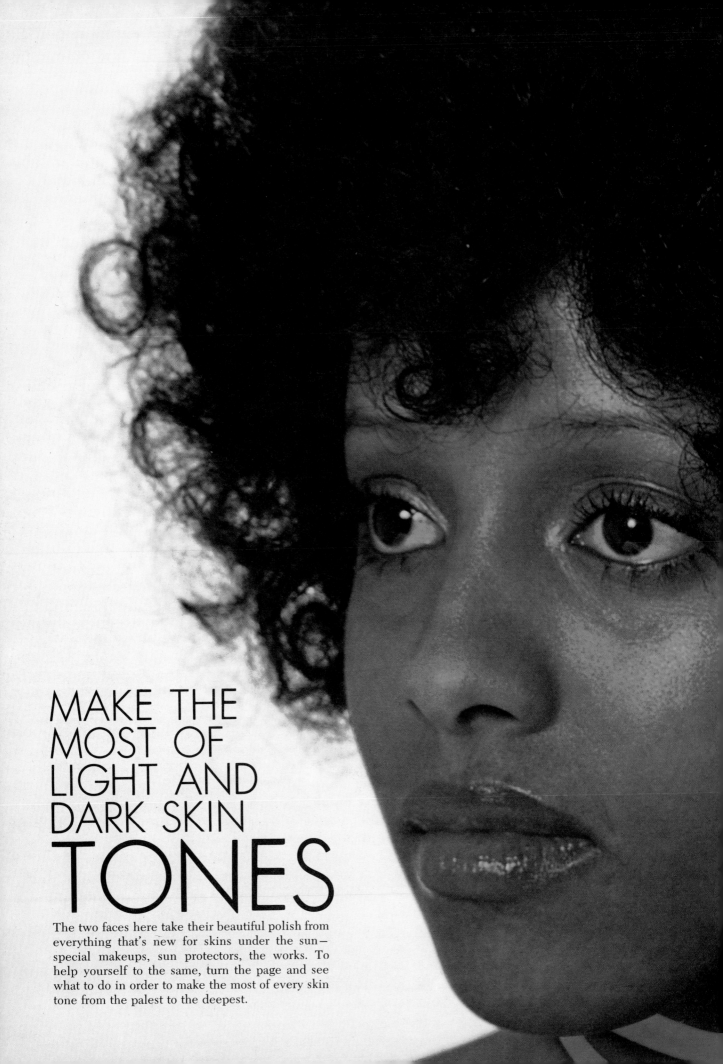

MAKE THE MOST OF LIGHT AND DARK SKIN
TONES

The two faces here take their beautiful polish from everything that's new for skins under the sun— special makeups, sun protectors, the works. To help yourself to the same, turn the page and see what to do in order to make the most of every skin tone from the palest to the deepest.

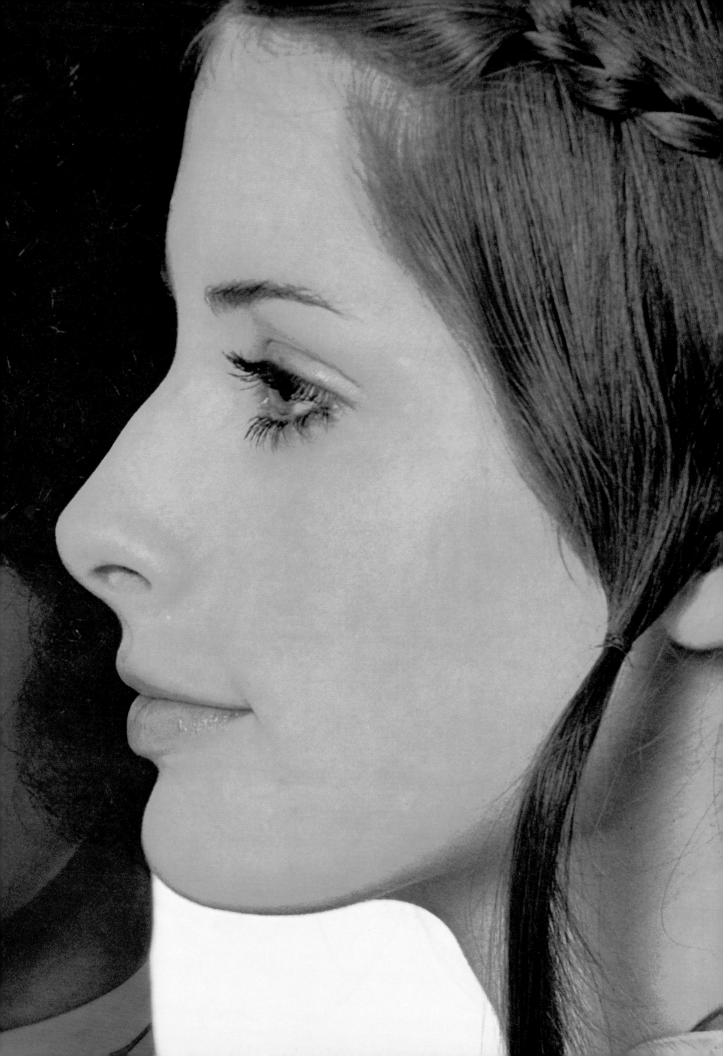

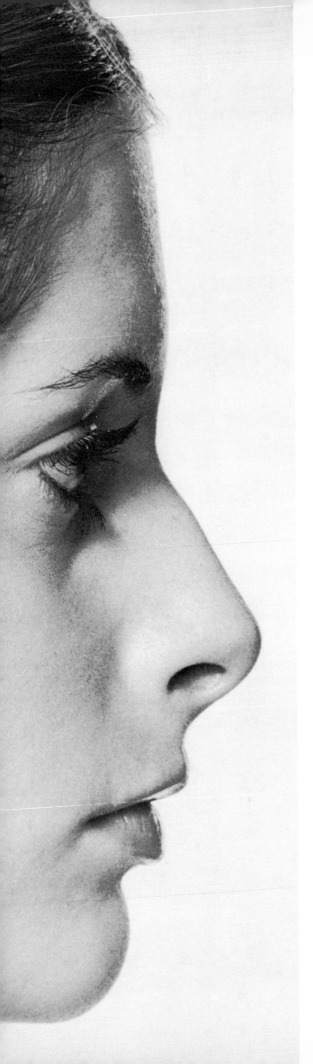

LIGHT SKIN TONES

Pale to Pink — Blushed to Rosy

If your skin tone is less than it should be, there's a lot you can do to improve it that you probably don't know about. If it's drab, you can give it life; uneven, you can smooth the shading; off-color, say too yellow or too ruddy, you can blend these tones out; or you can change tones — within certain ranges — simply because you want to. But you have to know how to take advantage of everything scientists and cosmeticians know about sun exposure and know about the subtlest new sun-protection lotions. Especially in summer, nothing affects skin tone more than sun. You have to know how to use the sheer new makeup that camouflages skin tones. The combination of sunscreens and these makeups is unbeatable.

Skin Tone Basics

Fair-skinned girls can usually be divided into three groups: very pale skin with almost no pink in it; a slightly blushed pink; and a full-blushed fairness. Fairer skins are usually not as much troubled by off-color undertones, such as sallowness or ruddiness, as olive or medium-dark-toned skins are. But if your skin does need correcting, here's how: To tone down too much pink, specially tinted under-makeup moisturizers in aqua or green so subtle the color never shows. They just counter the pink. For sallow or yellowish undertones, try rosy under-makeup moisturizer.

Sun Protection

The fairest skin obviously needs the most protection, especially the type that never tans, only burns. It needs the strongest sunscreens, the shortest exposure to sun. Don't pick lotions which merely lubricate skin and do not screen out the ultraviolet rays. These by law do not have to list ingredients. The lotions that help prevent burning will always list ingredients. Fair skins that do take a tan should use preventive screens too that list ingredients, but they usually don't need superprotective ones.

Makeup Correction

The palest-skinned girls don't have to look that way anymore. The new transparent bronzers in stick form or the gels in a tube are so sheer they can be worn on even the lightest of skins. They come in a range of shades from the very light tans to deeper ones and can be used for overall accenting or for evening off color. Always wear a moisturizer under bronzers which helps them go on smoothly.

DARK SKIN TONES

Olive to Caramel to Brown or Black

Skin Tone Basics

Dark-skinned girls have as many ranges of shades of skin as fair ones. Olive and caramel skins sometimes show pronounced sallow undertones, but the darkest of dark skins are mostly free of undertone problems. To combat the sallow tones, olive, medium-dark or caramel skin-toned girls can use an apricot undermakeup moisturizer. Less common to very dark skin tones is a ruddiness problem, which can be cut by using an aqua undermakeup moisturizer. Whichever undertone you're trying to avoid, avoid it too in eye shadow colors.

Sun Protection

A skin burns if it's exposed to the sun long enough, even the darkest. And, any skin dries out in the sun without lubrication. It's true that dark skin doesn't burn as easily as fair skin and can take more exposure to sun, but that's no signal to leave it unaided. Brown to black skin requires a mild sunscreening lotion or one that simply moisturizes and lubricates with emollients, without screening out ultraviolet rays. It's the olive-to-caramel-skinned girl, who doesn't want her tone to deepen, who needs a lot of protection. In fact, she should pick the same extra protective sunscreen as the girl who has the fairest of skins—see how to tell when you're buying a maximum sunscreen in the "Sun Protection" section for fair skin, opposite. And don't forget lip protection—a slick of shining gloss not only looks sexy but keeps lips from getting sun-damaged.

Makeup Correction

Girls with dark complexions usually don't need to add much color to their own. Instead, you'll probably want to buff and polish your own color and even out the tone if it's blotchy. The transparent bronzing gels or bronzing sticks are perfect for the darkest dark skins. The lighter shades of dark look especially beautiful buffed with deep amber or peach blush in powder, gel or stick form and sexy shines of lipgloss. A very pale olive skin usually needs a flush of deep rose to highlight the cheeks, or maybe even as an overall pickup.

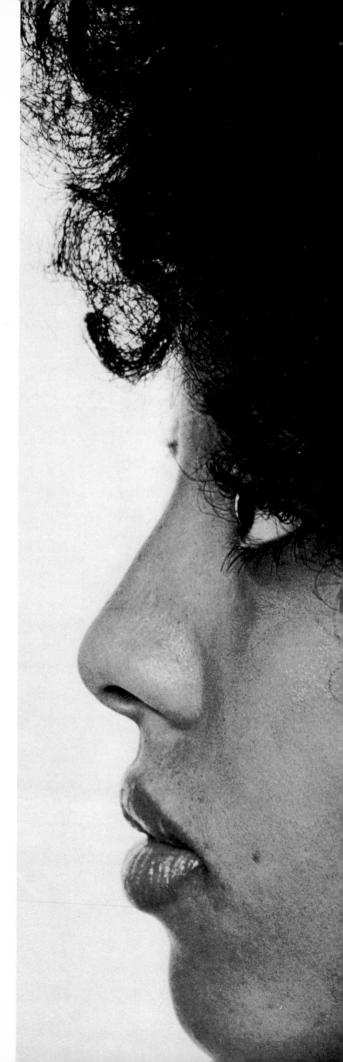

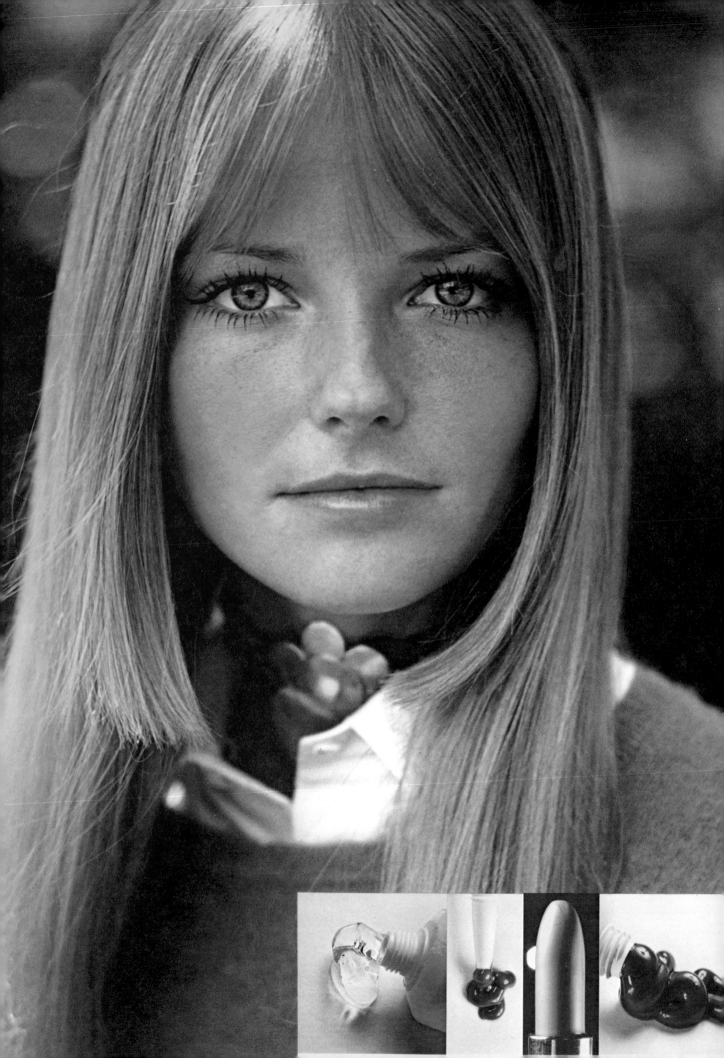

THE GAMES YOU CAN PLAY WITH
MAKEUP

You have clothes that are right for dinner at your mother-in-law's and others for dinner for two at a great restaurant. So why shouldn't you have different faces too? Like one for an eight o'clock class and another for a fantasy evening mood or for when you're feeling like an adventuress? That's why we've summed up some of the prettiest beauty ideas into four different interesting faces for you to try on. Actually, each one is a little mood picture in color and texture. And each one has two or three definite color focal points—eyes, cheeks and/or mouth—to give it life. Opposite you see one mood— healthy, glowing with rich tawny earth tones. On the next pages, you'll see three more entirely different ones plus a step-by-step how-to for each face. The fun of them is that any girl can wear any of them—the one opposite and the three following are all done on one model, Cheryl Tiegs, just to prove it. It all goes to show that if you're clever enough, the faces you wear can be just as revealing emotionally as the clothes you wear.

GLOSSED WITH TAWNY HEALTH

When you want nothing but the freshest gloss in tawny earth tones, wear this face. It has the exuberance of health—it's clean, unspoiled and absolutely natural. The two important spots for color focus here are the soft mocha mouth and the intense browned-pink cheeks. The look is done primarily with gels. The trick is to work quickly with them and to blend thoroughly. Apply to one section of the face at a time and continue to add more color until you get the color intensity and degree of glow you want. Start with a clear gel moisturizer blended all over the face and neck (1). (You can use a stick coverup for blemishes if you need to.) Then a tawny gel to give the face an all-over glow. We used a generous dab of bronze cheek gel on each cheek and blended it thoroughly for more intensified color. Do one cheek at a time and add color as you need it (2). For the eyes, brush mascara on upper and lower lashes. Powder lashes first and then apply two or three coats of mascara to give a luxurious effect. The finish is a dab of the clear gel moisturizer on the eyelids smoothed up to brows. Several coats of gel give a beautiful glossy effect (3). Finish the mocha-colored lips slicked with gloss (4).

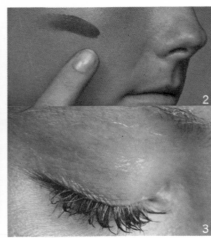

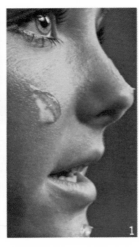

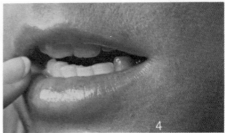

POWDERED COOL

The face opposite is cool, direct and approachable—no shine at all. It's the one to wear when you're feeling smooth and velvety. The look is done with translucent powder misted over unmistakably strong color. The main emphasis here is on deep rose lips, smoky teal-shadowed eyes, peach-brown cheeks; the translucent powder mattes the look but doesn't add any color of its own. To start, we blushed the cheeks with tan. Next, the translucent powder applied with a soft fluffy powder puff. The powder is patted on, not rubbed, and we used lots (1). Then, with a natural bristle powder brush, the face was brushed gently to remove excess powder (2). This should be done with quick short strokes so that you don't streak the blusher. For the smoky eyes, a grayish teal blue shadow. The color is brushed in the crease of the eye first and extended just beyond the outer corner (3), then smoothed with a cotton swab. With darker shadows like this, keep stroking till color is even. The color is brought around and under the eye, up to center of lower lid. Band of color under the eye should be narrow (4). A burnt rose see-through lipstick gives lips a deep blushed color (5).

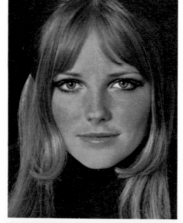

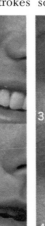

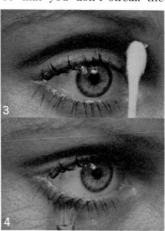

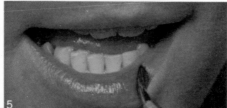

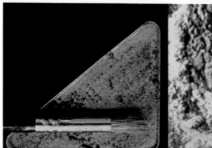

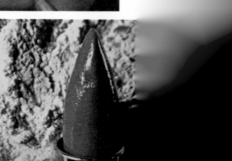

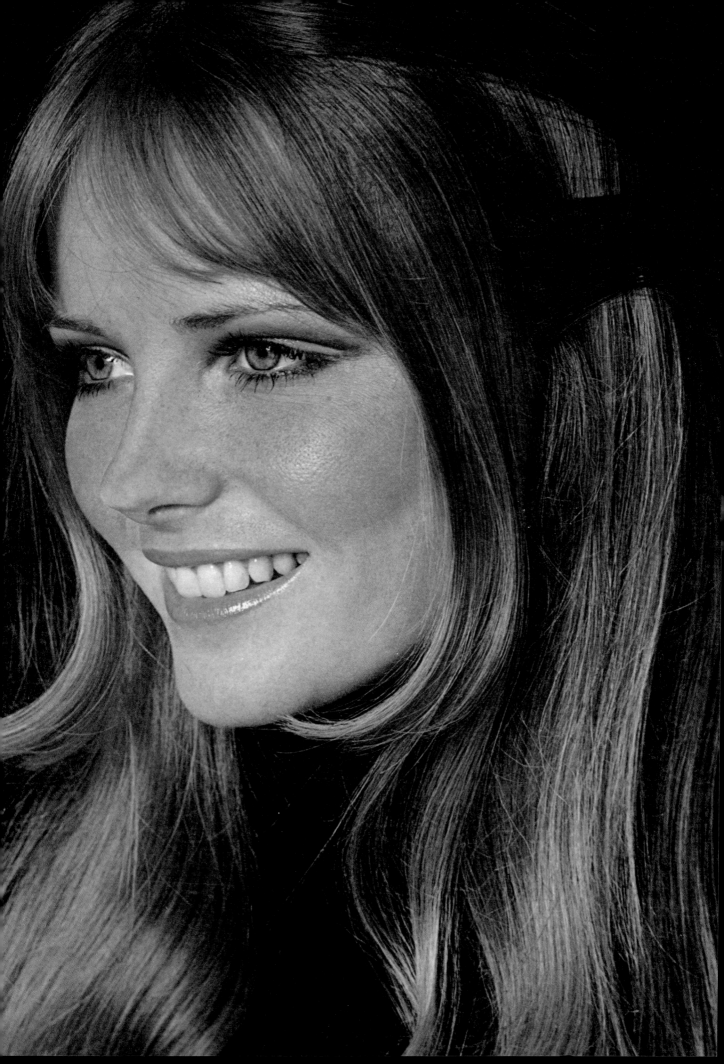

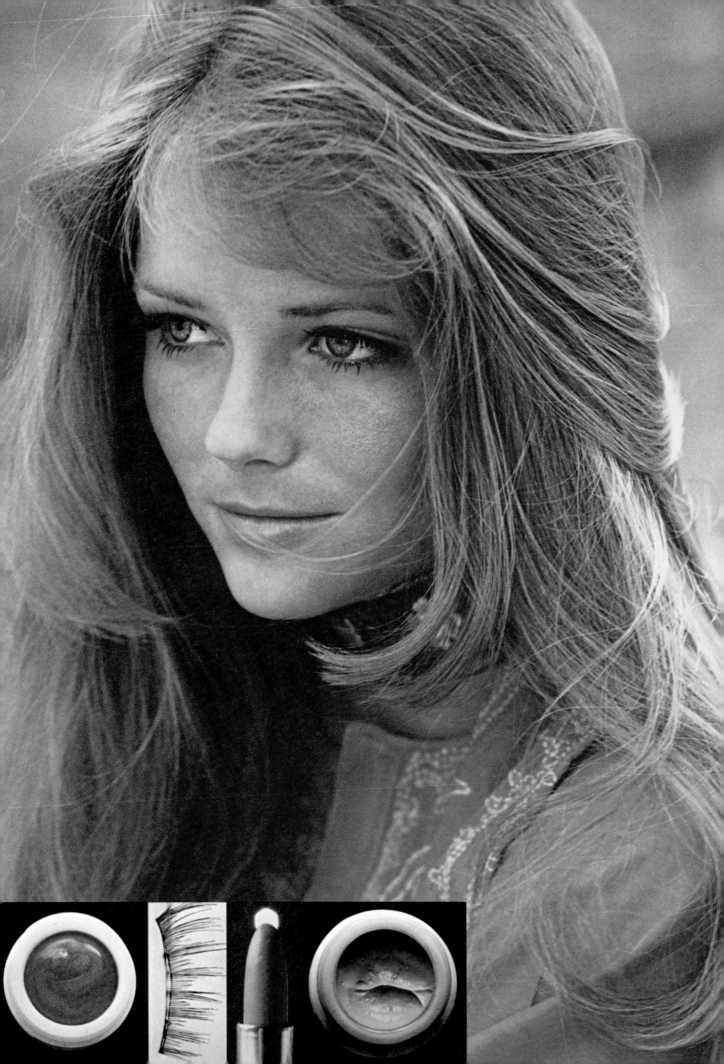

COLORED
REALLY
SUPER

The face opposite positively shimmers in vibrant but soft color. The cheeks are sparkled with a deep raspberry, the eyes are shadowed with pale violet and the mouth is a sensational super-bright lilac. The main focus is on eyes —swept with long plum-colored false lashes—and on the bright but soft mouth. This look starts with a moisturizer. The first color is a sparkling raspberry incandescent cheek blush (1). We misted the eyes with violet cream shadow blended from the center of the upper lid to the corner and extended beyond it slightly. Next, it's brought under the eye, fading at the center of the lower lid. Stroke over the color to even out the tone (2). The eyes get fabulous drama from long sweepy false lashes unexpected in burgundy. To apply these or any other lash, flex the back over your finger to soften it. Trim slightly. Apply glue and set in place with your finger, and stretch eyelid slightly with one finger at each corner to smooth (3). Mascara bottom lashes lightly with black. Color on mouth is a strong but soft, violet tone (4).

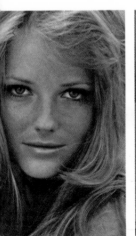

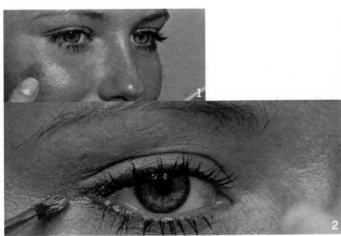

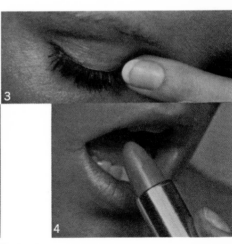

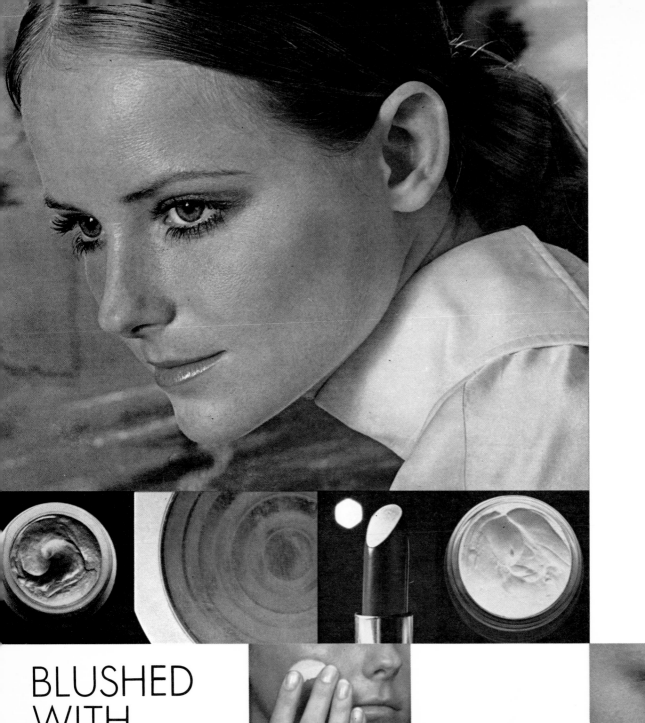

BLUSHED WITH PEARL

The luminous face above looks as though it were lit from within and that's the way you should feel when you wear it—all aglow inside. It has a pearled base with deep wine lips and blackberry shadowed eyes. The pearl blush comes from, first, a luminous moisturizer applied all over the face and neck for the subtlest pearl glow. Next, a lovely see-through rose blush on the cheeks (1). Soft pearled blackberry eye shadow goes over the entire lid and is extended slightly beyond the outer corner of the eye, around and underneath. This gives an aura of pearly color. The undereye color should fade away at the center of lower lid (2). Individual clusters of false lashes go on the bottom lids only—a nice balance to the shadow when applied this way: the longest clusters at the center of the eye, shorter ones at the corners. An off white frosty shadow is blended just under the brow for another pearly accent (3). The delicate but "in-depth" color on the mouth is a sheer wine lipgloss (4).

DOS & DON'TS
FOR PLAYING THE FACES GAME

Any girl can look super in any of these faces, but not without some know-how and a little fitting here and there. For example, if you're very pale and never tan, you can still wear the tawny look on page 146—see-through bronzing gels can do what the sun can't. But you will probably want to tone the cheek color down more than the girl who may already have a bit of tan or naturally darker skin. Just use less of the gel or blend it until the color is next to nothing. The point is to avoid stark contrasts. On the other hand, a dark-skinned girl whose lips naturally have a deep rose blush may want to cut the deep rose lipstain on page 149 by blotting it considerably. Take a look at the Dos and Don'ts here, then have fun learning the face games.

DO think of yourself as a painter who knows her art and wouldn't dream of starting on any unprepared surface, whether it's wood, plaster, canvas or skin. You have to prime it. A moisturizer does this for skin, helps makeup go on smoothly as well as protecting skin from the environment and from losing moisture.

DO remember that any makeup line that's harsh means trouble for your face—hard lipstick demarcations, hard endings of shadow (smooth with a cotton swab or brush), foundation lines. Everything should be soft-edged with no definite outlines. If you wear your hair back or up, carry makeup over entire neck and behind ears.

DON'T be timid about experimenting with foundation colors different from your own skin tone. Some makeups are so sheer and see-through you have a great range of shades to try. There are limitations, of course, but you can be much more adventuresome. When you're cosmetic shopping, try the store's testers on the inside of your wrist where the skin tone is most likely to be close to your face's. If you pick a deep bronze tone and you're quite fair, remember to blend the gel or stick in well and to use it sparingly.

DO keep your eyebrows a shade or two paler than your hair so that your eyes and mouth can come forward. Dark heavy eyebrows are overpowering to the new makeup looks.

DO realize that more color on the mouth doesn't mean a deep opaque color; the idea is sheer transparent color with depth. Think of lips wet with wine or the stain of fresh berry juice. Use lipgloss under or over these new colors to soften them. Gloss put on first is the most color-softening.

DON'T neglect this trick for using cheek gels—you'll get a sensational result. Start with a small dab of color and blend it quickly and well. Build up the color and the degree of gloss with several light coats. This gives you a tremendous color range with just one gel. The gels are quick-drying, long-lasting.

DO try on the sexy-eyes look you get from powdering your eyelashes before you mascara them. Flick on a bit of white talc or baby powder with your fingertip, and then mascara over this—terrific.

DON'T be afraid to try different textures in makeup. Some may work better on your skin than others. To keep the price of experimenting within your budget, here's a guide to help you know where to start. Gels work especially well on normal or oily skins. Very oily skins do best to stick to powder blushers and shadows and forget the gels or creamy ones. Oil- and cream-based makeups are great for drier skins. If you want to try gels but your skin is quite dry, use a bit more moisturizer than you ordinarily would have and you should have no trouble. If you love the look of stick blushers or bronzers but find their glow turns to shine too soon, carry a little package of facial blotters in your purse and blot away the shine.

DON'T be rigid about makeup. Just because lipgloss is supposed to be used on lips doesn't mean it won't look sensational glossed over your eyebrows, too, or just under the brow bone. Some girls find the most effective use for a product may not be what it was intended for. For example, a bit of cheek blusher under the brow bone or a slick of very pale translucent lipstick under the brow as a highlighter.

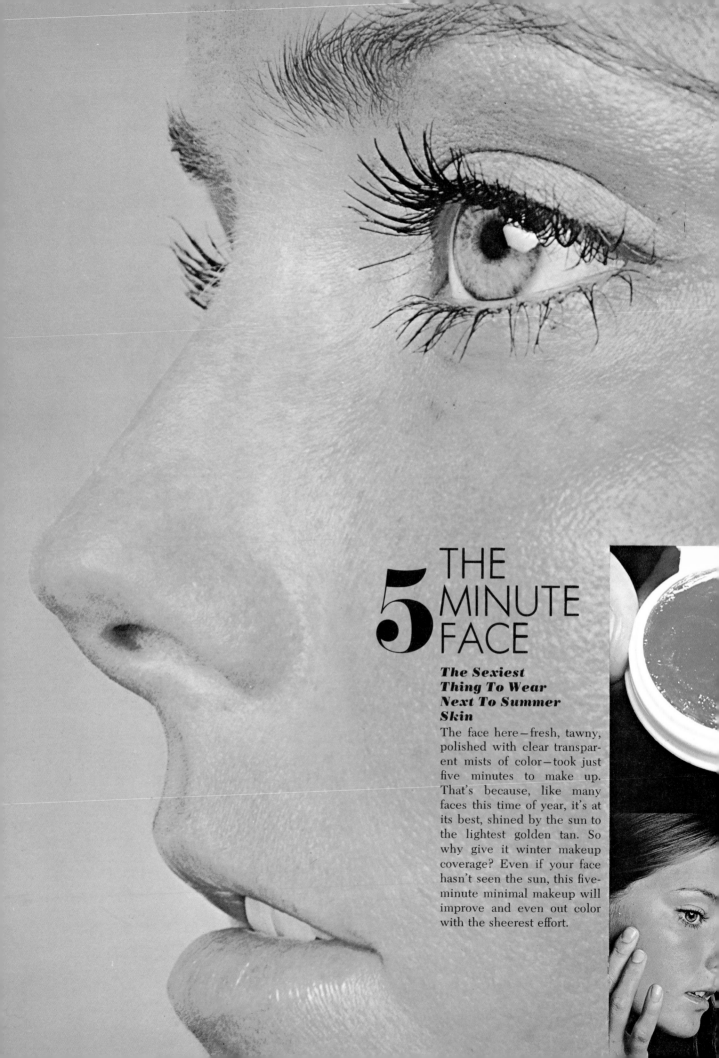

5 THE MINUTE FACE

The Sexiest Thing To Wear Next To Summer Skin

The face here—fresh, tawny, polished with clear transparent mists of color—took just five minutes to make up. That's because, like many faces this time of year, it's at its best, shined by the sun to the lightest golden tan. So why give it winter makeup coverage? Even if your face hasn't seen the sun, this five-minute minimal makeup will improve and even out color with the sheerest effort.

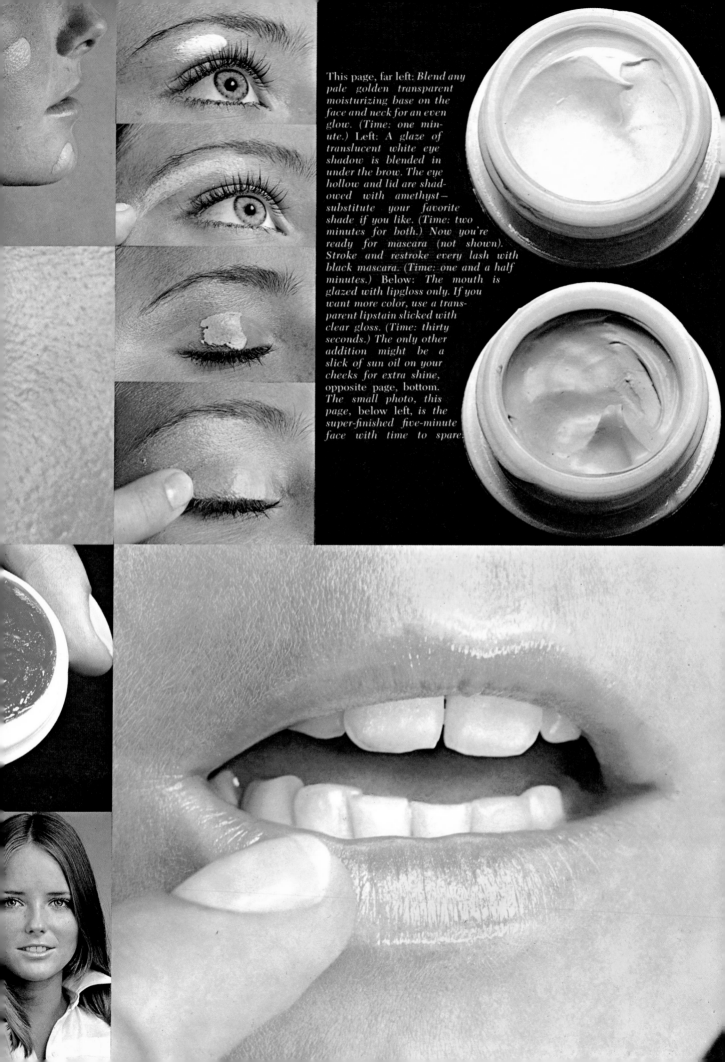

This page, far left: *Blend any pale golden transparent moisturizing base on the face and neck for an even glow. (Time: one minute.) Left: A glaze of translucent white eye shadow is blended in under the brow. The eye hollow and lid are shadowed with amethyst—substitute your favorite shade if you like. (Time: two minutes for both.) Now you're ready for mascara (not shown). Stroke and restroke every lash with black mascara. (Time: one and a half minutes.) Below: The mouth is glazed with lipgloss only. If you want more color, use a transparent lipstain slicked with clear gloss. (Time: thirty seconds.) The only other addition might be a slick of sun oil on your cheeks for extra shine, opposite page, bottom. The small photo, this page, below left, is the super-finished five-minute face with time to spare.*

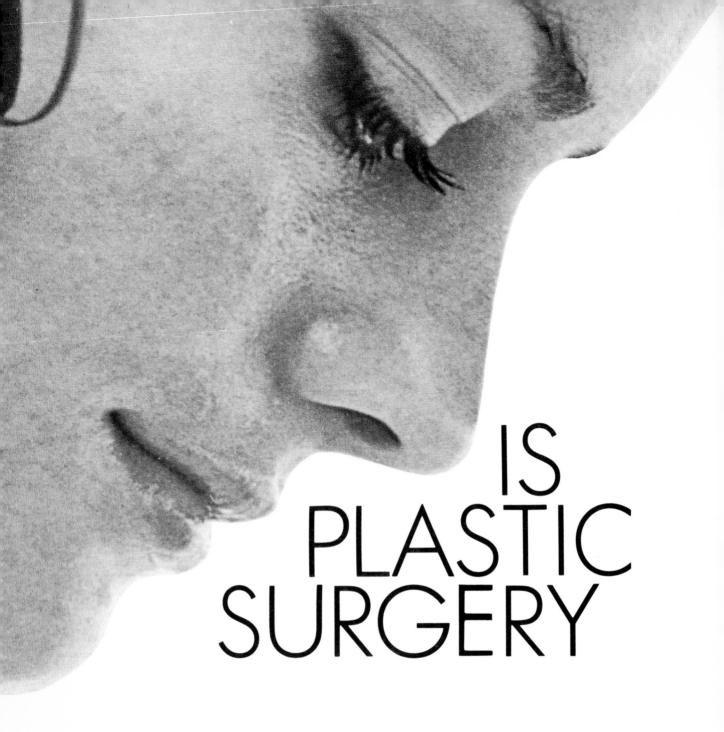

IS PLASTIC SURGERY

Correcting imperfect features by cosmetic plastic surgery is as acceptable a beauty treatment today as tinting your hair. However, it's not for everyone. Here are questions and answers that help answer your queries.

More and more young women are now reasoning that if nature has made an error in nose or chin-line or in ears that are set in less than classic style, there's no earthly reason not to correct it early in the game. Young actresses and models, with a professional stake in their facial contours, consult plastic surgeons as a matter of course, if the need is indicated. For non-professionals, especially in big metropolitan areas, such surgery has become as acceptable a part of the total beauty treatment as tinting, curling or straightening hair.

This doesn't mean that surgery is the answer for every girl who has, or thinks she has, a facial imperfection. Reputable plastic surgeons are quite fussy about whom they operate on, and generally examine the patient's motives carefully before accepting a patient.

"I don't need plastic surgery to get a job or anything. I just want to look prettier. Do I qualify?"

Probably. The simple normal desire to look your best is a healthy instinct, and you'll very likely pass. Doctors also like to know if you've thought seriously about the operation. Changing a feature is not something to do on a whim. You can't change it back if you don't like it. "The ideal patient," Dr. Blair O. Rogers, a New York plastic surgeon, said,

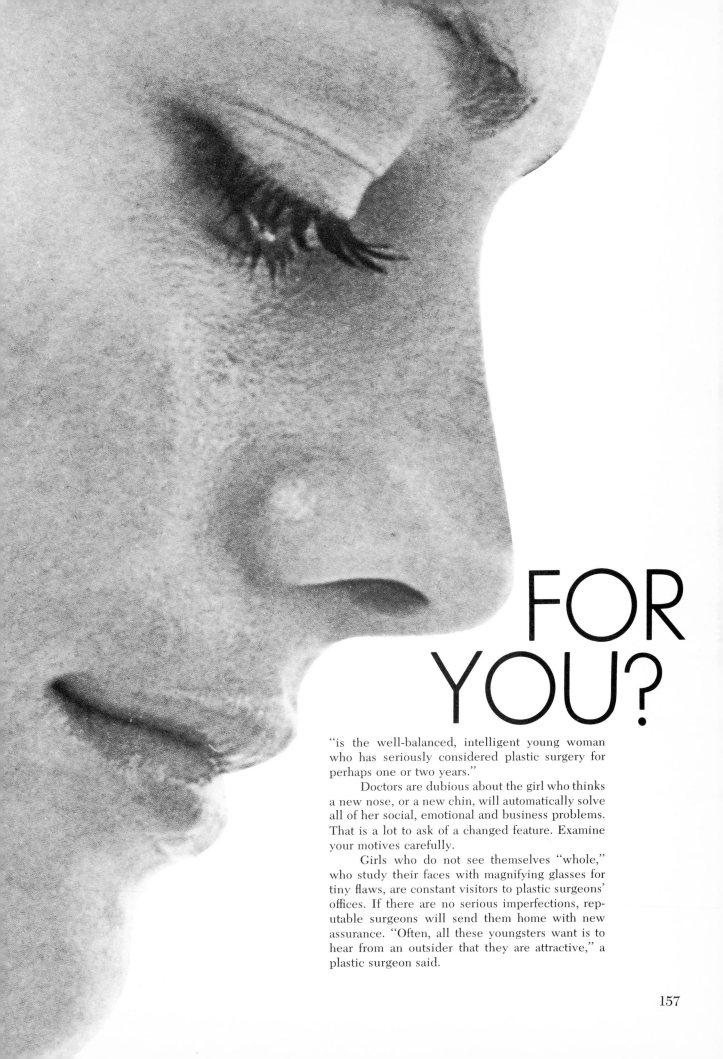

FOR YOU?

"is the well-balanced, intelligent young woman who has seriously considered plastic surgery for perhaps one or two years."

Doctors are dubious about the girl who thinks a new nose, or a new chin, will automatically solve all of her social, emotional and business problems. That is a lot to ask of a changed feature. Examine your motives carefully.

Girls who do not see themselves "whole," who study their faces with magnifying glasses for tiny flaws, are constant visitors to plastic surgeons' offices. If there are no serious imperfections, reputable surgeons will send them home with new assurance. "Often, all these youngsters want is to hear from an outsider that they are attractive," a plastic surgeon said.

Actually, it's not how a patient wants to see herself, but how the surgeon sees her, inside as well as out, that determines not only how she will look after the operation but whether he will perform the operation at all. He is a sculptor in bone and tissue, and won't put a tiny, tilt nose on a moonshaped face any more than a sculptor in stone would place a delicate hand on a warrior's arm. But there are countless women and girls who want to look exactly like their friends who have had cosmetic surgery. One girl has a nose or an ear or chin done and six of her friends call the doctor for an appointment. But on all of them the same cute, perfect little nose or chin shape will be meaningless. The whole face must hold together. That's why it's advisable to go along with a surgeon when he suggests a nose or chin shape that you think is less than ideal. Unfortunately, when a fee is involved, it's usually possible to find a surgeon who will do the job the patient wants, even if it's not the right job. This is one of the major complaints of ethical doctors.

Because understanding between patient and doctor is so important, reputable surgeons stress the initial consultations; some insist on a minimum of two before surgery. The need for rapport is particularly important during the post-operative period, when a patient must follow her doctor's instructions to the letter if the best possible results are to be obtained.

"What can plastic surgery accomplish?"

Essentially, plastic surgeons reshape an individual's own features into a new, more attractive form. Noses can be corrected (rhinoplasty). Large ears, ears that stick out, can be reshaped and flattened against the head (otoplasty). Receding chins can be brought out and jutting chins de-emphasized (mentoplasty). Bags beneath the eyes can be removed, even eye-lids can be reshaped by especially skilled surgeons—but these two areas don't usually concern the young. Unfortunately, little can be done about the contour of the lips. Nose shortening, however, often results in more space between nose and lips. And when the skin that has been pulled up by the unshapely nose is relaxed after surgery, the resultant lipline is often improved.

No surgeon can promise exactly what a face will look like after surgery, but he can give some idea by penciling in his plans on a preoperative photograph. Just as there is no guarantee or warrantee in life or medicine, there can be none in plastic surgery. Nor can surgeons predict the precise type of healing that will take place. In a nose operation internal scar tissue occasionally causes thickening of the skin of the nasal tip. This occurs very rarely. If it does, skillful plastic surgeons have methods of eventually correcting it. In ear operations, where the incision is behind the ear, and in those chin operations in which an incision is made in the chin fold, there is a remote possibility that keloids—weltlike overgrowths of scar tissue—may form. These are uncorrectable.

"How do I find a plastic surgeon?"

Plastic surgeons must be selected carefully; if one does a poor job, you may not get a second chance.

A certified plastic surgeon has satisfactorily completed as many as eight years of study and practice after graduation from medical school. At least three of these years are spent in general surgery.

In choosing your surgeon, first consult your family doctor. If he has no suggestions to offer, contact your County Medical Society, or check the list of plastic surgeons in the *Directory of Medical Specialists.*

Don't expect plastic surgeons to be as numerous as obstetricians. New York plastic surgeon Dr. Herbert Conway points out in a 1967 issue of *Plastic and Reconstructive Surgery* that two-thirds of all plastic surgeons in this country are located in ten states—New York, California, Texas, Ohio, Illinois, Pennsylvania, Florida, Michigan, Mississippi, and New Jersey. And 30 percent of all plastic surgeons in the United States practice in New York and California.

"How much does plastic surgery cost?"

Highly respected plastic surgeons in New York quote fees of $500 to $1,500 for rhinoplasty, $400 to $750 for otoplasty and $350 to $750 for mentoplasty. Fees vary slightly from area to area. As one plastic surgeon explained, fees are gauged, too, according to the doctor's reputation, the number of years he has practiced and his position in his hospital's hierarchy.

There is a consultation fee in addition to the surgeon's fee. Patients, especially those a surgeon does not accept, sometimes question the consultation fee. They feel they are "shopping" for a commodity, forget they are receiving the advice of a trained specialist.

Tacked onto these charges is the expense of before and after medical photographs, and in rare cases, plaster casts that help the surgeon work out the blueprints of new features. And, of course, there are hospital fees. All expenses—and the possibility of insurance coverage—should be discussed fully and frankly with the plastic surgeon.

"What is the best age for plastic surgery?"

Many plastic surgeons believe that the earlier nose, chin and ear surgery is performed the better the results. Younger skin is more elastic; unshapely noses tend to become more so as they mature. However, some surgeons prefer not to operate on young women until they are out of the skin-blemish stage, up to nineteen or twenty. "The average girl is considered fully grown at sixteen or seventeen," said one surgeon. "She is, internally, but her skin isn't and her sebaceous glands may still be overly active. As long as a girl's complexion is poor, a surgeon will get less ideal results."

"How painful is plastic surgery?"

The answer appears to depend on your threshold of pain and anxiety. A booklet published by the American Society of Plastic and Reconstructive Surgeons notes "there is little more than minor discomfort." Yet some, perhaps overly sensitive women, have rated surgery "uncomfortable" to "painful."

"It's like a broken bone," explained one surgeon. "Once it's splinted, it doesn't hurt." The area can be tender for a while, he pointed out, especially so if the patient is rough or careless with it.

"What happens at the hospital?"

Actually, there is no set routine. A surgeon designs each operation to meet each person's specific problems. The patient is usually admitted to the hospital the night before surgery is scheduled and is given mild sedation. There is additional sedation before she is wheeled into the operating room. Most surgeons prefer to use local anesthesia. Chances of bleeding are reduced; there is less chance of nausea that would disturb the newly shaped feature; and the patient can respond to the surgeon's instructions to move certain lip or facial muscles if necessary.

The actual operation, in the case of a nose, lasts about ninety minutes. The injection and the subsequent cuts are made inside the nose. The nose is then "degloved," i.e., the skin is lifted from the bone and cartilage framework underneath, which is then reshaped. Next, the skin is taped to the corrected framework, thereby molding the nose into the desired form, and covered by a splint, which is applied to hold the bones in their new position.

In a chin operation, the incision is made either in the chin fold, where it's not visible, or deep inside the lower lip. An implant—either of the patient's own cartilage or, more likely, of silicone—shaped to the correct size is then inserted, and an external adhesive strip is often applied to stabilize it. If an ear correction is being made, the incision is made behind the ear, the skin is separated from the back of the ear, the cartilage is "rolled back" with stitches, any excess cartilage and skin are removed and a bulky headdressing is applied over the ears to maintain the new shape.

Occasionally, nose and chin are corrected during the same operation.

After nose operations, patients are usually discouraged from looking into the mirror for a few days. There may be considerable swelling and discoloration around the eyes.

Anywhere from the fifth to the seventh day the splint may be removed. But it may be several weeks before the nose settles into an acceptable shape. It may take another six months to a year for it to settle permanently into final shape.

Secondary work may be necessary and it's no cause for alarm. According to Dr. George V. Webster, a plastic surgeon in Pasadena, California, "minor corrective surgeries are necessary for about 4 or 5 percent of rhinoplasties." Writing in *Plastic and Reconstructive Surgery*, Dr. Webster pointed out that these corrections can often be performed in the office and that no additional charge is made for them. Another doctor explained that this secondary work was occasionally called for, not because of any mistakes on the operating table, but because not even the best plastic surgeon can always anticipate nature's various healing processes.

"Will I have scars?"

After a nose operation, there will be scars but they will be inside the nose and not visible. Occasionally, it is necessary to leave minute external scars around the nostrils. After an ear operation, the scars are in the creases behind the ears (both are done at the same time) and are scarcely visible unless the ears are pulled forward. In chin surgery, the scars are inside the mouth or hidden in the chin fold.

"How soon can I return to work?"

Students often try to schedule surgery for school recesses. Many career women do it on their two-week vacation. Several surgeons emphasize that patients can return to work or school by the eighth, ninth, or tenth day provided they have fairly sedentary jobs, aren't ballet dancers or physical education majors.

The patient who has to stay out longer is the exception. She may have extremely thick skin or an expecially long nose. In both cases, adhesive tape supports may have to be left on for a longer period. Everyone has seen women with bits of adhesive over their nose tip. If they have understanding employers and aren't overly sensitive themselves, there's no reason why they can't return to work or school with the tape in place.

"I have scars from an automobile accident. Can plastic surgery help?"

Probably it can. Post-accident work is called reconstructive, rather than cosmetic, plastic surgery and is definitely covered by most insurance plans. It may be advisable to call in a plastic surgeon, if one is available, immediately after the accident, but this is not always possible. Actually, scars from an accident are treated by plastic surgeons from four to six months after the accident. Reconstructive work is most successful after scars have had a chance to settle. Even if a plastic surgeon does the original work, it may be necessary to have scars worked on again six months later—depending on the nature of the injury.

"I want to have my nose fixed. But I'm afraid of what my friends will say."

This is understandable. It's quite likely that when you first venture out with your new nose you'll get a few stares and what you may interpret as unfeeling questions from some tactless souls. Simultaneously, you'll undoubtedly get some appreciative stares you weren't getting before from strangers, which is marvelous for the ego.

Remember, the new, prettier you is bound to cause comment, but that what you may interpret as criticism is simply curiosity and interest. And it will pass quickly. Your friends, the people you work or go to school with, will accept your new face very quickly and turn their attention to other things. They're much less interested in it than you are, you know. Meanwhile, the trick of getting through the first, self-conscious period: Keep smiling, and affect a confidence you may not feel. Act like a beauty, and you create the illusion of beauty. But you've got even more going for you—with your new face, it won't be an illusion.

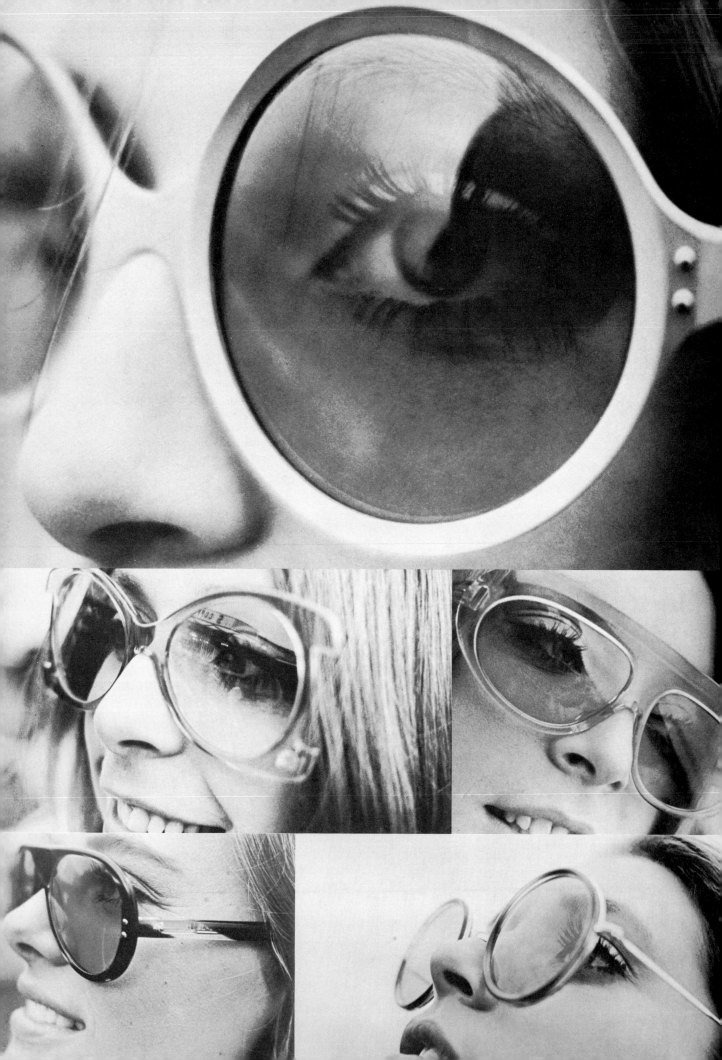

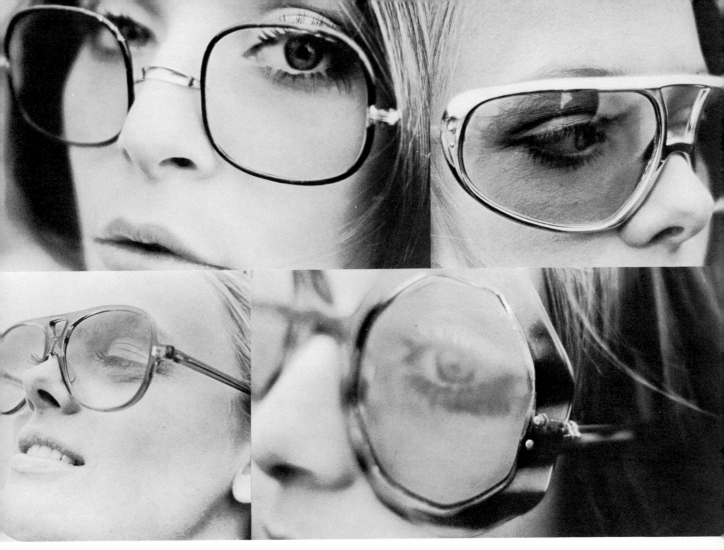

DOS & DON'TS

for getting
more fashion out of
your glasses

DO treat "serious" glasses like a fashion accessory. Because you wear them all the time is all the more reason to have frames and lenses with some chic.

DO search for an optometrist who has the new shapes. Many are afraid to experiment, so find the most fashion-conscious; it's worth the extra trouble.

DON'T typecast yourself as the "tortoise" or any other type. Have different-shaped frames with different-tinted lenses. It's really not an extravagance, since you wear them all the time, but an investment in good looks.

DO wear pretty glasses to disguise circles and dark shadows from lack of sleep. Beauty glasses are the best cover going and add color to your face.

DON'T disregard the shape of your face when you pick out your beauty glasses.

Keep these rules in front of you:

Square face — *pick large square or rectangular frames so that the lower outer corners of the frame protrude past the cheekbones. This distracts from the squareness of the jawline and gives the illusion of a more oval face.*

Long face — *wear a vertically deep frame so that it covers more of the length of the face and therefore leaves less of it showing.*

Small short face — *a narrow rectangular little frame is best because it will leave more face showing.*

Round face — *the best frame is horizontally wide and vertically narrow, preferably oval in shape. This tends to put an obvious horizontal line at eye level, which makes the lower two thirds of the face look thinner and longer.*

Oval face — *any frame goes for you.*

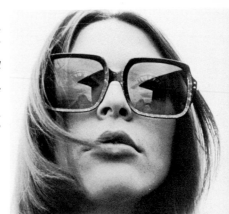

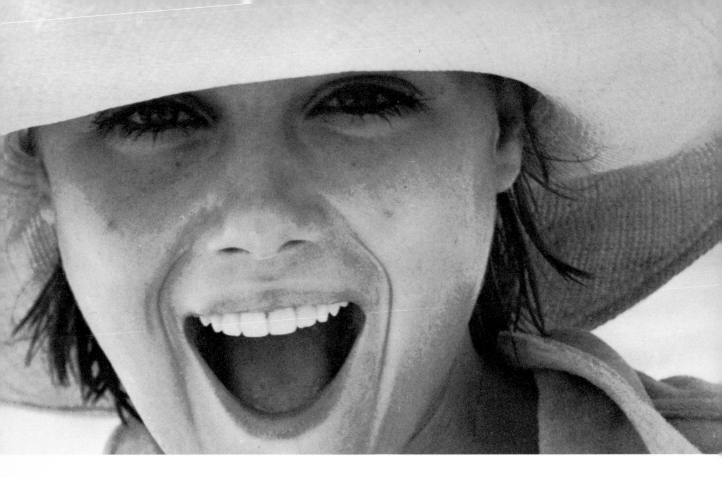

ARE YOUR TEETH A DON'T

Orthodontics used to belong to the early teen years only—a gleaming set of braces simultaneously the status symbol and cross-to-bear of adolescence. No longer. Faulty alignment of teeth can, and should, be corrected at any age. The techniques are the same (for postadolescents, some may take a little longer) and modern techniques make anything— well, almost anything—possible.

The sooner you start, of course, the better. Structural teeth problems grow more pronounced with age, can lead to other problems: teeth crowding each other every which way provide places for food particles and increase the chances of tooth decay and gum problems. Bad bite can lead to loosening of teeth, erosion of bone, gum diseases. Missing teeth, badly positioned teeth, can affect facial structure, can hasten the advent of side-of-the-mouth wrinkles.

No need to live with obvious faults either. Sandy Dennis may look marvelous with buck teeth; you, perhaps, do not. An orthodontist can fix them. And this kind of correction pays off psychologically as well as aesthetically; orthodontists today realize, as do plastic surgeons, that living with correctable faults can be psychologically damaging.

The basic corrective technique is teeth-straightening using the familiar braces, although these days they're much more comfortable. These may be removable or permanent. Don't use either, or both at different times. This kind of straightening takes about two years for adolescents, a little more or less, depending on the type and amount of correction required, for someone older. There are also biteplates, and headgear to wear only at night.

Beyond this, modern orthodontists have at their command a complex of techniques to solve a complex of problems. They are able to redirect or graft gum tissue, to graft bone, to splint or suture a tooth into position, add a cap or jacket to anchor the suture for invisible straightening.

Formerly unsavable teeth can be salvaged by root therapy; an impacted tooth can be brought down. Orthodontists work with plastic surgeons for major structural changes—a receding jaw, for example. "Interceptive orthodontics" means just what it sounds like: by using X rays and knowledge or rate and pattern of growth, dentists today can spot a problem coming on and solve it before it happens.

Orthodontists are artists as well as craftsmen. Caps or jackets hide malformed or damaged teeth (newest and most effective are porcelain baked on gold), and dentists today are careful about matching tooth color, not only to other teeth but to age—teeth darken slightly as you grow older. They try to approximate nature by artful use of small irregularities and imperfections to avoid a "false teeth" look or a smile that resembles, as one doctor put it, "A box of Chiclets laid out in a row."

Modern dentists look at the whole woman, realize that the health of her teeth ultimately depends on, and affects, her total health. They will, for example, discuss general health and basic nutrition with a patient at the same time they discuss oral hygiene.

The cost of orthodontics is not excessive, prorated by time. There's a set fee for diagnosis, $35 to $100, depending on what's needed in the way of X rays and casts. Average treatment takes about two years and costs roughly $1,200 to $1,500, depending on the complexity and amount of treatment required. It's worth it. Your dentist or hospital can recommend an orthodontist; there are orthodontic clinics in all major cities, either attached to hospitals or municipally run.

A brief case history of straightening

The braces below gave her the maximum movement and grip in the shortest possible time. She wore them for 8 months; the complete treatment will take 15. Each case varies in length, depending on the state of the teeth, crookedness and crowding.

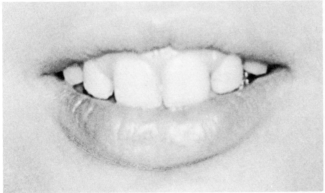

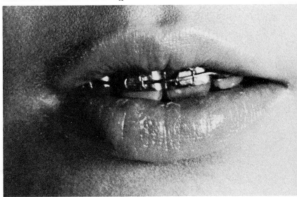

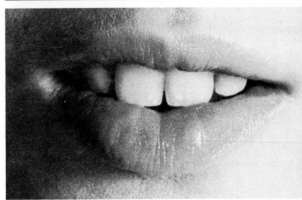

A year ago, this eighteen-year-old model began having her teeth straightened. Above, you see them before—protruding, too long over her lip. They closed unevenly, and as she grew older the bone around them would have become weakened.

The spaces you see between the teeth, right, will disappear in about six months time. They were caused by the braces and they will close up by wearing a removable appliance.

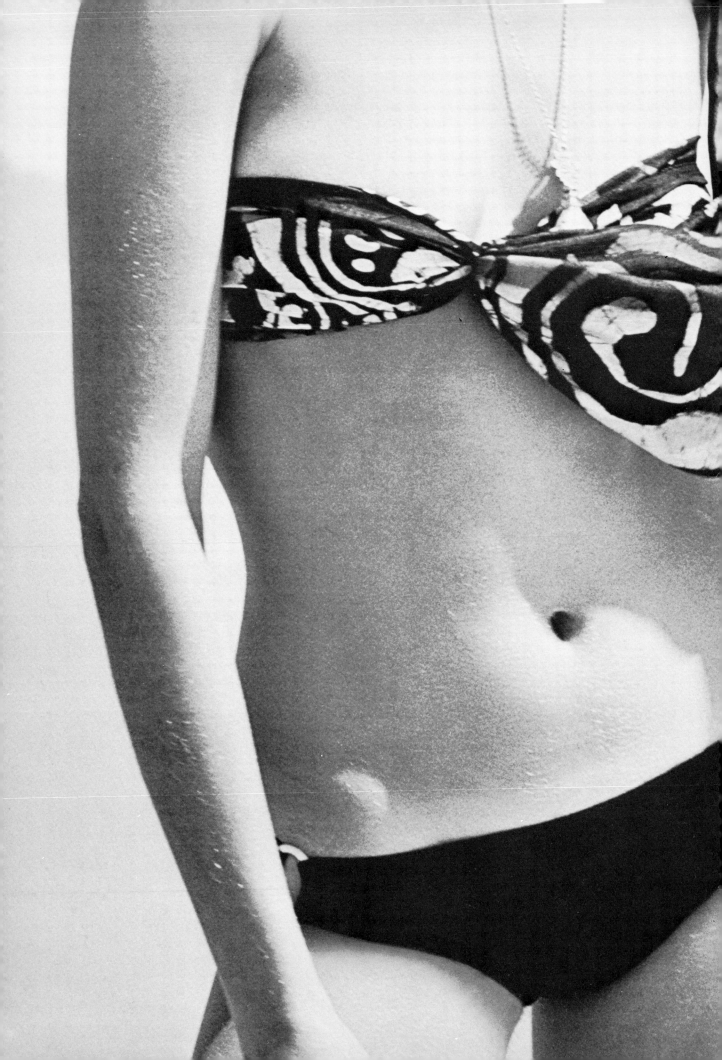

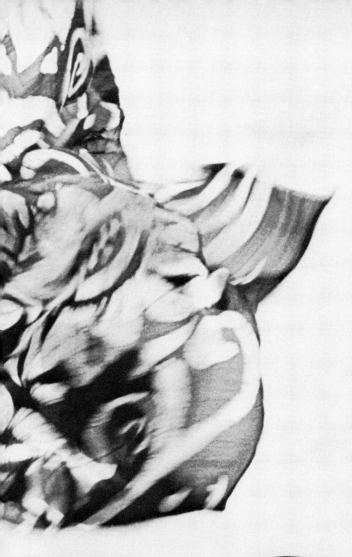

BODY

HOW TO

GET A BEAUTIFUL ONE
OUT OF THE ONE
YOU'RE STUCK WITH

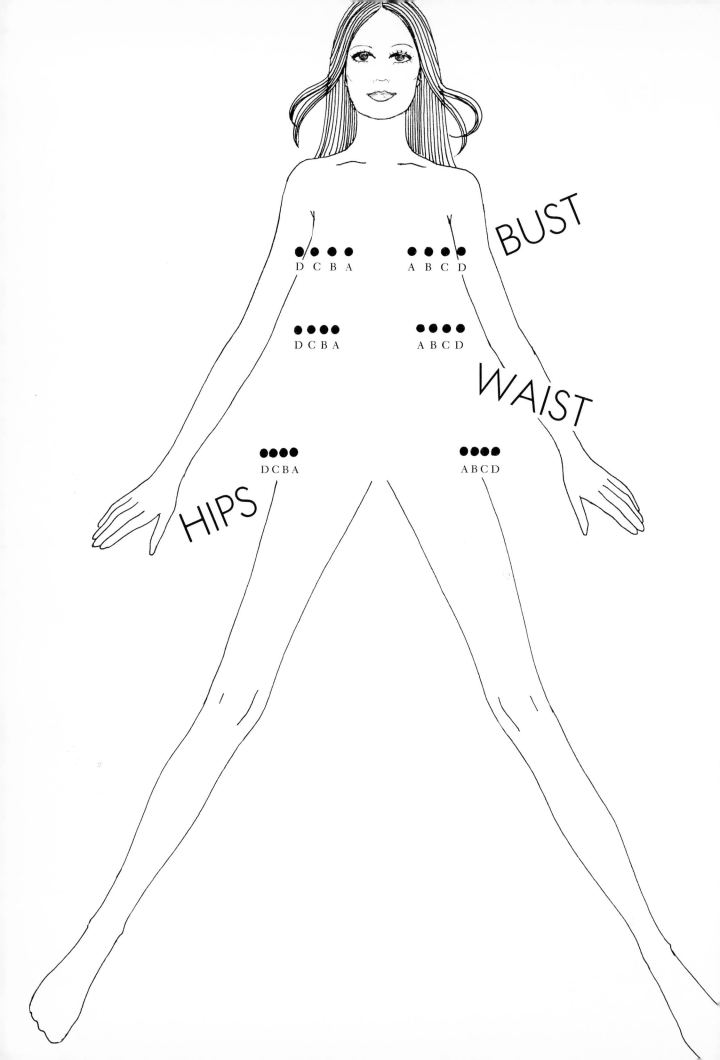

BUST

D C B A   A B C D

D C B A   A B C D

WAIST

D C B A   A B C D

HIPS

THE BODY TESTS

There's scarcely a girl or woman in America who at some time or other in her life hasn't needed to improve her figure. Overweight and poor muscle support are her two biggest worries, but childbirth, psychological and metabolic changes, and, of course, illness all make their marks. In this chapter it's the two big enemies we want to fight, plus dealing with some of the psychology that goes into getting and keeping your body in great shape. That does not necessarily mean a model's figure. It means realistically the best possible figure for you, not a superstar's or anybody else's, but yours. It's the individual proportions between the parts of your body that count enormously, your own particular bone structure and distribution of fat.

Following are two tests to help you determine a realistic figure goal for yourself, or, if you have already reached it, to reassure you and keep you there. The first test has to do with your proportions and locating the trouble spots. The second is the simple pinch test to determine overweight.

PROPORTIONS TEST

Find your figure trouble spots by filling in this drawing, opposite. Measure bust, waist, and hips. Then, using chart below, find the right letter for each measurement. Say you have an "A" bust, "B" waist, and "B" hips. Draw from A to B to B on each side of the figure. (Use heavy black pencil for best effect.)

Just for fun here's a spot check on a group of young women who were in beautiful shape and took the test. You might want to compare your own measurements with theirs, which although a far cry from a model's ideal assure the girls who have them good looks in and out of their clothes.

Bust	Waist	Hips
31"–32" A	21"–22" A	32"–33" A
33"–34" B	23"–24" B	34"–35" B
35"–36" C	25"–26" C	36"–37" C
37"–38" D	27"–28" D	38"–39" D

Height	5'3"	5'5"	5'8"
Bust	32"–36¼"	33"–36½"	34"–37"
Waist	23"–25½"	24"–27"	25"–27½"
Hips	33"–37"	34"–37½"	35"–37¾"

THE OVERWEIGHT TEST

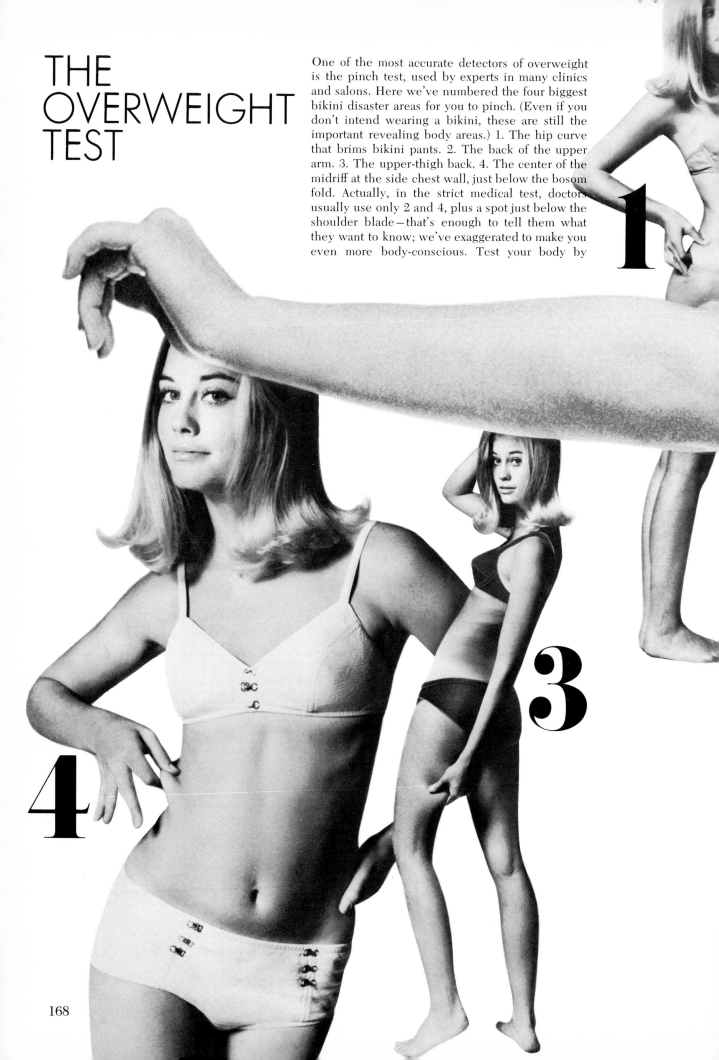

One of the most accurate detectors of overweight is the pinch test, used by experts in many clinics and salons. Here we've numbered the four biggest bikini disaster areas for you to pinch. (Even if you don't intend wearing a bikini, these are still the important revealing body areas.) 1. The hip curve that brims bikini pants. 2. The back of the upper arm. 3. The upper-thigh back. 4. The center of the midriff at the side chest wall, just below the bosom fold. Actually, in the strict medical test, doctors usually use only 2 and 4, plus a spot just below the shoulder blade—that's enough to tell them what they want to know; we've exaggerated to make you even more body-conscious. Test your body by

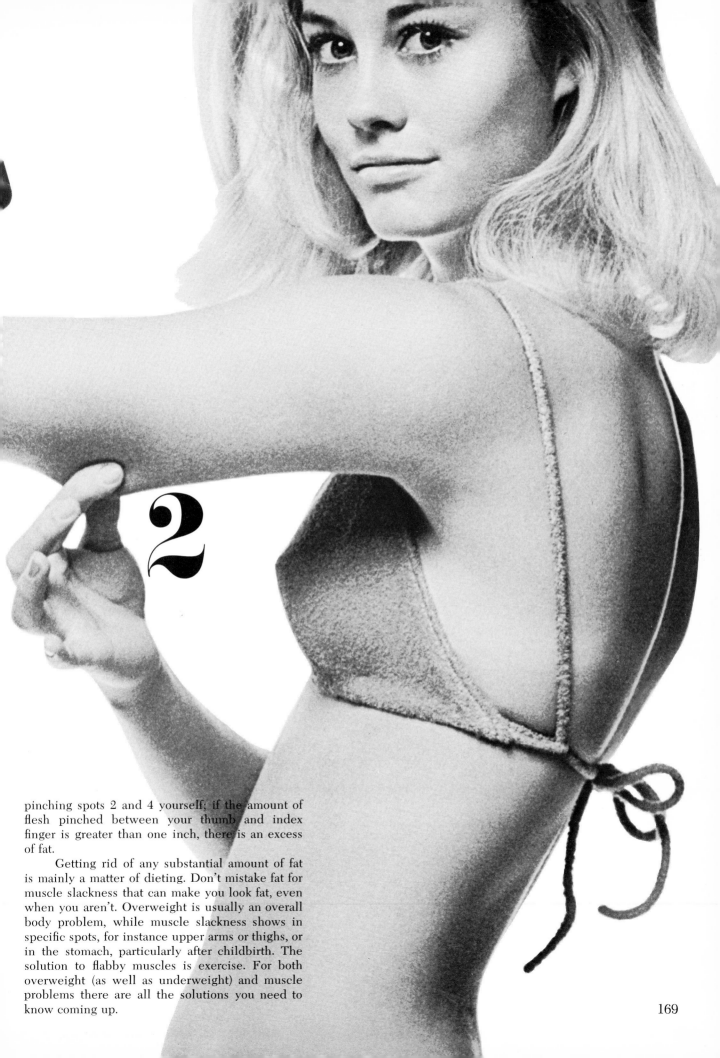

2

pinching spots 2 and 4 yourself; if the amount of flesh pinched between your thumb and index finger is greater than one inch, there is an excess of fat.

Getting rid of any substantial amount of fat is mainly a matter of dieting. Don't mistake fat for muscle slackness that can make you look fat, even when you aren't. Overweight is usually an overall body problem, while muscle slackness shows in specific spots, for instance upper arms or thighs, or in the stomach, particularly after childbirth. The solution to flabby muscles is exercise. For both overweight (as well as underweight) and muscle problems there are all the solutions you need to know coming up.

169

YOUR WEIGHT CHART

If after the pinch test you still yearn for the facts of overweight in hard cool numbers, check yourself on this chart. These weights are medically prescribed and taken from the Metropolitan Life Insurance Company's booklet "Four Steps to Weight Control." You may find them a few pounds more lenient than today's fashion ideal. Most women look better if they keep below the maximum figures given here.

Age: For girls 18 to 25 subtract 1 pound for each year under 25. For women 25 years old and over:

Height with 2" heels	Small frame	Medium frame	Large frame
4'10"	92–98	96–107	104–119
4'11"	94–101	98–110	106–122
5' 0"	96–104	101–113	109–125
5' 1"	99–107	104–116	112–128
5' 2"	102–110	107–119	115–131
5' 3"	105–113	110–122	118–134
5' 4"	108–116	113–126	121–138
5' 5"	111–119	116–130	125–142
5' 6"	114–123	120–135	129–146
5' 7"	118–127	124–139	133–150
5' 8"	122–131	128–143	137–154
5' 9"	126–135	132–147	141–158
5'10"	130–140	136–151	145–163
5'11"	134–144	140–155	149–168
6' 0"	138–148	144–159	153–173

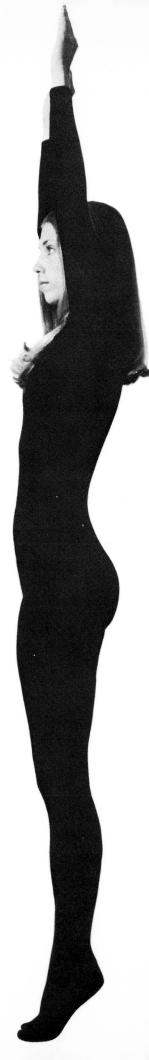

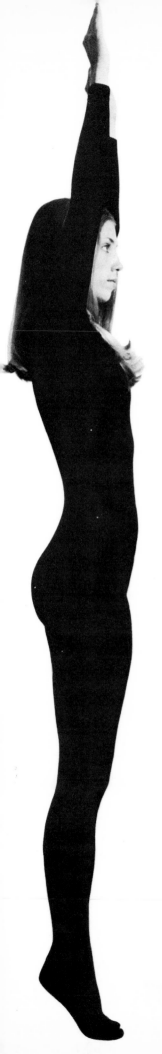

YOUR CALORIE CHART

To maintain or to reduce to the following weights
your caloric intake a day should be:

Weight	Maintaining calories	Reducing calories
105–109	1920	1200
110–114	2000	1300
115–119	2100	1400
120–124	2190	1450
125–129	2250	1500
130–134	2300	1550
135–139	2400	1600
140–144	2500	1650
145–149	2600	1700
150–154	2700	1750
155–159	2800	1800
160–164	2900	1900
165 and over	3000	2000

NEW-THINK DIET
AND EXERCISE

A plan that works whether you want a quick drop-down of 5 pounds; or something more—5 to 10 pounds; or still more—10 to 25 pounds. Worked out by GLAMOUR editors with Dr. Morton Glenn.

New-think diet and exercise doesn't start with old-think rules applied rigidly to everyone; it looks at the total weight-loss situation, finds out all there is to know about it, then applies the rules to the individual case—that's yours—to see if they work. If they don't, then it adapts them so that they do. It is based on the new-think way of solving problems that's going on now in business, research and politics. Here, with Dr. Morton Glenn, an internist who specializes in weight control and nutrition, we applied its fresh, sound methods to weight loss. Dr. Glenn is also a professor of clinical medicine at New York University School of Medicine.

The single measure of new-think applied to anything from corporate business reform to dieting and exercise is does it work? This plan certainly does.

Because it is simply an exaggeration of a good eating habit. At the end of the diet you simply drop the exaggeration and are left with the good habit which can last for life and which is the only way of maintaining a weight loss anyway. This is a practical program that you can stay on without suffering, unlike the old-think ones with their strict menus or the monotonous one-food crash plans that were *supposed* to work but so often didn't because nobody could stand them for long. Don't expect from this new-think diet a daily program of just what you can and can't eat, do expect to be able to make an intelligent, informal and satisfying choice from a great variety of things that you like to eat.

The same is true with exercise; you have to develop it into a habit, something that you do at fixed times during each week or day, like washing your hair. It need not be any more demanding or exhausting than that.

But before starting to set up your own new individual diet or exercise plan, you have to look at the total picture. Know all the facts. That's the first step in new-think.

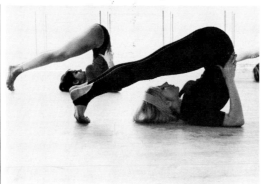

One hour of active exercises burns up 200 calories, but it takes the loss of 3,500 to remove 1 pound.

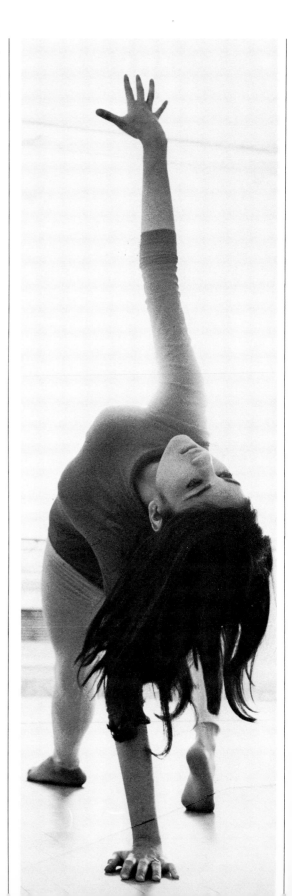

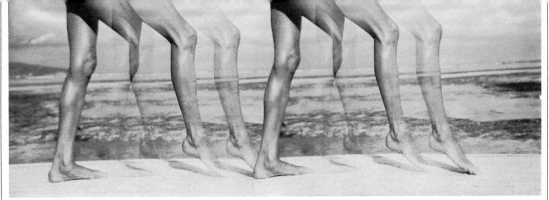

If you walk 1 mile to work or classes every day and 1 mile back, in 35 days you can lose 1 pound—and your appetite will not increase by doing this amount of exercise.

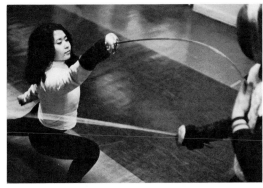

There are only two ways of reducing: either you take in fewer calories or expend more.

That means you eat fewer calories or work more of them off by exercise or some other expenditure of energy. It is theoretically possible to change your weight by exercise, but it is really impractical because it takes too much exercise over too long and steady a period. Besides, the entire framework of our lives makes a loss of weight by exercise too difficult.

But that is not at all to imply that exercise is irrelevant in a body-shaping system. It has to be seen in its proper perspective. For example, if you chopped wood for three hours every day, you would show some appreciable sign of weight loss, but very few people can chop wood three hours every day. And when you think about sports—new-think. You drive to the golf course, and once there you're attended by caddies. Swimming is only of value as exercise the minutes you are swimming, not the rest of the time when you are lying in the sun or, again, driving to the beach. Lying in the sun or motoring, you are using up fewer calories than you would be if you were standing or walking, holding your body upright. When it comes to calisthenics, enough to make any significant weight loss takes too long and is too difficult. Sometimes, too, really strenuous exercise makes you want to eat more. And,

if you are fat, you probably have a tendency to want higher-calorie foods and drinks than other people.

Exercise does, however, have its value. It is necessary for toning up. Muscles are kept tight, and as a result your figure is kept better—but exercise does not tighten skin, or subcutaneous tissue. The cardiovascular system, too, keeps in good tone with a moderate amount of exercise. Actually the exercise of walking can result in the loss of enough calories to count. For instance, if you usually take a bus or subway to the office, you might walk 1 mile of the way instead. That would mean a loss of 50 calories a day, and if you walked 1 mile each way, to and from the office, then 100 calories. If you did this regularly each day, in 35 days you would lose 3,500 calories, which is equal to 1 pound of weight. And—this is important—you could do this with no increase of appetite from the exercise. Actually, if you were to double your walking time, you could double the loss, but that wouldn't be wise psychologically. You would probably give up that much walking. Four miles a day is a lot; it would tire you and wouldn't be practical.

Always keep in sight exactly what exercise does and doesn't do. Dr. Glenn recommends modern dance and fencing because they use most of your muscles and they are done in classes with others, which helps to keep them from becoming lonely and boring; or exercise

classes at your local YWCA or reputable gym. You'll need about 2 45-minute classes a week; and if you're thinking of doing more, it would be better to increase the number of sessions rather than the length. It isn't good to overstrain, either physically or psychologically. Always stop when you feel you could do a little more, then exercise won't seem exhausting. If you think you can make a success of at-home exercises, there's every kind to pick from on pages 208–211. A tip Dr. Glenn offers for doing any at-home exercises is to do them daily and start at an easy level, then build up. If you're touching your toes, begin with only 3 times the first week so you won't feel worn out or stiff, and you'll be *able* to and *want* to do more later.

With any active exercise, 200 calories an hour are lost, but only if you are active all 60 minutes of the hour. To lose 1 pound, which, remember, is 3,500 calories, you would have to do a 1-hour session twice a week for 9 weeks. With that small loss you can see that the basis of any real weight loss has to be diet, not exercise.

New-think dieting means looking at your total weight situation, not just losing pounds but forming a good eating habit you can live with and enjoy all your life. Old-think dieting is taking on a rigid and monotonous deprivation which may accomplish the weight loss you want, but not for long because the diet is too hard to stick with. As Dr.

You are not likely to lose more than
2 pounds a week on an average, but many
lose 3 to 5 in the first week alone.

Morton Glenn pointed out at the beginning of this plan, a good diet is simply an exaggeration of a good eating habit. After you have lost the amount of weight you want to, the way you can maintain it is by dropping the exaggeration and continuing with the good habit.

For women between 18 and 35 years old who are relatively active, a good eating habit is a well-balanced diet stabilized at 2,300 calories daily after they have lost the amount of weight they want. During the weight losing the daily calorie intake should be limited to 1,200. Dr. Glenn's plan is simple: "The highest-calorie main-course portions that most people eat," he said, "are beef, pork and lamb. If you concentrate chiefly on chicken and fish, you'll lose. When you do have beef or lamb, make sure the portions are small and lean. Do you know that 1 pound of porterhouse steak is 1,600 calories while 1 pound of fillet of sole is only 360 and 1 pound of chicken, 380? A 1-ounce meatball of prime-grade beef, the size of a walnut, is up to

100 calories or equivalent to over 5 lumps of sugar in calories." The chart below lists some more pretty dramatic contrasts between low and high calorie foods that will help you learn how to count calories to your advantage. For instance, look at what happens on the chart when you put chicken in a potpie with sauce and pie crust—it zooms up. Keep rich sauces off your meats, poultry and fish. Keep cream out of your soups; instead have light broths. Keep away from the high-calorie snacks; substitute raw carrots, celery, radishes, tomatoes. Switch from regular soft drinks to the low-calorie soda pops. Instead of pies, cake and ice cream for dessert, eat fruits. Start each day's diet with a breakfast with protein in it—an egg or cottage cheese, a slice of dry toast, tea or coffee without sugar or cream, and orange juice. To these diet tips add what you can learn from a simple dieting booklet or pamphlet that has a calorie-counting chart in it. The Metropolitan Life Insurance Company puts out an excellent one, *Four*

Comparative calorie chart for some usual main-course meats, poultry and fish

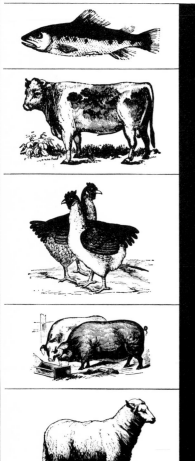

Fish	Bluefish, baked or broiled	3 oz.	135 calories
Shrimp	Fresh	3 oz.	75
Crabmeat	Canned or cooked	3 oz.	90
Beef	Rib roast, cooked without bone	3½ oz.	262
Hamburger	Lean ground, broiled	3 oz.	185
	Market ground, broiled	3 oz.	245
Steak	Sirloin, broiled, lean and fat	3 oz.	330
	Lean only	3 oz.	173
Chicken	Broiled flesh and skin without bone	3 oz.	185
	Breast, fried, with or without bone	½ breast	215
	Potpie, about 4½″ diameter	8 oz.	485
Pork	Roast, oven-cooked, no liquid added		
	Lean and fat	3 oz.	310
	Lean only	2.4 oz.	175
Ham	Smoked, lean and fat	3 oz.	290
Lamb	Chop, broiled, lean and fat	4.8 oz.	405
	Lean only	3 oz.	140
	Leg, roasted, lean and fat	3 oz.	235
	Lean only	3 oz.	130

Steps to Weight Control; so do most state health departments. Almost any library will give you a responsible list of diet books.

But realize that a good diet requires something more than arithmetic.

Just because two foods have the same calorie count they might not have the same nutritional value. An orange has roughly the same number of calories as one bonbon-size piece of chocolate candy, but it is better to eat the orange because it is more nourishing. It is better, too, to substitute watercress or fresh uncooked spinach for lettuce in a salad because both contain more nourishment than lettuce. You'll learn in no time from one of the booklets to distinguish high-nutrition, low-calorie foods.

The next consideration is how much you want to lose.

We've broken the new-think plan into three categories of weight loss —5 pounds and under, 5 to 10 pounds and 10 to 25—so that you can see how long each loss will take and some of the things to expect day by day and week by week as your metabolism adjusts to the dieting. If you are new-thinking about any loss over the 10-pound line, you ought to check in with your doctor first to be sure that you are in good general health. Don't embark on *any* weight loss at all if you are not in good health—unless your doctor advises it.

For anyone confused about the amount of weight she should lose, there are charts in most of the diet pamphlets, but some tend to be a little more generous in their estimates than current fashion is. You may want to weigh a few pounds less than they advise. If you find yourself in the easy 5-pound-and-under bracket, you can probably manage the loss in three weeks. To try to reduce any more rapidly would mean going on an unrealistic diet that would not allow you to live your usual life, and that would be unhealthy. The average loss on this plan is 2 pounds a week. Some women, in fact many, may achieve a loss of 3 to 5 pounds in the first week alone. But that's no signal to stop dieting. The first week is usually associated with water loss of a couple of pounds, which is why you appear to have lost weight when you actually haven't. This happens without the use of diuretic pills. In the third week, however, the body metabolism readjusts and the water you have lost returns. What takes place when you cut down on your food is that you automatically cut down on the salt in your diet—and salt is the thing that controls water retention and loss. You may have heard that just before your menstrual period there is a need to restrict salt in your diet, but there isn't in any of these three weight-loss categories unless you are an excessive salt user (by Dr. Glenn's definition one who salts before she

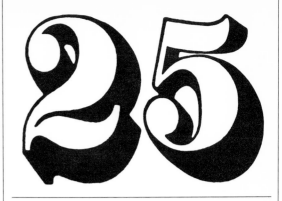

and up to

It will take about 10 weeks to lose 20, about 13 for 25. You'll lose least in the third week—it's quitters' week—but if you get over it, you'll probably stick to your diet.

tastes) or unless you really have a water-retention problem that has been established by your physician.

In the 5- to 10-pound bracket, you are not likely to lose more than 6 pounds in the first 3 weeks, and it will—on the 2-pound-loss-a-week average—take 8 weeks or more to accomplish the 10.

For anyone who needs to lose more than 5 to 10 pounds the diet-

"The biggest problem with all overweight people is that they are self-indulgent instead of self-centered. They have to learn to feed their needs instead of their desires," said Dr. Morton Glenn.

ing method is the same but, of course, concentrated over a longer period of time. To lose 20 pounds will take about 10 weeks, and probably 3 more to achieve the 25-pound reduction. The third week is the week you lose least—the week, too, that water balance restores itself. It is what Dr. Glenn calls quitters' week, but, he said, if you can get through this one, you will probably stick to the diet. The important thing in this group is not to stop before you've reached the definite goal you've set for yourself. To reach a 20- or 25-pound loss takes a whole season of your life. But the real compensation—besides the weight loss itself—is that if you have been able to diet successfully for that length of time, you are well on the way to having established a good eating habit that won't desert you for the rest of your life. That is, after all, the goal of all new-think dieting.

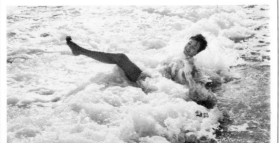

pound loss

You probably won't lose more than 6 in the first 3 weeks—on the average of about 2 a week. It will take about 8 weeks to lose all 10.

The basis of any substantial loss in weight is diet and not exercise.

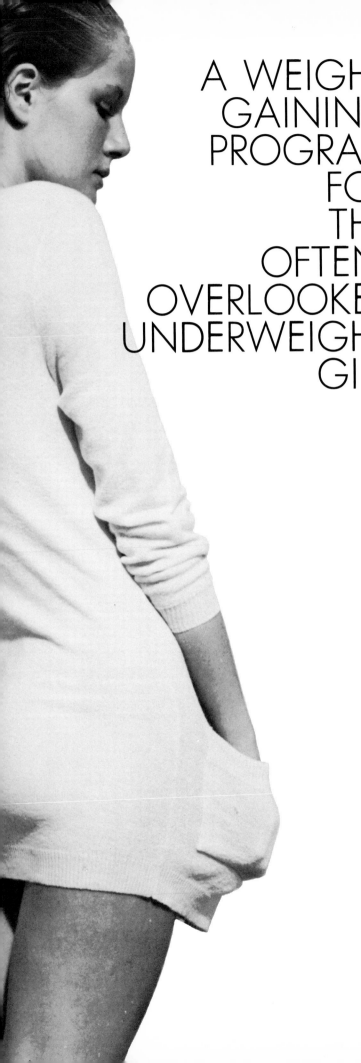

A WEIGHT GAINING PROGRAM FOR THE OFTEN-OVERLOOKED UNDERWEIGHT GIRL

A weight specialist once said that he had never come across anyone in his entire practice who ever thought twice before answering the question "Would you rather be overweight or underweight?" The answer was unthinkingly, instantaneously, unanimously "Underweight." Nevertheless, underweight is a problem. The far fewer number of underweights than overweights in our population, plus their greater social acceptability and our ideal of a slender figure, obscure the fact that trying to gain when you're too "skinny" takes as much effort and willpower as trying to lose.

If you weigh 10 percent or more under the ideal on weight charts, or if you look in the mirror and see no curves, only skin and bones, you're probably in need of a diet, a weight-gaining one.

First step is telephoning your family doctor for an appointment. Underweight is associated with poor health, so the importance of that first step cannot be emphasized enough.

If a thorough medical reveals no body mal- or misfunctioning, your doctor will probably put you on a high-calorie diet. You are too thin because you take in fewer calories than your body needs to maintain your desired weight.

There may be, and probably are, underlying reasons for this. You tend to lose your appetite under tension (unlike the fat girl who eats under tension), and you often skip meals. In case histories, one underweight girl disliked just about everything on anyone's menu and another had unpleasant memories associated with food. Some skinnies don't really want to start gaining because they're afraid of fat.

Whatever the reason for your too-bony frame, you've made up your mind that it's time to gain a few pounds. Muster your willpower and set yourself on a determined regimen.

First, make a decision to never, repeat—never, skip a meal. Three meals a day, twenty-one meals a week, are a must. Learn something about calories, too, and which foods have the most. Since one of your problems is getting food down, the best trick is to make sure you get the maximum number of calories per bite.

Plan each meal as you normally would but include high-calorie rather than low-calorie foods. Dr. Morton B. Glenn, an internist specializing in weight control and nutrition, suggests that you plan to have either beef, pork or lamb at every meal. Protein is the mainstay of any diet and should be the main course of any meal and these are the proteins with the most calories attached. Add a soup, vegetables, dessert, whatever—but make sure each item is high-calorie rather than low. As Dr. Glenn said, it's ridiculous for the underweight person to waste her appetite munching celery.

The thing to remember about snacks is that they must not interfere with those carefully planned, calorie-laden three meals per day you've already determined to get down. Better to skip the gooey four o'clock sundae than to have no appetite for dinner at seven. And, if you can get a snack down too, do. But be sure it is a high-calorie one.

One common mistake for the weight-gainer is trying to increase the amount of food she eats to the highest possible point the very first day. This is likely to prove so difficult and really sickening that she'll give up immediately.

Don't worry about eating great quantities. Eat the same amount but more calories; gradually increase portions.

You probably won't have to actually count calories. Dr. Glenn has found that people do much better when they think about types of food rather than the exact number of calories they are consuming daily. But if counting is easier for you, you can determine, with the help of your doctor or from charts predicting daily calorie needs, how many you'll need. For example, a moderately active twenty-five-year-old girl, five feet five inches tall, needs 2200 calories each day to maintain her desired weight. By adding 500 to that she'll gain.

If you do count calories, learn something about food and good eating habits, too, so that six months or a year from now you won't have to start all over again after losing what you gained. Dieting "is simply an exaggeration of a good eating habit. At the end of the diet you . . . drop the exaggeration and are left with the good habit which can last for life. . . ."

If you've been underweight for long, you undoubtedly know that appetite stimulants exist and that some perfectly reputable doctors use them. Dr. Glenn, while recognizing their possible value in special cases, does not recommend their use by the average dieter. Medical research has not proven that they really do increase one's desire for food. Their apparent effect may be all psychological. At best they are a crutch that you're going to have to drop sometime; then you'll have to develop a good eating habit anyway if you have any hope of maintaining your proper weight.

Unfortunately, there is no known way to direct newly acquired pounds to specific areas. You're more or less stuck with the basic shape you inherited. But exercise can help you control the size of certain parts of your body. Exercise tightens and strengthens muscles and a moderate amount of it is required for good health. It can help the weight-gainer in two ways: first by increasing the size of particular muscles—in the arms or legs, for instance—and second by increasing your appetite. Don't overdo it, though, so that you either become too tired to eat or use up all the extra calories you've managed to get down.

Be sure, too, to get the proper amount of sleep and try to gain control over that tension that made you lose your appetite in the first place. Let this be your last resolution to shape up.

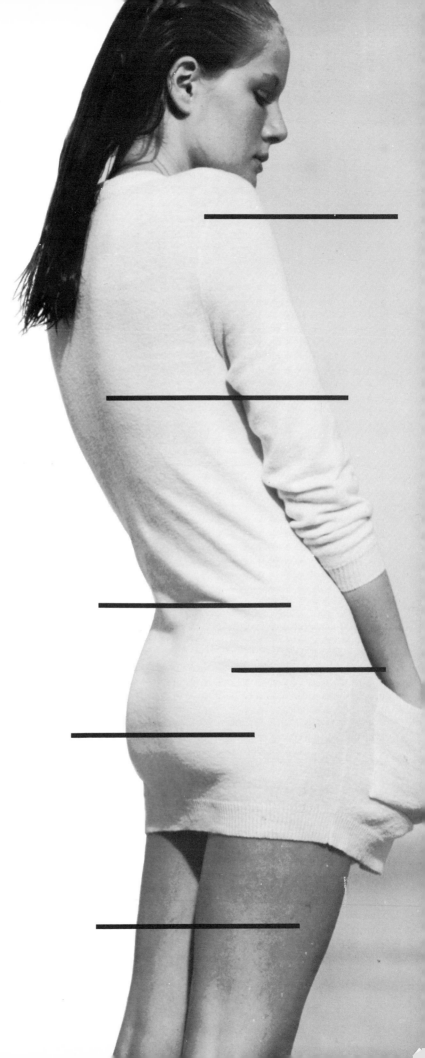

COUNTING YOUR CALORIES

Take this quiz to see how well up you are on calories. In each pair of foods, check the one with the *lower* calorie count:

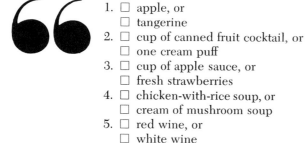

1. ☐ apple, or
   ☐ tangerine
2. ☐ cup of canned fruit cocktail, or
   ☐ one cream puff
3. ☐ cup of apple sauce, or
   ☐ fresh strawberries
4. ☐ chicken-with-rice soup, or
   ☐ cream of mushroom soup
5. ☐ red wine, or
   ☐ white wine
6. ☐ five dried prunes, or
   ☐ one peach
7. ☐ slice of white bread, or
   ☐ slice French bread
8. ☐ swordfish steak, or
   ☐ codfish steak
9. ☐ gin-and-tonic, or
   ☐ Tom Collins
10. ☐ beef tongue, or
    ☐ roast beef
11. ☐ one pretzel, or
    ☐ three double Ry-Krisp crackers
12. ☐ broiled salmon, or
    ☐ broiled flounder
13. ☐ ladyfinger, or
    ☐ slice of gingerbread
14. ☐ Camembert cheese, or
    ☐ Roquefort cheese
15. ☐ fig newton, or
    ☐ brownie
16. ☐ big porterhouse steak, or
    ☐ two strips of bacon
17. ☐ *caffè espresso*, or
    ☐ *café au lait*
18. ☐ one anchovy, or
    ☐ one shrimp

19. ☐ cup of corn, or
    ☐ ear of corn
20. ☐ big dish of squash, or
    ☐ baked sweet potato
21. ☐ crackerful of black caviar, or
    ☐ two green olives
22. ☐ two cucumbers, or
    ☐ large dish of green peas
23. ☐ pear-half sprinkled with cinnamon, or
    ☐ fresh banana
24. ☐ medium-sized baked potato, or
    ☐ small dish of lima beans
25. ☐ sour cream, or
    ☐ sweet cream
26. ☐ big slice of watermelon, or
    ☐ half a cantaloupe
27. ☐ cream cheese, or
    ☐ pot cheese
28. ☐ nectarine, or
    ☐ apricot
29. ☐ one fresh fig, or
    ☐ medium bunch of Concord grapes
30. ☐ tomato juice, or
    ☐ lemonade
31. ☐ one serving of chipped beef, or
    ☐ slice of pizza
32. ☐ custard cream pie, or
    ☐ apricot pie
33. ☐ one Danish pastry, or
    ☐ dish of frozen custard
34. ☐ cheese soufflé, or
    ☐ omelette
35. ☐ one popover, or
    ☐ small piece of pound cake

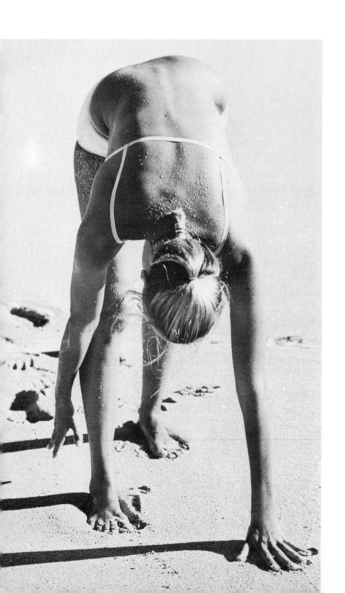

Answers to the calorie countdown

(Give yourself one point for each correct answer.)

1. A tangerine has 35; an apple, 75.
2. Surprise! A cream puff has 125 calories. A cup of canned fruit cocktail has 175.
3. A cup of fresh strawberries has 55 calories; a cup of apple-sauce, 185.
4. A bowl of chicken-with-rice soup has 100 calories. Cream of mushroom soup, 183.
5. Most red wines have 73 calories a glass. White wines are usually less dry; average glass, 85 calories.
6. A large peach contains 46 calories. Five dried prunes, 120.
7. A slice of French bread has 54 calories. A slice of white bread, 65.
8. An average-sized codfish steak has 100 calories to swordfish steak's 223.
9. A gin-and-tonic, 75; Tom Collins, 180.
10. Three slices of beef tongue have 160 calories. Three slices of roast beef, 287.
11. Three double Ry-Krisp crackers, 63; a pretzel, 72.
12. A serving of broiled flounder has only 80 calories; broiled salmon, 204.
13. A ladyfinger has fewer calories (37) than a slice of gingerbread (180).
14. An ounce of Camembert cheese has 85 calories; an ounce of Roquefort, 111.
15. A fig newton is a lower-calorie snack (56) than a brownie (141).
16. Two strips of bacon have 95 calories; a big porterhouse steak has 513.
17. You can sip *caffé espresso* without counting calories. It hasn't any. *Café au lait* (half strong coffee, half milk) has 40 per cup.
18. A shrimp has 2, an anchovy, 10.
19. An ear of corn, 50; a cupful, 170.
20. A big helping of squash has 36 calories; a baked sweet potato has 185.
21. Two green olives have 14 calories. A crackerful of black caviar, 35.
22. Two cucumbers add up to a cool 50; a big serving of green peas, 110.
23. A pear-half sprinkled with cinnamon has 47; a banana, 88.
24. A medium-sized baked potato (no butter) has 95. A small dish of lima beans, 100.
25. Surprise again—one tablespoon of sweet cream has 50 calories to sour cream's 58.
26. Half a cantaloupe has 35 calories. A big slice of watermelon has 120.
27. An ounce of pot cheese has 14; an ounce of cream cheese, 105.
28. An apricot, 18; a nectarine, 38.
29. A fresh fig has 30 calories; a medium bunch of Concord grapes, 55.
30. Tomato juice (50 per glass) has half as many calories as lemonade.
31. A serving of creamed chipped beef, 175 calories; a slice of pizza pie, 245.
32. A slice of custard cream pie has 265; a slice of apricot pie, 328.
33. A dish of frozen custard has 150 calories; a Danish pastry has 200.
34. An omelette, 106; cheese soufflé, 280.
35. A popover has 60 calories; a small piece of pound cake, 130.

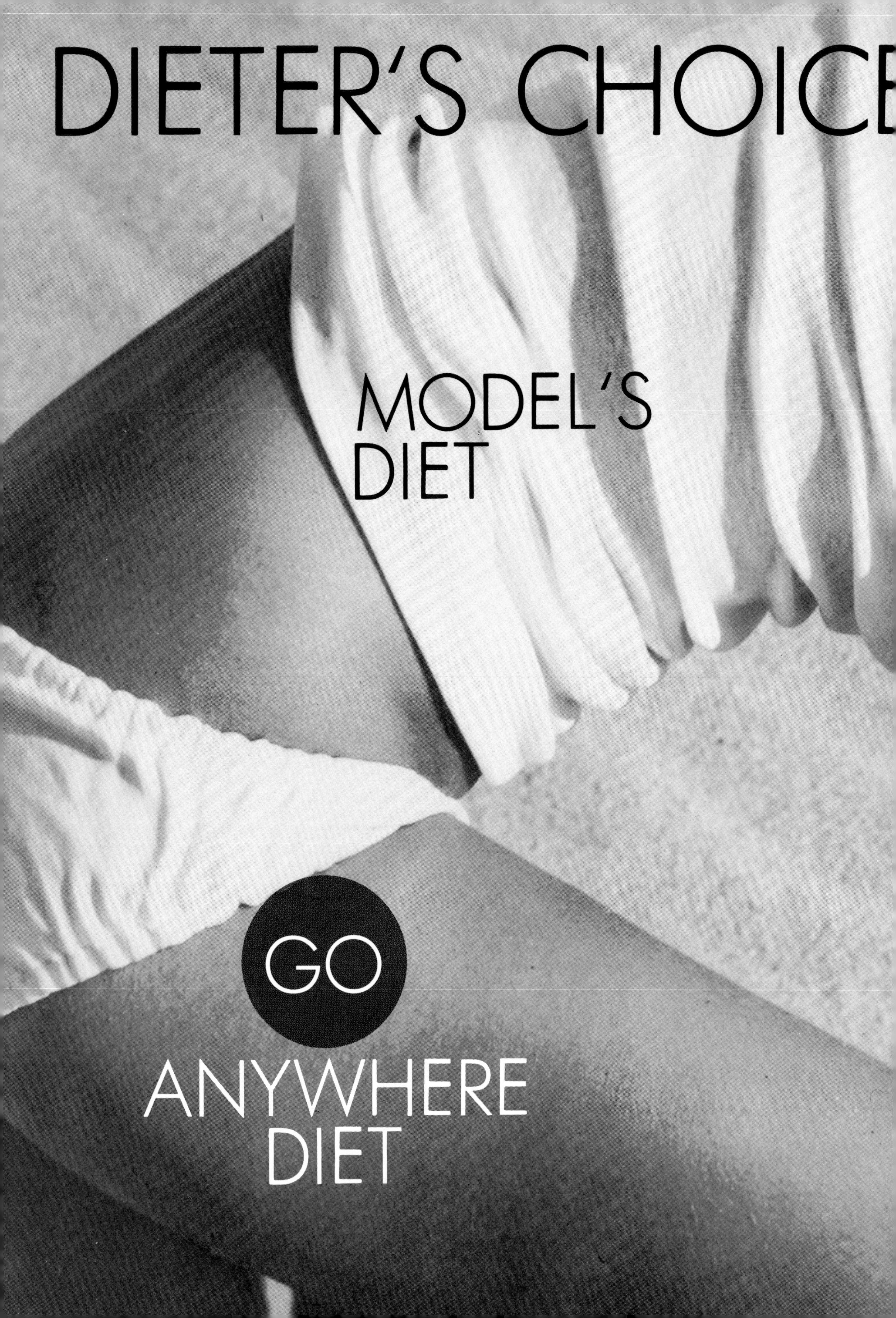

DIETER'S CHOICE

MODEL'S
DIET

GO
ANYWHERE
DIET

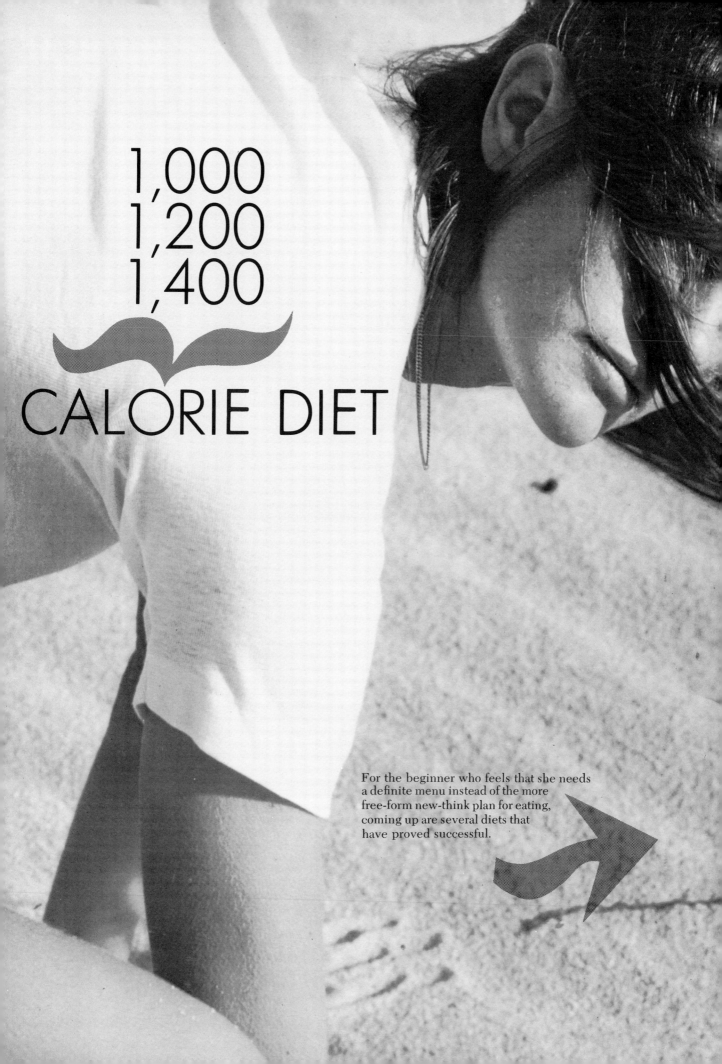

1,000
1,200
1,400

CALORIE DIET

For the beginner who feels that she needs a definite menu instead of the more free-form new-think plan for eating, coming up are several diets that have proved successful.

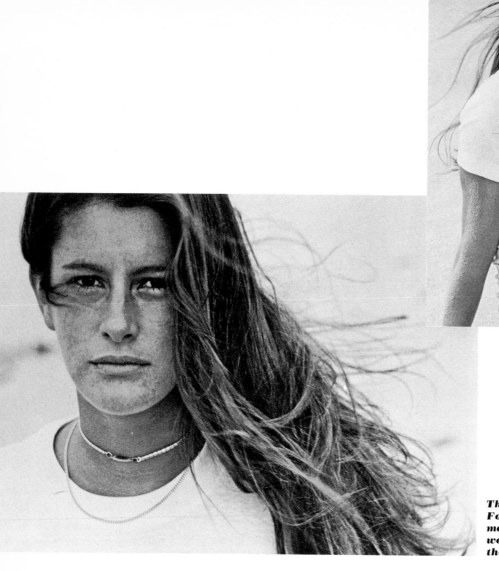

This is the regimen that Eileen Ford, head of one of the most famous modeling agencies in the world, puts her girls on when they need to lose weight.

THE MODEL'S DIET

breakfast	lunch	dinner	snacks
Either: *Grapefruit juice, grape-fruit half, cantaloupe half, or a medium piece of watermelon* *One or two boiled or poached eggs* *Black coffee (with artificial sweetener)*	*Either:* *Broiled hamburger or hard-boiled eggs* *Raw tomato and raw carrot*	*Either: Tomato, vegetable, or grapefruit juice* *Either: Broiled lamb chop, steak, chicken, fish, or chopped beef; or roast lamb, beef or chicken* *Either: Spinach, string beans or tomatoes* *Lettuce with lemon juice or vinegar and vegetable oil* *Grapefruit half* *Black coffee*	*Hard-boiled eggs* *Carrot sticks* *Tomatoes* *Celery* *Cucumbers* *Skim milk* *Fruit juice* *Vegetable juice*

1,000-CALORIE DIET

Breakfast
Unsweetened fruit or juice, ½ cup
1 egg
1 slice whole-wheat or enriched white bread, no butter
½ cup skim milk
Coffee or tea, no sugar

Lunch
Meat, fish, chicken or cheese, 3 oz.
1 portion green salad
1 portion leafy green or yellow vegetable
1 slice whole-wheat or enriched white bread, no butter
1 portion unsweetened fruit
½ cup skim milk
Coffee or tea, no sugar

Dinner
Meat, fish, chicken or cheese, 3 oz.
1 portion green salad or vegetable juice
1 slice whole-wheat or enriched white bread, no butter
1 cup skim milk
Coffee or tea, no sugar

1,200-CALORIE DIET

Same as 1,000-calorie diet except ½ cup whole milk is substituted for skim milk at lunch; 1 cup whole milk for 1 cup skim milk at dinner. Also at dinner, add 1 portion unsweetened fruit. A sample 1,200-calorie menu:

Breakfast
Grapefruit juice, ½ cup
1 poached egg
1 slice whole-wheat toast, no butter
½ cup skim milk
Coffee or tea, no sugar

Lunch
Broiled flounder, 2 oz., with lemon wedge
Asparagus tips on lettuce with pimiento garnish
½ cup beets
1 slice whole-wheat bread, no butter
1 fresh peach
½ cup whole milk
Coffee or tea, no sugar

Dinner
2 rib lamb chops
1 portion green salad
½ cup baked acorn squash
1 slice whole-wheat bread, no butter
½ cup apple sauce (unsweetened)
1 cup whole milk
Coffee or tea, no sugar

1,200 is the usual amount of calories set by doctors but you can hurry pounds off with the more stringent 1,000 menu or lose more slowly with the more generous diet of 1,400.

1,400-CALORIE DIET

Breakfast
Unsweetened fruit or juice, 1 portion
1 egg
1 slice whole-wheat or enriched white bread
1 pat butter or fortified margarine
½ cup milk
Coffee or tea, no sugar

Lunch
Lean meat, fish, chicken or cheese, 3 oz.
1 portion green or yellow vegetable
—or 1 portion salad, such as 2 oz. tuna fish, 1 hard-cooked egg, lettuce and tomato
1 slice whole-wheat or enriched white bread
1 pat butter or fortified margarine
1 portion unsweetened fruit
½ cup milk
Coffee or tea, no sugar

Dinner
Lean meat, fish, chicken or cheese, 3 oz.
1 portion green salad
1 portion vegetable
1 slice butter or fortified margarine
1 portion unsweetened fruit
1 cup milk
Coffee or tea, no sugar

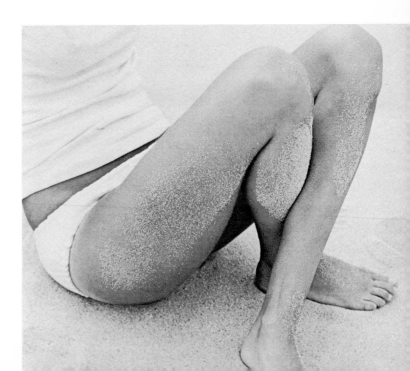

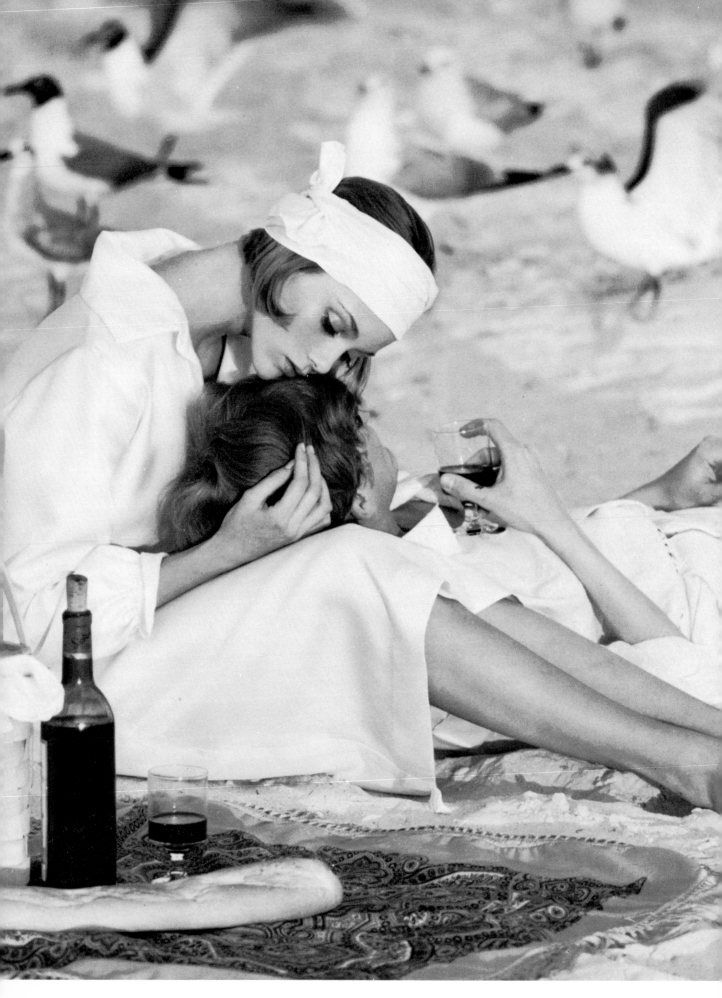

HOW TO
DIET
ANYWHERE
YOU GO

by Dr. Morton B. Glenn

You can diet in any situation, even when you misinterpret a menu and get a totally unexpected food. Leave your food scale, as well as your measuring cup, at home, but take these basic principles and suggestions away with you. They are all based on actual experiences of mine and of my patients who have traveled extensively. They worked for them, and they can work for you.

For most of us, the morning is the easiest time to control appetites. As the day progresses, watching your diet becomes increasingly more difficult. There are reasons for this. Usually you have more time on your hands in the evening, and what better way to fill this time than with food.

It is a very common practice to compensate for fatigue by eating. But most of all the problem is one of HIDDEN HUNGER. In most people, the blood sugar level begins to fall about four hours after eating.

The stomach is also quite empty by then. If you are preoccupied with whatever you are doing, you may pay little attention to this hunger. Later, when you become so hungry that you can't ignore it, it is difficult to control your appetite. The answer is to prevent the development of this hidden hunger.

Prevention must start early in the morning. If you eat breakfast, lunch about four hours later, and then have an afternoon snack if necessary, you will reach the difficult time of the day without excessive hunger. I am always asked by a new patient whether it might not be better to cut down on calories by skipping breakfast and even scrimping on lunch

if possible. My answer is that most people with a weight problem will eat more calories in the evening because of hidden hunger than they will save during the day.

Do not skip breakfast or lunch. Eating then will mean less eating later, and fewer calories in all.

A continental breakfast is quite different from the typical American breakfast. You can, of course, order orange juice and eggs, but be prepared to pay for them. The usual continental breakfast is rolls or bread with butter, coffee and hot milk and perhaps jam or marmalade—sometimes juice.

In France and Italy the continental breakfast is often included in the price of the room, and it is pleasant to have it served there. At breakfast, the best appetite control is achieved by eating protein, and in most of Europe cheese is the best source. The simplest, pleasantest and most economical solution to the problem is to shop for local cheeses yourself (and it's fun to try the specialties of each country). Order your continental breakfast and substitute cheese for the butter and jam. Do eat bread— one slice is enough—or a croissant. If it's your first trip to Europe, you may be surprised by the taste of the coffee. In France and Italy it's dark and strong, in England it's likely to be made with chicory, and many Americans have difficulty getting used to it. Tea is readily available; or you can take along your favorite brand of instant coffee and order hot water.

The most important single thing that you can do to maintain weight control is to choose the proper main courses.

You don't have to gain weight while traveling, and you can even lose. There is no need to let a trip ruin your figure, and there is absolutely no need to let a diet ruin your trip.

The lowest-calorie main courses are fish and poultry; the highest are beef, lamb, and especially pork. Be an explorer with fish and poultry dishes wherever you go.

Compare fish dishes all over the U.S.—each section has its own. The French, Spanish, and Italians do wonderful things with chicken and fish—they are much more available in the Latin countries than red meat. When you think that half a pound of filet of sole has less than two hundred calories, it is worth trying, isn't it? Of course, sauce does add calories, but if you have only enough to season, you will still be ahead on calorie count.

European beef and lamb have fewer calories than their American counterparts because European animals are considerably leaner. But this results in a less tasty meal, which is one reason rich sauces are used so often in Europe. If you do want meat, order veal as often as possible. It is lowest in calories of the meats.

Next to your choice of main courses, portion control is probably the most important part of calorie control. As a rule, portion servings in Europe are small, and if you learn to be satisfied with the small portion, you will have a built-in safety check on your eating habits. Traveling in the U.S., don't eat all of everything on your plate. If you are determined enough to choose a low-calorie food, it is ridiculous to turn it into a high-calorie food by having a portion that is too large. "Just this once" is the beginning of total defeat for the dieter.

Multiple-course meals can mean a large caloric intake unless you're careful. *Keep the portions small*, and don't be a plate-cleaner. Taste everything—you don't have to forego the great restaurants which are one of the great pleasures of travel—but leave some food on the plate. Explore new and different foods, but watch those portions.

In Europe you may become involved in unusual eating schedules. In Madrid, don't be surprised if you have dinner between 10 and 11 P.M. Of course, you *can* eat at 9—but you might be dining alone.

If you plan to follow local custom and wait a long time between meals, protect yourself from going overboard at the next meal by drinking tea or coffee and eating fresh fruit (sold everywhere throughout Europe in shops, on the street, at railroad stations and stops). In order to avoid long delays in eating while you are traveling, as soon as possible after boarding a train make a reservation in a dining car. It is the custom. Try not to skip meals, and never double up on a meal because you haven't eaten in a long time.

There is another custom that can trap the dieter: the long nonworking lunch hour. The longer you stay, the more you're tempted to eat. And in Europe the waiters don't hurry you; it is usually the Americans who rush the waiters.

I will never forget going to a restaurant in Copenhagen that is famous for its sandwiches. We had nothing but sandwiches and were still waiting for the check three hours after we arrived. When we left the restaurant, we saw a man eating a frankfurter (without the roll) as he walked along, and immediately thereafter we saw a young woman doing the very same thing as she rode on her bicycle. We assumed that this was their protection against the three-hour lunch.

Many Europeans have their large meal at midday, and you may be tempted to do the same. This is fine if you then have a light evening meal. But you will probably still want your large meal in the evening, and if you have *two* large meals, the outcome will be disaster! Force yourself, even if a large lunch is included in a tour price, to have a light one. American-style snack bars are cropping up in many parts of Europe. If you prefer local food, I suggest an omelette, particularly all over France, and seafood in the Scandinavian countries. If you like yoghurt, it's available on many menus and is especially good in Greece and Turkey. However, one of the great ways to have lunch in Europe is to go native: Buy the ingredients in a grocery store. But shop before noon, because in the warmer countries shops close at noon for a few hours. Cheese and bread are excellent and quite inexpensive. In France add jambon de Parme, a delicious lean, smoked ham, and a bunch of grapes for a festive picnic lunch. A delightful lunch in Greece is a large green salad with feta cheese. It is also one of infinite variety, since no two Greeks make a salad the same way.

The sour rye of Germany, the dark breads of Eastern Europe, the brioche and croissants of France and the shortbread of Scotland—taste them all, but don't stuff yourself. Restrict yourself to one slice of bread or half a roll at breakfast and again at lunch, but don't touch bread at dinner. And give your pat of butter to a thin friend. When it comes to Italian pasta, eat it as a bread substitute at lunch—or as a meal if it contains meat or fish—but eat only half a portion. And be stingy with the grated cheese.

Be aware of how food is cooked. The French use butter, the Italians olive oil, the Germans lard, etc. There is nothing you can do about the cooking procedure, but you can order those foods that are least likely to require fats and oils in their preparation.

A corner bakery or a dessert table laden with

pastry can sorely tempt anyone whose salivary glands are in good working order. Choose fruit instead. If you don't have a single pastry on your trip, your fun will really not be curtailed one bit. Every restaurant serves fruit. The red oranges of southern Italy are great, the melon in Spain fabulous, and the fraises des bois (wild strawberries) of France have no equal. For variety, try a meal without dessert once in a while.

If you happen to have the opportunity to eat at one of the famous restaurants here or abroad, it can be an unforgettable experience. This is the one circumstance in which I would find it perfectly understandable if you went off your diet. Let the maitre d'hotel guide you in your selection. Try a new food even if it does look fattening, but don't relax portion control. Whenever one talks about great restaurants, it is natural to talk about wines. You can have some alcoholic beverages without losing ground in your diet. The best rule is to restrict yourself to less than seven drinks per week, whether they be wine, champagne, Danish beer (and every country has its characteristic beer) or brandy. It really doesn't matter what kind of wine you drink, but do avoid the sweet ones. If you are sensible about your eating and stay under seven drinks per week—even if you have three at one sitting—you should have no weight-gain problem. But save the drinks for the special meals and the special social events. And never, never eat less food in order to drink more.

The "tired-feet problem" is one which can plague the dieter. Every day traveling, you will walk and walk and walk. Between car rides, bus stops, plane hops and boat trips you will walk—and walk! Then you will probably sink into a chair at the nearest café, preferably outdoors. And obviously you just can't sit at a café without ordering something. If you are tempted to combat your fatigue with food—STOP! At a time like this have a cold diet drink or coffee or tea without cream or sugar. If diet drinks are not available, one of the best things to order in Europe is fresh lemon juice and water, a refreshing drink frequently ordered by Europeans. Carry a liquid sugar substitute in your bag at all times and make a lemonade. Or order a small bottle of mineral water—Vichy or Perrier in France, or San Pellegrino in Italy.

Traveling invariably requires a certain amount of eating while you're in transit. Airplane travel of any great distance almost always includes one major and often one minor meal. The saving grace of airline meals is that the portions on the tray are small. However, the balance is good, and you are never hungry after eating. With the portion con-

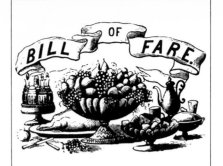

There are three dangers among European foods: bread, pasta, dessert.

trol built in, all you have to do is avoid the potatoes and pass up the dessert (which is usually quite rich). Some flights, however, can be so brief that often there is no time for more than coffee. Don't eat the accompanying pastry or snacks. Most trains that cover long runs have dining cars with reasonably good food choices, and this should produce no problem. But if you are traveling by ship, difficulties can arise. There is a tendency for ship lines to keep their passengers constantly busy eating. But they have one "weight saving" custom: bouillon is readily available. Drink it whenever you're hungry, and when the "fourth meal" is being served, just remember how you want to look on your night of arrival.

It would be unfair not to discuss the greatest eating disaster that can befall the European traveler—although it has little to do with dieting. It happens mostly in restaurants where you are doing your best to speak the language as a native. After you order and are feeling quite pleased with yourself, it happens! The main course that you thought was chicken turns out to be octopus. Of course, you can insist that everyone at the table taste your dish and get rid of most of it this way, or you can try it. You may find that you like it. (Octopus, incidentally, is high in protein and low in calories, and Greeks and Italians consider it a great delicacy.) But if it's still a little more than you're able to cope with, settle for a slowly eaten roll—this is the time to make an exception to the "never eat bread at dinner" rule.

Enjoy. Enjoy eating everywhere. Do not let calorie-guilt lessen the fun of your vacation, but do follow the positive rules about your dieting. If you are willing to pay the same attention to your eating as you do to your grooming, you too can be one of those well-turned-out, slim Americans enjoying all the world has to offer.

In Madrid, don't be surprised if you have dinner between 10 and 11 P.M. Of course, you *can* eat at 9—but you might be dining alone.

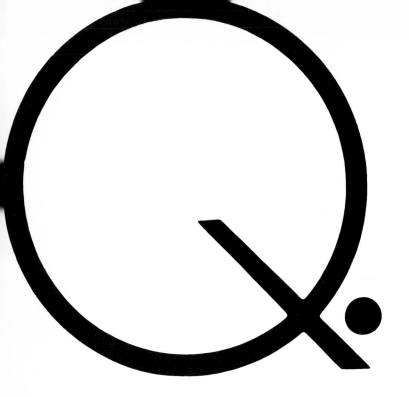

QUESTIONS YOU MIGHT HAVE ABOUT DIETING

(Answered by
a panel
of doctors,
weight experts
and beauty
editors)

Why are you eating more?

Overweight is a personal problem. The causes are personal. The incentives to solve it are personal. The difficulties in losing weight are perhaps the most personal of all.

If you are overweight, you probably know it. Facing the fact is the first step. And it may be the only one needed before you start in with determination on a weight-losing regimen. But this is rarely the case. If just deciding to diet and then

doing it were so easy, you wouldn't be overweight right now. Usually there is an additional step, a hard one to take: finding out why you're overweight.

The physical (or metabolic) reason is simple. Your intake of calories is greater than your expenditure of them, and those that aren't used up are stored as fat.

This happens, of course, when you increase the amount of food—or certain kinds of food—that you eat and do not compensate for the difference through exercise. But it also happens if you decrease your exercise while your eating habits stay the same. And this is so often the sudden and unexpected plight of young women in their late teens or early twenties who have just passed from the hyperactive stage of adolescence into a less-active college or married-life routine.

Why are you eating more? Why are you exercising less? Our modern way of life is at fault to a great extent.

We ride when we should walk; we eat because food is so available. Often, we overwork, and eat to "keep going"; we undersleep, and eat to compensate for fatigue.

Dr. Raymond Ellis Dietz, a physician who specializes in the treatment of obesity, feels that a lot of the problem can be traced to what we now consider a normal way of life: bulk buying at the supermarket and the filled-to-capacity home freezer. Do you still have to walk a few blocks to buy an ice cream cone?

Dr. Ervin Barr, another obesity specialist, calls it "civilizationitis," which he lists, along with metabolic and psychological factors, as one of the basic causes for our overweight population. (Both doctors are members of the American Society of Bariatrics, a group of physicians who either specialize in or limit their practice to treatment of obesity and demand strict standards of treatment.)

Your parents may be a big part of your problem. Dr. Dietz maintains that in families where one parent is obese, 60 percent of the children will be; where both parents are, 88 percent. It's usually a matter of environment, of family eating habits that are hard to break, even when you become an adult.

Parents can be at fault in another way. If they feel inadequate in their role, or feel guilt because they're not playing it properly, they may ply their children with food instead of love, understanding, advice and guidance. Not only a bad emotional pattern but a bad eating pattern is established.

Now that we've let you blame society, and perhaps your parents, for those extra pounds, it's time for you to assume some of it. Why have you let yourself stay overweight?

It may be simple ignorance of what and when you should eat. In that case, your doctor will usually give you a basic, balanced weight-losing diet or you can follow the New-Think method on page 172.

But usually the whys are more complicated. Take another good long look at yourself in the mirror and scrutinize yourself from top (is your hair unwashed and uncombed?) to bottom (are your heels run down?). Overweight and bad personal habits usually form a vicious circle. The fatter we get, the more careless our other personal habits become—and around we go until we've gained a few more pounds, our posture sags, our depression grows and we've gained still more pounds.

But the circle can be broken and it's usually broken with pride.

Start with the simpler things—your hair, your posture, your clothes, your general grooming. Try to boost your morale even before you start dieting. Stand tall. Those excess pounds won't look as bad upright.

Now begin your diet, definitely under a doctor's supervision if your goal is ten pounds or more. It sounds easy, but we know it isn't. You'll probably be off to a soaring start; however, there are, unfortunately, often many psychological factors involved in overweight, factors that can slow down your best efforts. Understanding them can be a painful process, but understanding is about the only way to conquer them.

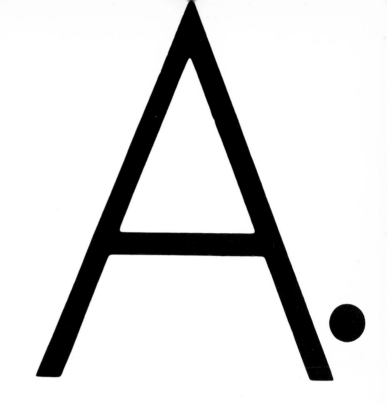

Have you an overweight problem that's psychological?

Most are, in varying degrees, and here's what can be done about them.

Case A, as far back as she could remember, has heard her mother talking about the difficulties of childbirth. We can't go into her mother's hang-up, though it's serious enough; the point is: What did it do to A? It made her become grossly overweight. She hid from the attention of boys and soon found that the safest hiding place was behind a barricade of fat—chiefly because A was deathly afraid of marriage and pregnancy. But when her doctor first asked her why she couldn't lose weight, she didn't know.

Case B's mother and father divorced, and B married a few years afterwards. She loved her husband, and they were, on the surface, quite happy. But growing inside of B was the gnawing fear that her marriage, too, would end on the rocks. So she, too, retreated from life to inside the refrigerator. In her longing for security, she went "back to the baby bottle."

C was going to be married, and she was about ten pounds overweight—and since she was just five feet tall, those ten pounds really showed. She had, incidentally, been overweight since early adolescence, and no one, neither her parents nor her family doctor, had taken her in hand. ("It's only baby fat—she'll outgrow it," was the familiar excuse.) But C wanted desperately to be a slim bride, so she went to a specialist and followed his instructions to the letter. She made it—to the pound—two days before her wedding day. But her fiancé made it, too—to parts unknown, on the wedding eve. C gained back all the weight she had lost, with dividends.

D wanted to have a baby but learned she couldn't. She balked at suggestions of adoption. Within a matter of months she gained twenty pounds. To her, food was, of course, a solace, but the psychological reason went deeper. Under the patient guidance of her doctor, she realized she was gaining weight to simulate the appearance of pregnancy.

Let's look at one more case: This girl was married to a young and attractive doctor who had just started his private practice after years of study and internship during which she was his morale as well as financial booster. Suddenly, he didn't need her as much, at least not in the tangible ways she was used to. Also, his hours away from her had to increase—hours at his office, the hospital, professional meetings. She retreated into a little private fantasy world of neglect and rejection. Her new companion was food.

As Dr. Leonid Kotkin, author of *Eat, Think and Be Slender*, explained, "In normal people, hunger means a need for food. In fat people, hunger implies more than food alone. It is a hunger for security, a hunger for affection, a hunger for power, a hunger for happiness."

Whether it is nagging parents, fear of poor grades, an unhappy romance, fear of men, frustration in marriage, sex or job, an inadequacy complex, or any one of many other problems that plague people during their lives, eating can often give them relief from it.

Dr. Raymond Ellis Dietz, a bariatrician (the name coined for obesity specialists), feels that compulsive eating, even compulsive eating that begins in adulthood, can usually be traced to childhood—to rejection, to unstable and tense home atmospheres, to loneliness, to the sense of not measuring up to the mark.

It's hard to outgrow those feelings; they usually grow more deeply into us. Then obesity, as Dr. Dietz puts it, "may become a shield to ward off men's advances, a retreat to avoid competition or an expression of self-punishment or hostility."

"Knowledge," wrote Kotkin, "is not sufficient without understanding." You know why you should lose weight—the social reasons, the health reasons—but do you understand why you haven't? Try a moderate dose of introspection and a big dose of honesty.

Here's what you'll probably discover: The reasons you're carrying those excess pounds will lead you to the reasons why you want to lose them. You just reverse a negative reaction to life to a positive motivation to enjoy it. Try it: You're overweight because you feel insecure; you want to lose weight to feel secure. You feel neglected; you want to lose weight to gain attention. Fear does add another complication, i.e., you're afraid to lose weight because then you'll be expected to compete on a normal level. But, remember, you will lose weight gradually, giving your self-confidence time to grow to the point where you'll want to be noticed—as your figure shrinks to the point where you'll want to be noticed—as your figure shrinks to the point where you will be. Try spelling out your goal, not in terms of pounds but in terms of pleasure, happiness, all the rest of your life.

You may need help. Lots of people do. But you have to find the right person to help you, and it's probably not your parents or your husband. Most likely they're too involved in your problem to see it clearly. Also, they may not want to; the searchlight might reflect back on them. A doctor is usually the answer, a doctor who will take time to help you understand your problem not just hand you a printed diet and give you the canned pep talk about self-discipline. In some cases, psychiatric help is needed; it's supportive therapy.

As bariatrician Ervin Barr points out, "Dieting has to be planned. There's a part of you that wants to be fat—your feelings—and a part that wants to be thin—your brain. So you have to plan your diet within rigid boundaries. Leave nothing to spur-of-the-moment decisions, leave nothing to chance. Then when your pride is in the forefront, when self-denial becomes a greater pleasure than self-gratification, you have it made."

What is the advantage of a high-protein diet?

Protein has higher "staying" power than carbohydrate and holds off hunger pangs a little longer. Fat has the highest staying power, but it's loaded with calories and is also a potential danger to our circulatory systems. Protein causes the greatest rise in metabolism, which means the expenditure of caloric energy, or "burning up fat." And protein foods generally contain less calories in the first place.

So, the core of your high-protein diet should be meat, fish, poultry, eggs, cottage cheese and skimmed milk. Round it out with vegetables (but skip the starchy ones) and fresh fruit. Because of the chemical interactions in the body, it's also necessary to include fat. However, cut down drastically on the amount that you eat consciously. The fat you eat unconsciously (look again at that carefully trimmed steak) is probably more than adequate. Doctors also advise eating some carbohydrate (starches and sugars), again for reasons of chemical balance. But they emphasize that only minimal amounts are necessary.

Does the timing really affect dieting?

There are sound reasons behind the three-meals-a-day adage. One is chemical: spreading meals over the day keeps the metabolism elevated. The other is very human: if you skip breakfast, you'll be so hungry that you'll either compensate at lunch or resort to a midmorning snack—and it won't be a carrot stick.

Snacks, of the right variety, are in fact an important part of a sustainable diet. Doctors realize that when you're hungry you're unhappy; that the unhappier you get the more you'll think about food; and the more you think about food the greater chance that you'll eat something you shouldn't. So keep your refrigerator full of celery, carrots, radishes and fruit juice; your shelves stocked with bouillon. Take an apple to your office. Take a bag of apples. If a craving is unmanageable, here's a suggestion: Let's assume that chocolate sundaes are your downfall. Eat nothing but chocolate sundaes for one or two days. As long as you eat nothing else, you probably won't go too far over your calorie limit. And you may never want another chocolate sundae.

Today, there are so many commercial aids to dieting, so many substitutes for our calorie-laden pleasures, that there's less and less excuse for giving in to a sudden "craving." There are dietetic soft drinks, salad dressings, jams, diet-packed fruits and vegetables, ice milk and dietetic gelatin mixes. The dietetic soft drinks—with usually only one or two calories per bottle—are perhaps the most useful aid of all, since they satisfy both thirst and the craving for something sweet.

Which diet will fit your needs best?

Essentially, going on a diet must always be a do-it-yourself proposition: no one else can supply the willpower for you. Various kinds of help are available, though, from calorie charts to doctors and diet clubs. The question, once you've decided to lose weight, is: what kind of help will you need?

If you're trying to shed just a few pounds, you can probably dispense with all help, including calorie counting. Dr. Seymour Lionel Halpern, a New York internist and nutrition authority, said: "For someone who needs to lose ten pounds or less, I rarely recommend going on a strict calorie-counting diet. It usually will suffice to follow three basic rules. Cut out altogether all the obviously fattening foods. Eat smaller portions of everything else. And cut out between-meal snacks. If you must have a bedtime snack, have something like an apple —or delay having your dinner-time dessert."

The average person following this non-diet diet will lose a pound a week quite painlessly. Dr. Halpern believes that many people who diet and fail to do so because they crash-diet instead of settling for more gradual results.

For those with more serious—or more stubborn—weight problems, dieting under a doctor's supervision may be the answer. Like any long-term medical treatment, this can be expensive. The doctor, however, provides not only medical advice and a diet tailored to your own tastes and needs but the continuing moral support many people seem to require. Doctors to beware of: the ones who dose patients assembly-line fashion with quantities of possibly dangerous diet pills. Your family doctor or local medical society can supply the name of a reputable diet specialist.

Some restricted diets, especially those of the faddish type, can be dangerous for people with certain diseases, including undiagnosed diabetes. A checkup is always a good idea, although Dr. Halpern feels that a young person under thirty-five in good health, who has seen a doctor fairly recently, can safely diet away as much as twenty to twenty-five pounds without asking medical advice—as long as the diet chosen is a sound, well-balanced one.

Compulsive eaters, driven to overeat by their own anxieties, can sometimes be helped by psychotherapy. But this is an alternative to consider only if you have other serious emotional problems.

For people with a really big weight handicap—those who must lose forty, fifty, and even a hundred pounds—who can't afford a private physician, there are obesity clinics in most large cities, run either by the board of health or by teaching hospitals. They are usually excellent, providing medical supervision, a sound diet and regular follow-up sessions to keep you going. However, many clinics have long waiting lists and require patients to attend during stipulated daytime hours.

Diet clubs are doing a booming business. The biggest of them, Weight Watchers International, has about a million members, and there are similar smaller operations springing up everywhere. The weight-control club is really the fat man's Alcoholics Anonymous. At weekly meetings members weigh-in in private, and their losses or gains are called off later before the group. There's a pep talk by a once-fat lecturer, whose stock-in-trade is his or her own success story, and a discussion period during which those who have gained weight have a chance to confess their dietary sins. People with less than ten pounds to lose aren't usually allowed to join the diet clubs—they might demoralize other members. Very often the club is the last resort of the truly obese person. He gets from it the companionship and encouragement of people who are in the same boat—and perhaps even a social life.

"Most of our members are experienced weight-losers," said Ruth Maislin, one of the founders of the country's second-largest club, Weigh of Life. "They've tried every fad diet and pill and have never failed to lose weight—but always gained it back. We try to provide them with an eating program they can live with for life."

In Dr. Halpern's opinion, the clubs are useful for some individuals, but he has important reservations about them. First, some don't *require* members to have medical checkups, though they usually recommend it—and for the substantially overweight person chances are fifty-fifty that some medical complication is present. Then, lecturers are laymen trained by laymen, and sometimes no doctors or nutritionists are available as consultants. And members are dealt with en masse, not as individuals. For example, some clubs insist that members follow a single rigid diet—no substitutions allowed. It's usually a good high-protein diet, but if it says you must eat fish five times a week and you loathe fish, you're simply out of luck. Rigid diets do produce results more quickly, but they're harder to live with in the long run.

These, then, are some of the choices available to dieters. The trick is to pick the one that suits your particular needs.

Are you under some of the usual misconceptions about diets and dieting? Test yourself here.

Dieters can so easily be trapped in a maze of fact and fallacy. Because intensive study into the causes and cures for overweight is relatively recent, new theories, some only half-substantiated, crop up with increasing frequency, and usually they only compound the dieter's confusion.

Here are some of the statements most commonly made to doctors by their overweight patients. Some are outright misconceptions; others waver between true and false.

It's dangerous for me to diet quickly. Obviously, if you go on a prolonged starvation or crash diet, it's dangerous. But a quick diet per se is not. A lot depends on how much you have to lose. If

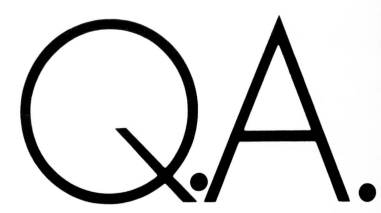

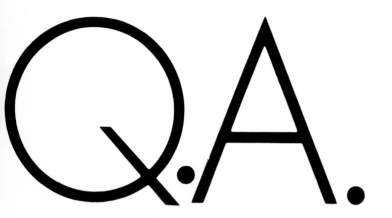

Q.A.

your goal is five pounds (and you're healthy), you can cut down drastically on your calorie intake for a limited period—perhaps fast for a day occasionally. The important thing to realize is that it is only a short-term project, not a healthy pattern, and that after you've lost five pounds you will have to be more careful, consistently, about how much and what you eat. (Also remember that the first large loss in weight may be largely salt and water. Your weight can actually go up a bit temporarily after the salt-and-water balance is re-established.)

Although a few doctors maintain that certain people simply cannot lose weight except by the quick-reduction method because they need to see fast results in order to sustain their determination, most diet experts favor the long-range approach. And for sound reason.

Dieting is re-training. If you diet too quickly, you won't allow yourself enough time to change your habits. And the chances are that as soon as you lose the desired weight and return to "normal" eating, the pounds you lost will reaccumulate very quickly. On the other hand, if your weight loss is spread over months, you will probably find that your automatic eating pattern has changed.

Dr. Seymour L. Halpern, a New York internist and specialist in nutrition, has observed this result among his patients: When they drop from a 3,000-calorie to a 1,000-calorie-a-day diet and maintain it over a prescribed period of time and are then told that they can increase it to 2,000 calories a day, they usually settle spontaneously at a calorie level under the one permitted.

I'll lose weight if I eat only the "healthy" foods. Unfortunately not. Steak is a healthy food, but one ounce of fat-trimmed beef has 75 calories. So if you eat a one-pound steak, you've already gone well over the 1,000-calorie level. Fruit juice is good for you, but one cup has from 80 to 100 calories; so do ten oysters. The fine print in most of the eat-all-you-want-to diets says "carrots, celery, diet colas, etc."

*I can't lose weight; I have a glandular prob-*lem. The thyroid gland (it determines metabolism rate or the speed with which we use up calories) has taken the blame for everything from lack of willpower to lack of honesty.

"There is no one," says Dr. Halpern, "who can't lose weight on an appropriate diet." Although overweight is a complex subject, one rule stands: If calories taken in are less than calories expended, weight will be lost. Even in instances of actual glandular obesity—estimated at the *highest* at 5 percent of obesity cases and usually as low as 1 percent—there is a level of caloric intake, says Dr. Halpern, that will cause weight loss.

Eating one big meal is as good a way to diet as eating three small ones. Wrong on all counts. In the first place, if you skip breakfast and lunch, you'll probably be so hungry that you'll consume more calories during that one end-of-the-day meal than you would have if you'd spread them out. Your stomach doesn't "shrink," causing your appetite to decrease; what happens is that you have a higher hunger level and a lower satiety level, probably because of the reduction in blood-sugar content.

Then there's the psychological reason for overeating after you've starved yourself all day. You're tense, nervous and irritable; once you start eating it's hard to stop until you go to bed, since food is acting as a sedative.

Also, your body doesn't dispose of, say, 1,200 calories eaten at one sitting as well as 400 calories three times a day. Tests have shown that if a person who needs 2,000 calories a day to maintain a consistent weight eats 2,500 at one meal, there is a substantial weight gain; if the 2,500 calories are spread over three or more meals, there is only a slight weight gain.

I'm inactive and listless because I'm overweight. The odds are that you have reversed cause and effect. You're overweight because you're inactive and listless. Of course, carrying those extra pounds certainly makes you less energetic, but studies have shown that the tendencies to avoid exercise, to sleep longer, in general to follow a lazy physical pattern, are characteristic of people who become obese. An overweight young woman probably moved at a snail's pace even before she became overweight. If you're serious about long-term figure and weight control, run, don't walk, from the nearest refrigerator.

How can you possibly diet at college or in a boarding school?

Although a tendency to gain weight when you go to school is a common problem you cannot only avoid it but actually lose weight, even if your school is buried in the country and you must eat every meal on campus or not eat at all.

The conditions are certainly not ideal. College meals are usually of the nourishing, hearty variety with no allowance made for special diets; college chefs don't use skimmed milk or artificial sweeteners, and they seem addicted to fried foods and cream sauces. Here is a typical college dinner menu to show you what you'll be up against:

> V-8 Cocktail, mixed green salad, breaded veal cutlet with tomato sauce, baked potato, broccoli, hot rolls, coconut layer cake, coffee, tea, milk.

Also, you're under new pressures, academic and emotional, which will probably increase your urge to eat. But we're assuming you have the motivation, a normal amount of self-control and just need practical advice.

If your school's menu is typical, you'll find it's top-heavy with cream soups, desserts, breads, butter, potatoes and rice. So the basic rule is: Be selective. (And it's one that can be applied, in some degree, to any fixed-menu situation.)

If you've been eating approximately the same kinds and amounts of food at home, you can lose at least five pounds during your first month on campus if you follow either of two guidelines: skip entirely at least two starchy or fat items on the menu (one should be dessert); or eat only half a normal serving. You have to use judgment here to balance your college diet against your usual one at home; it may be necessary to skip potatoes *and* bread *and* dessert consistently for dinner, even cut down somewhat on the size of your portions at the same time.

Now, the secondary rules:
1. Substitute artificial sweeteners for sugar in tea and coffee.
2. Never have second helpings of *anything*.
3. Eat slowly. This is one of the best devices. If you've served yourself a half portion, you won't be staring at an empty plate while others are still eating; if you're trying to eat only half of what you've been served, it's easier to allow your dinner plate to be taken away if everyone else's is empty.
4. Don't eat between meals unless you have the facilities to keep a supply of low-calorie snacks. Here's a suggested list (some require refrigeration, others don't): carrots, cucumbers, tomatoes or other low-calorie vegetables or fruits; canned diet-pack fruits; bouillon, chilled or hot; tomato juice (chilled in cans on the outside windowsill in winter); melba toast, low-calorie crackers, in moderation.
5. Stick to low-calorie soft drinks.
6. At breakfast, eat the cereal, not the toast, rolls or muffins (that eliminates the temptation of butter and jam).

There may be times when a lunch or dinner menu is hopeless—everything is smothered in sauce or gravy, even the lettuce is precoated with mayonnaise. Don't go to the meal. It won't hurt you occasionally to have a bouillon-and-Ry-Krisp dinner or a can of liquid diet. Suffer a bit; you'd feel worse if you ate the asparagus hollandaise and creamed seafood.

When you're dieting at college, you have to use every trick; be aware that every calorie counts. But don't try to count calories. Accuracy under uncontrolled conditions is impossible.

It might help if you make an across-the-board decision to eat no potatoes and no desserts or no bread and butter and no desserts; then you won't have to make that decision every day. But if you feel you must have a potato occasionally (every diet, to be successful, must have some flexibility), eat a small baked potato. It's worth only about 80 calories, but if you add a pat of butter, that doubles the caloric content—so don't. The same strategy applies to desserts: eat the gelatin and leave the whipped cream; eat the filling and leave the pie crust.

If you get tired of cereal in the morning and want to substitute a slice of toast, that's relatively harmless—about 60 calories. But with butter, it's at least 140.

Even if salads are pre-tossed with dressing, eat them anyway because of their nutritional value (except lettuce, which is low in vitamin content); however, if they aren't, skip the dressing (one tablespoon of salad oil has 100 calories) and use lemon juice (you can buy plastic lemons filled with juice that are less awkward than fresh ones to bring to the table). If you have a sandwich for lunch, you can neatly turn it into an open-face sandwich and eat only one piece of bread. Cut all of the fat off your meat; scrape off all the gravy.

A final word of caution: Be particularly careful on weekends. The days are freer, with more opportunities to eat, and the evenings are longer and more sociable, the time for long talks and midnight snacks. During the daytime, try to be as active as possible; stay involved in college projects. At night, ally yourself with a group of friends who also want to perfect their dancing, their guitar playing—anything to divert you from potato chips.

After a month you'll feel you have won against tremendous odds. And you'll be right.

How can you cope with husband, fiancé, mother, sister, roommate and hostess when you're dieting?

When you're dieting, you're likely not to get much help from people. In fact, the people who logically should be your staunchest allies can be your stoutest enemies.

They'll tell you that you're starving yourself, that you're ruining your health. They'll recommend fad diets or tell you about some machine that will do it all for you.

They may make a huge joke of it (the Falstaff hang-up), and unless you can muster a good sense of humor about being overweight, and not many fat people can, their ridicule can be quite destructive. Or there is a perversity in human nature that will often make even your best friends—yes, your beau or husband—try to break down your determination, often unconsciously. As Dr. Leonid Kotkin pointed out in *Eat, Think and Be Slender*, perhaps your willpower makes them feel guilty about their own weight problems; perhaps they are afraid of your becoming physically competitive and challenging; perhaps your being overweight makes them feel superior.

Just the normal course of family and social life is at odds with the pattern of a serious diet. You have to make the adjustments. When your friends and family don't encourage you, it's time to work out a way to foil their "good intentions."

Parties are difficult; so is the whole hospitality syndrome of our society. If you're the hostess, it's a little easier; no one is pressing you to eat your own hors d'oeuvres. But when you go to a party or out to dinner, your hostess, even if she's your best friend, may be your potential enemy. Her role is to make you eat and drink; yours is to resist her. Saying that you're on a diet is not usually going to protect you. In fact, the very word can trigger a barrage of insistence. You've probably heard it again and again: "Why, couldn't we all lose a few pounds, but this is a party. Besides, I made these myself. . . ." Each time the food is passed you feel like you're the number-one target. But if no one knows you're on a diet, you're already ahead in the game. It's only when you call attention to the fact that you aren't eating that other people notice it. This is invariably true at a large party. At a small one, it may be more difficult, especially if your hostess feels that food is the only synonym of hospitality. But you can *look* as though you're eating steadily and manage with a few tricks to eat practically nothing. Butter a piece of bread, return it untouched to your plate; start to take a forkful of cake from your plate, then absent-mindedly put the fork down. The varieties of ploy are endless.

If you've already talked about your diet, if your "no, thank-yous" aren't quietly accepted and you're really pushed to the wall, you may have to embarrass your hostess mildly so she will realize your seriousness. You might try something like: "My doctor . . . everything is probably all right . . . but . . . did warn." Or if your hostess persists in talking about your diet, simply say "I'd rather forget it."

But these are only occasional problems. Doing the cooking day after day and meal after meal at home needs tactics too. Not eating the children's cookies is simply a matter of willpower, but having to fix and then sit down to dinner with a husband who loves to eat heartily is an endurance test. To win it, you have to set rigid rules. Your husband, even though he may approve of your dieting, is probably going to be bored with the means. Dieters *can* be social nuisances. So spare him the details or he may become so unsympathetic that he drives you to the refrigerator in frustration.

In general, try making what you eat appear as similar to your husband's dinner as possible; you won't feel deprived and he won't be constantly reminded of the fact that you are. Plan menus that can be calorie-laden, but optionally; avoid those that have the calories built into them, i.e., broccoli with hollandaise but not creamed broccoli; beef with gravy but not sauerbraten; strawberries with cream but not strawberry mousse. For every calorie-rich food your husband likes, keep its dietetic coun-

terpart, if possible—mayonnaise, salad dressing, jam, soft drink, canned fruit, etc. If he likes his hamburgers fried, fry them, but broil yours. Fried chicken for him; broiled for you. Tasting food while you're cooking is another problem. There are only two solutions: Don't do it at all and take a chance on your seasoning instinct; or have one tasting session for everything fattening that you must cook fairly consistently. Measure every ingredient carefully and make a note of it so that from then on you can go by the book, not the taste buds.

Also, plan your meals ahead. This kind of menu-juggling is difficult on the spur of the moment.

If you live at home with your parents and your mother isn't too sympathetic about your diet, eat very small portions and not of everything, then be firm about not eating any more. (The difficulties of dieting at college were discussed on page 193.) Mothers can be very persistent about food; they feel it's part of their duty to make you eat and that's why so many children are allowed to become fat in the first place. Get your doctor to back you up, if possible; your family is probably really concerned that your new eating habits are bad for your health, and if you're on a long-term fad diet, they're probably right. But if your diet is a sane one, try explaining that your overweight makes you very unhappy; if that doesn't work, just be stubborn. When you're dieting, in fact, stubbornness may be your only true ally.

What foods make up a balanced diet?

What nutritionists call the "basic seven foods": 1) green and yellow vegetables which provide vitamin A, vital for growth, vision and healthy tissue in various internal organs; 2) citrus fruits and tomatoes, which provide vitamin C for good teeth and gums and for healthy blood vessels; 3) potatoes, other fruits and vegetables, which offer vitamins A and C and needed minerals; 4) milk and cheese, which give protein to help build and repair tissue, and calcium to strengthen bone structure; 5) meat, fish and poultry, which are rich in protein, iron (for your blood) and B vitamins, which aid appetite and digestion; 6) whole grain enriched bread and cereals which provide B vitamins, protein and roughage; 7) butter and fortified margarine, which contain vitamin A, a guard against infection.

Can those extra pounds you've gained just be because of water retention and not real fat?

It's hard to talk to anyone about dieting without the subject of water retention coming up. It's one of the most misunderstood scapegoats in the overweight situation. Too many women blame too many pounds on it. You've probably heard—and it is true—that *some* women can gain up to nine or ten pounds practically overnight because of their body's tendency to retain water. But is water the cause of *your* weight problem? To what degree does it affect your weight? How does it really work?

For most women water retention, medically called edema, is a relatively normal by-product of other body processes. The basic reason for it is the body's need to balance salt with water. It is usually caused by one of three things: 1) excess salt in the diet, 2) a woman's stepped-up hormone level at a particular time during her menstrual cycle, 3) an artificially stepped-up hormone level caused by some kinds of birth control pills. Or it can be, in severe form, the symptom of a serious heart or kidney problem. Any woman who suspects this condition should see her doctor—if only for the comfort of finding out, as she probably will, that she is wrong.

Excepting, then, the cases of severe edema, whom does water retention affect? how much? and what can be done about it?

A person who uses lots of salt regularly will spend a sizable part of each day with excess water in her tissues and thus will weigh a few extra pounds. The heavier a person, the more pounds will be involved, but in 95 percent of the cases, according to New York internist Dr. Morton B. Glenn, the number of pounds involved is less than five. And in the majority of cases, it is under three. There are people, however, who are excessive water retainers even on moderate amounts of salt. They may carry as much as six to ten or more extra pounds in water weight. If you suspect you are one, have your doctor verify or else eliminate your suspicions. To do this, he may simply put you on a bland diet for forty-eight hours to find out how much weight you'll lose. If you are an excessive retainer, he will probably put you on a more or less permanent low-sodium diet.

Water retention due to too much salt in the diet happens, of course, to both men and women. Some women have the additional problem of experiencing water retention just before menstruation or at some other regular time during their monthly cycles even though their salt intake has been normal. The reason for this is an increased amount of the female hormone, estrogen, in the body. Estrogen, according to the well-known Boston gynecologist, Dr. Robert W. Kistner, prevents the kidneys from excreting salt in the usual manner. The retained salt attracts water and is recirculated. It is deposited in the tissues, causing them to swell. There is a weight gain and a woman feels uncomfortable.

This condition occurs naturally when the body produces estrogen to bring on menstruation and usually disappears after the period begins. The same condition also can be caused by certain birth control pills—those with a high estrogen content. The best solution is probably for a woman's physician to prescribe a different pill—one containing the lowest amount of estrogen. In either case, using a diuretic to help the body eliminate salt and water

and/or sticking to a low-sodium diet might be helpful.

Water retention, then, is not really as significant a contributor to weight problems as it is often set up to be. It may add pounds, but does not contribute to obesity by adding fat. It may be responsible for a bloated feeling and may cause some minor swellings—rings, bracelets, belts, shoes, may feel tight, for instance.

Water retention is significant in weight control primarily because weight-watchers are scale-watchers. Every pound or two of extra weight when you've been especially faithful to your diet can be disheartening enough to prompt disaster. However, if you're aware of the problem and its controls, perhaps you won't let it happen.

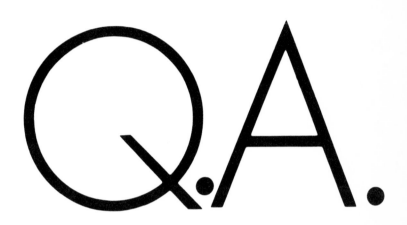

ARE HEALTH FOODS HEALTHIER?

We have been a food-conscious nation for a long time. For many years interest was focused on calories; now, along with the troubled ecology, the interest has shifted to health. People are concerned about the nutritional value of processed foods as opposed to organic foods; about vitamins for which all kinds of wonders are claimed—from curing colds to increasing sexual potency; about macrobiotic diets; about the dangers of chemical sprays and more. There is a mass of information about all these concerns, and for almost every statement a contradictory one can be found. To try to make sense out of all this, GLAMOUR sponsored the discussion below with the four experts above, all of whom are very involved with nutrition.

ADELE DAVIS
"I've never found out yet what a good basic diet is, and I've been in the business for forty years."

Her best-selling nutrition books are considered extreme by many doctors but are bibles for a lot of people.

DR. LEO LUTWAK
"Nutritionally it doesn't make any difference whether you eat white, brown, stone-ground or any other kind of bread."

A professor of clinical nutrition at Cornell University, Dr. Lutwak is also a physician, biochemist, and nutrition consultant for the National Aeronautics and Space Administration.

LILLIAN ROXON
"It always seems that vegetarians, especially old people who've been vegetarians for many years, are terribly healthy."

A journalist, Lillian Roxon, who writes a column about health in *Fusion*, a rock magazine, and says that the purpose of her column is to "get kids away from hard drugs and into health instead."

DR. THOMAS WADDELL
"The people who are truly malnourished in the United States can't afford to think about organic foods."

A specialist in infectious diseases, Dr. Waddell was a participant in the decathlon event in the 1968 Olympics, served part-time as physician for the team. He has written several articles on food and drug abuse among athletes.

Roxon: In this discussion I really represent the average confused consumer and I'd like to start off by asking about bread—white bread versus whole grain bread. I go out of my way to find whole grain, stone-ground bread and I wonder whether I'm wasting my time.

Lutwak: Nutritionally and physiologically it doesn't make any difference whether you eat white, brown, stone-ground or any other kind of bread. Bread is an insufficient food, man can't live on it alone. But then he doesn't have to—he gets his nutrition from other foods. White bread, however, does have supplemental nutrients. It is enriched; it has protein and calories.

Davis: But the enrichment does as much harm as it does good. There was a study in 1942 in which rats that were fed enriched flour died sooner than rats fed plain white flour. There's no biotin, no choline in the white bread. All sorts of B vitamins are missing. Saying we don't eat *just* white bread is not a reason to eat it. It's just an excuse for a sloppy diet. Instead of a really good diet we accept many unnutritious foods because we don't eat any of them alone.

Lutwak: There is no known information that any of the chemicals in bread that you mention, Miss Davis, are required by man. There have been very extensive studies done in the last twenty to thirty years which show there is no requirement for choline or for biotin.

Davis: There have been hundreds of studies that showed the opposite.

Lutwak: Bread, as it is sold in the store, is made of flour that has gone through the process of milling which removes certain chemical substances like phytates, normally present in whole grains and impossible for man to digest. These phytates in whole grain bread probably do more harm than any other substance which is normally found in the so-called natural food diet. They prevent the body from absorbing and utilizing, among other things, iron, calcium and magnesium.

Davis: Only when calcium and iron are extremely deficient can you detect decreased absorption.

Roxon: It seems that more studies of bread have been done with rats. Why not humans?

Lutwak: Much work has been done on humans

with bread. The experiment essentially has been done for us in underdeveloped countries such as India and some of the Latin American nations where the sole or major component of the diet is grain. People in such places do very poorly. The death rate is extremely high; people mature very late and die fairly early. Children are of short stature and both children and adults are more susceptible to diseases. This is evident again that man cannot live on bread alone or on any one food alone.

Roxon: I'd like to ask about the artificial foods which have vitamin supplements in them. The astronauts took Tang with them to the moon. A lot of people are drinking Tang because they think that if the astronauts did, it's better than orange juice.

Lutwak: The reason Tang was used for vitamin C is that Tang is a powder and it can be reconstituted. The diet on the Gemini program required foods that could be completely dehydrated. You cannot obtain a stable concentration of orange juice by freeze-drying. They could just as easily have taken pure ascorbic acid, but Tang has flavor; it was a way of providing a flavorful drink that astronauts were willing to take. One of the requirements of any good diet is that it is palatable and acceptable to the individual. The other is that the diet include a range of foods that fulfill the normal requirements for bodily nourishment. If you happen to like goat's milk, then drink goat's milk. If you like Tiger's Milk, then drink it. What counts is that you wind up with a balanced diet.

Roxon: As long as you mentioned goat's milk, there's a point I'd like to ask you about. When I came to this country the cottage cheese tasted rancid and stale to me. About a year ago I tasted goat's milk cottage cheese and it tasted very fresh.

Lutwak: It's the problem of overpopulation. When you have a large population which you have to provide for by centralized means, you have to prepare large quantities of food. We prepare large quantities of cottage cheese and much smaller quantities of goat's milk cheese. Cottage cheese, by the way, has nothing magic about it, despite Mr. Nixon's statement that he eats it.

Roxon: I don't think that anyone thinks that it's magical. But meat is expensive and I'm trying to keep my expenses down. Cottage cheese is protein in a cheaper form than steak.

Waddell: In terms of protein, you can't survive on cottage cheese. Cottage cheese is still deficient in certain essential amino acids.

Roxon: Is meat absolutely necessary in a diet?

Lutwak: No. You can replace it by the proper balance of mixtures of other proteins. This is being done in many countries. Haiti is among them.

Roxon: There's a whole new issue which people have become concerned about in the last few months, the questions of hormones and antibiotics in animal meats.

Waddell: The hormones and antibiotics aren't very healthy. We have an ecological crisis and a lot of things are being brought out in the open. We're discovering that we don't know a lot about problems that are being raised. The problem that the antibiotics given to animals creates is not that we ingest the meat with the antibiotic—antibiotics are not that stable—but that certain bacteria are becoming more resistant within the animals themselves because of the indiscriminate use of antibiotics, and these bacteria in turn may affect human beings.

Roxon: But wouldn't it be better if meat didn't have any antibiotics in it at all? You can buy it like that in organic food stores.

Waddell: Yes, but we talked about that before. With the increase in population, you have to increase the size of animals. And you can do this by giving them antibiotics and hormones.

Davis: I think that there are nine countries that will not import our meat anymore. Our steers are at the point where you can sometimes express milk from them because of the estrogen they're getting.

Lutwak: But that estrogen is not present in the food that you eat. That estrogen is stored in the fat of the animal and generally we don't eat the fat of the animal.

Davis: An awful lot of people do.

Roxon: Dr. Lutwak, you spoke of mass distribution of food. Now I'm speaking of an individual. If an individual can afford to buy from an organic store which has products that do not contain these additives, are you against it? I'm asking you now as my doctor.

Lutwak: I'm not against that, if you want to and you can afford to. But I think it is unnecessary.

Waddell: You don't think that you're malnourished, do you, Miss Roxon?

Roxon: Well, I don't know. Miss Davis' book, *Let's Eat Right to Keep Fit*, made me think I was.

Waddell: The people who are truly malnourished in the United States can't afford to think about organic foods. To me beriberi was only a word that I'd seen in a book in medical school until I went to South Carolina. Down there in Strom Thurmond country, where people have never seen physicians before, I saw beriberi. I saw human beings infested with worms that I didn't think existed in the United States.

Roxon: I know that these people would be better off having white bread with additives, rather than no bread at all.

Waddell: Rather than eating cornstarch. You know that the pregnant women there still eat a box of cornstarch a day? The problem for them is food—not organic food.

Lutwak: Today I stopped and looked at one item of food in two stores in Palo Alto. In a regular chain supermarket, large Grade A eggs were 59 cents a dozen. Health food eggs, across the street, were $1.75 a dozen.

Roxon: And there is no difference in nutritional value between the two?

Davis: There is one thing: the organic eggs are supposed to have more vitamin B_{12} and to have quite a different hormonal makeup.

Lutwak: Chicken hormones! What kind of hormones do chickens produce that the mammal requires! Chicken hormones are probably treated as foreign toxic substances by the human body.

Waddell: The two kinds of eggs are nutritionally comparable, as are plants growing in chemically fertilized soil, or organically fertilized soil. A plant growing in soil needs certain nutrients and it needs sun. If those nutrients are not in the soil, it won't grow. Whether it is grown in chemically fertilized soil, or organically fertilized soil, it has the same requirements.

Lutwak: There is one difference which I've found. The best-tasting carrots I have eaten were either grown in organically treated soil, or grown in a laboratory in a pure water culture with pure analytical grade chemicals added. And these are two diametrically opposed cultures. Ironically, you can grow the best-tasting fruits and vegetables, the best-looking with the best flavor, by pure organic culture and pure inorganic culture. But the commercially grown products are what make it possible for a New York child to have an orange every day. In 1931, an orange was a rare occasion, something that was seen only as a Christmas gift. Now varieties have been developed which keep well. Unfortunately, keeping quality and flavor-quality usually don't go hand in hand. But the nutrient quality is the same.

Roxon: I'm worried about insecticide sprays. Do any of you wash vegetables with plain water? Or do you wash them with something stronger? I know that they spray celery a lot. I usually wash it in a solution that I buy in a health food store. Now I don't know whether I'm wasting my money or not.

Lutwak: You're wasting your money. If you ate only celery for seventy-five years, you might, provided by some miracle you lived, accumulate enough stores of insecticides in your tissues to be of some damage. The more insecticide-sprayed food that is eaten in a population, the more that will be present in the fatty tissues of the body. As long as it remains there it is non-toxic. People who go on massive reducing regimens sometimes produce symptoms of toxicity. Generally, most of the stuff turns over slowly and remains stored for long periods of time.

Davis: Is this true of all sprays or only DDT?

Lutwak: It's true of those sprays that are fat soluble, which include most of the sprays that are used.

Davis: What about dieldrin?

Lutwak: Dieldrin is very rapidly destroyed in the liver—in both the human and various animals.

Roxon: Miss Davis wants us to eat a lot of liver, but we read that insecticide poisons are stored in the liver.

Waddell: The liver is a good clearing source not only for toxicants but for lots of things—for bacteria, for viruses. The blood supply passes through the liver continuously and all sorts of things are removed. Some of these detoxified materials may persist in the liver for some time, but for the most part they are excreted in the urine. If someone should eat animal liver, which has been exposed to toxins, they're getting them in their detoxified form. Therefore, they aren't harmful.

Roxon: Dr. Waddell, do you get your liver from an organic food market?

Waddell: I get it from the supermarket. This scare about liver is one of those areas of misinformation.

Roxon: Dr. Lutwak, you and Dr. Waddell say we are misinformed. Why don't we read about your point of view?

Lutwak: You read about it, but you don't remember it. What sticks in people's minds is the spectacular, the dramatic, the all encompassing. When someone says that they don't know, people tend to ignore it. When someone says that the information is hazy, or that there is no evidence, or the information is negative, people ignore it. If someone comes out with a positive statement, it's remembered. Let's take Linus Pauling and vitamin C for example. He came out with a very strong statement that vitamin C prevents and perhaps cures or helps cure the common cold. It is exceedingly difficult to disprove this because there are no controlled studies. Human experimentation is very difficult to design and carry through. But the burden of proof is really on Linus Pauling to prove that vitamin C works. However, you're under the impression that it does work because he made this statement. There are two effects that very large amounts of vitamin C have in the normal or in the ill patient. One, it produces diarrhea.

Roxon: It hasn't with me.

Davis: It hasn't with me either.

Lutwak: And secondly it produces a remarkable volume of urine. These are the principal effects. Now some individuals with kidney problems who take large doses of vitamin C will produce a urine concentrate with crystals sufficient to possibly do permanent renal damage. I'm tremendously upset by the publicity that Mr. Pauling's book has received because I think there are a large number of people who are taking these fantastic quantities of vitamin C.

Waddell: The most gross abuse of vitamins that I have ever seen in my life has been propagated on athletic teams. Up at South Lake Tahoe where we trained, they had cups lying around of chewable vitamin C, and I calculated that some of these kids had eaten as much as thirty grams of it a day. This is an enormous amount. And I can tell you most definitely that they were not void of the possibility of getting colds. They showed up in sick call with respiratory infections. I pointed this out to Linus Pauling. In fact I went to a lecture of his recently where he had to defend his book to a group of researchers. And they literally tore him apart. None of us came out of the conference convinced that vitamin C had anything to do with affecting the common cold one way or another. His studies are biologically naïve. He's basically a chemist and he knows very little about controlled studies in human beings. I agree that the medical profession has been somewhat remiss in doing these studies, but it's not easy to design a study which is going to prove vitamin C effective when you're working with two hundred varieties of the common cold.

Lutwak: You brought up a point about these bowls of vitamin pills lying around. Physicians are becoming very concerned about the excessive use of pills. They feel medication should be given only when it is essential and for as short a period of time as possible in order to avoid drug abuse.

Davis: Studies have shown that a hospitalized patient gets as many as thirty-two drugs a day.

Lutwak: A hospitalized person gets as many pills as is required for treatment and then it's stopped. In the current edition of *Let's Eat Right to Keep Fit*, Miss Davis, you state that you take a total of thirty-one pills a day. And then, when you feel that your nutrition is below par, you take additional pills totaling another fifteen after each meal. Furthermore, you recommend, for treatment of various addictions such as alcohol, providing plastic containers of pills at the table so that people can help themselves. What you're doing is substituting addiction to pills for addiction to alcohol. I don't care what the pill contains, whether it is a placebo or a vitamin or a hormone or digitalis or what will you—if a pill is unnecessary, a pill should not be prescribed. Medication is medication, and I think we should try to avoid medications wherever possible.

Davis: If you'll check my book, you'll see that I usually take only eight nutrient pills a day.

Roxon: You don't feel that any vitamin supplements are necessary if you eat a good basic diet, Dr. Lutwak?

Lutwak: You're absolutely correct.

Roxon: Do you think that too, Miss Davis?

Davis: I've never found out yet what a good basic diet is, and I've been in the business for forty years. I don't think that we can keep healthy on the foods that we have now, and I think the fact that we have so many sick people proves it.

Lutwak: The American public is living longer now than any other population in the history of the world.

Davis: With so many people on tranquilizers, what kind of health do we have?

Lutwak: People are surviving and living very full lives to a much later age than they ever did before. In the old days that Miss Davis recalls in her book, when people ate natural foods, people also died young of diseases like pneumonia for which there was no cure. They didn't live long enough to become sick with the diseases of aging; our population becomes sick with the wear and tear of time on the body.

Roxon: But it always seems that vegetarians, especially old people who've been vegetarians for many years, are terribly healthy.

Waddell: This is how nutritional neuroticism is started. So and so is a vegetarian and he is always so chirpy. He eats like a bird, he looks like a bird, he sounds like a bird. And people pick this up and it's very dangerous. A lot of this is coincidence, and a lot of the studies which lay people cite are coincidental. A lot of Pauling's studies on vitamin C are coincidental. And maybe he has one less cold a year and that's fine, but it is coincidental. And maybe he has one less cold because he's getting older and he's becoming more immune throughout the years.

Actually I think that our minimum daily require-

ments of vitamins and minerals are exceeded on a daily basis. I look at the labels and most of the things I eat are supplemented in some way. I see minimum daily requirements on cereal. I see that milk is fortified. Vitamins and nutrients are added to practically everything I eat.

I hate to keep referring to the Olympic team but the urinals in South Lake Tahoe were pungent with vitamin C. It was my suggestion that they save the stuff, crystallize it and send it to India, where it could be of some use. Let me tell you what was given the athletes, aside from the fact that the kitchen was open twenty-four hours a day, and you could eat as often as you wanted: one fellow was eating as much as four pounds a day of meat not to count the amount of vegetables and potatoes and starches and cans of food supplements which were provided and which we took to our cabins to eat as snacks. I was falling into the same thing; I was becoming nutritionally neurotic. We were provided with $20 bags of vitamins, minerals and enzymes. This form of nutrition regarding medicine and training was designed by lay people. These are not medical decisions.

Roxon: Were there any bad effects?

Waddell: I know of no way of measuring this. Sure, people got sick with ordinary infections. If they cut themselves, they'd bleed like everyone else, and sometimes they'd get infected. Some fellows developed ulcers from the anxiety of trying to make the team. There were as many psychological problems as one would expect in this type of population where kids have been working for this all their lives. And psychological problems can manifest themselves in physiological ways as most Americans know. So it's difficult to say whether their diet was producing these manifestations. But the most serious illness I saw up there was some venereal disease.

Roxon: Is there any basis for believing that if you're eating the right foods, you won't get venereal disease as quickly as you would if you were in poor condition?

Lutwak: This is absolutely untrue. You get VD if you're exposed, regardless of the state of your nutrition.

Roxon: In Miss Davis' book she says that cancer is a degenerative disease caused by poor diet. What do you think?

Lutwak: Some doctors believe cancer is a viral disease, and others believe that it is an upset in the DNA transcription. There is no evidence that nutrition and cancer are directly related, except that the nutritional requirements of the organism increase after the cancer has appeared. Cancer cells use a larger amount of nutrition and less effectively.

Davis: I would disagree with that very heartily. When native races which have been on pretty good diets without any refined food were investigated, it was found that cancer had not occurred.

Lutwak: Cancer is chiefly a disease of old age and the native populations that have been investigated have a median age of about thirty to thirty-five; it is the rare individual in these populations who lives beyond the age of fifty or sixty. Therefore one would not expect to find cancer. For significant instances of cancer you need a fairly long-lived population.

Davis: I believe in none of this nonsense at all. May I point out that the major cause of children's death is leukemia nowadays. It is not an old-age disease.

Lutwak: Leukemia is not a major cause of death. And secondly there is no relationship of leukemia to the nutritional history of the mother and the infant.

Waddell: The major cause of infant mortality is diarrheal-gastrointestinal disease.

Davis: I've heard older physicians, those who were in training twenty or thirty years ago, say that in those days leukemia or any form of cancer in small children was unknown.

Lutwak: They were undiagnosable years ago. Today we can diagnose leukemia earlier. In the past infant deaths were listed as spontaneous deaths, or death of unknown cause. No one did the investigations that are done today. Now parents are very well trained to bring their children to the physicians the minute any symptoms occur; diagnoses are made much earlier. One cannot compare death rates of diseases that were undiagnosed years ago.

Roxon: There is a school of thought which believes, as Miss Davis does, that vitamins can be used to cure certain diseases.

Davis: Most people who have come to see me through the years have been ill. They've gone from one physician to another and they still had the problems they started out with: arthritis or maybe multiple sclerosis or some other fairly serious thing that doctors couldn't cure, and that did clear up beautifully with good nutrition. And that's why I've recommended larger amounts of vitamins than these two doctors do.

Lutwak: There's the whole matter of confusing the symptom with the disease. Some vitamin deficiencies may produce some of the same signs or symptoms exhibited by other diseases. Vitamins, ever since they were discovered in the early 1900's, have been suggested off and on as the cure for virtually every disease known to man. And most of these cures have fallen by the way.

Waddell: I have yet to see a vitamin deficiency in a middle-class person who didn't have a hormonal problem.

Lutwak: Well, the only other cases that I have seen it in are chronic alcoholics, patients with chronic malignancies and patients who have had gastrointestinal surgery, where the gut no longer functioned properly.

Roxon: What about people who smoke marijuana? That's again supposed to use up a lot of vitamin C.

Lutwak: There have been no studies completed on marijuana and vitamin C. But there are studies I know of underway at the National Institute of Health and at the Veterans Hospital at Palo Alto.

Waddell: To date, there is no documentation of scurvy, the vitamin C deficiency disease, in kids who have been on pot.

Davis: There have been instances of scurvy in the macrobiotic diet.

Lutwak: Yes, the macrobiotic diet is another fad approach, and there you can expect to find anemias and virtually everything else.

Davis: A few people have supposedly died from scurvy on the macrobiotic diet, haven't they?

Lutwak: No, but there have been many complicated problems. The first girl that I saw who had been on a macrobiotic diet for a year had profound anemia. She had a marked iron deficiency, a marked ascorbic acid deficiency, a marked protein deficiency. It's mostly a grain diet and grain is relatively deficient in everything. To go back to the first statement made here today: you can't live on bread alone. You need a balance of foods.

Unlike the populations of Haiti and other poor countries, for many people here in the United States to suffer from a lack of protein or other requirements is unnecessary. We have good cheap sources of protein. You can walk into any supermarket and it stares you in the face. Cheese is one of the best foods known to man. And meats. We hear that meats are no good for you, some meats are better than others. Meat is meat. If you're paying large amounts for meat, you're getting luxury flavored foods, you're getting meats that are tenderized. We ought to learn how to cook meats better. Ground beef is one area where there is a lot of misconception. There is really no protein difference in 59 cents a pound ground chuck or $1.10 a pound ground sirloin. You get approximately the same amount of protein per dollar. Learn how to cook chuck and pour off the fat. All cooking methods, to a certain extent, are destructive of nutrients in foods. But all cooking methods also make nutrients more available.

Roxon: People aren't better off eating raw things if possible?

Lutwak: No. If you eat certain foods raw, you don't get any of the nutrients.

Davis: For example, with raw carrots you get 1 percent of the vitamin A or the carotene. You get 33 percent from cooked carrots. The nutrients are inside the cells and it's hard to break the cell walls down by chewing.

Lutwak: Could you say what you think a good diet would be?

Davis: You can't summarize a good diet for any one person. People have different requirements. An adequate diet is one that supplies at least the minimum daily allowances of all the nutrients—of which there are forty. I feel that it's very important to have whole grain bread and it simply is not true that you get everything in the white bread and the processed foods. It depends on what kind of health you want.

Lutwak: I think what it boils down to is this: eat what you like, prepared as you like, and do everything in moderation. Don't go overboard in any one area.

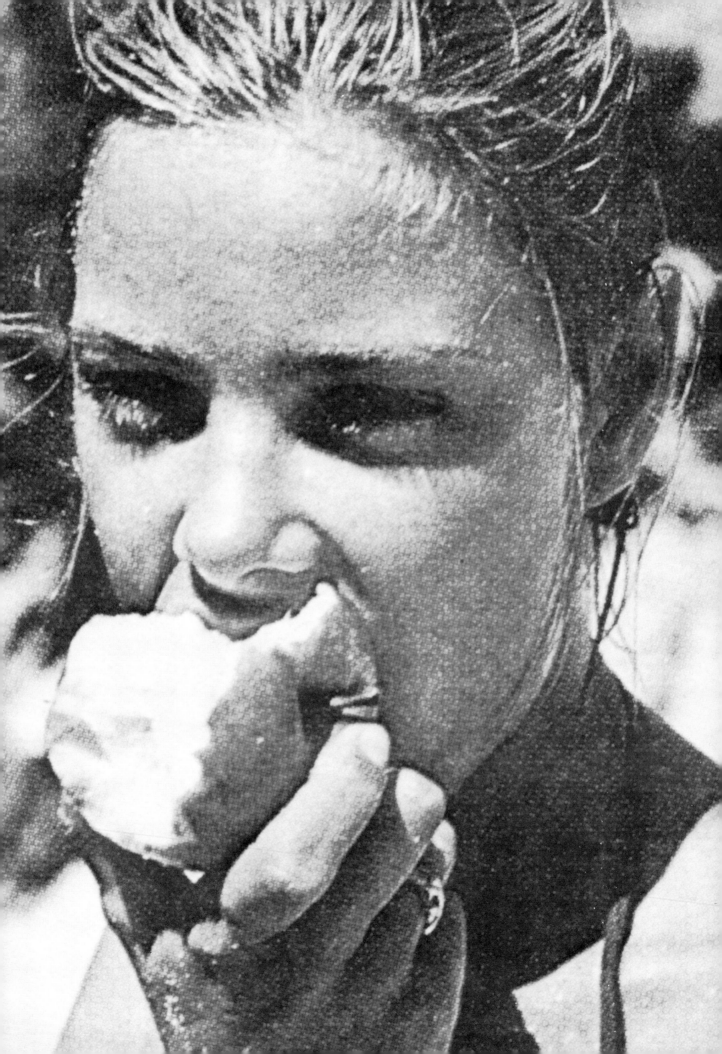

SUDDENLY YOU'RE OVERWEIGHT

by Flora Davis

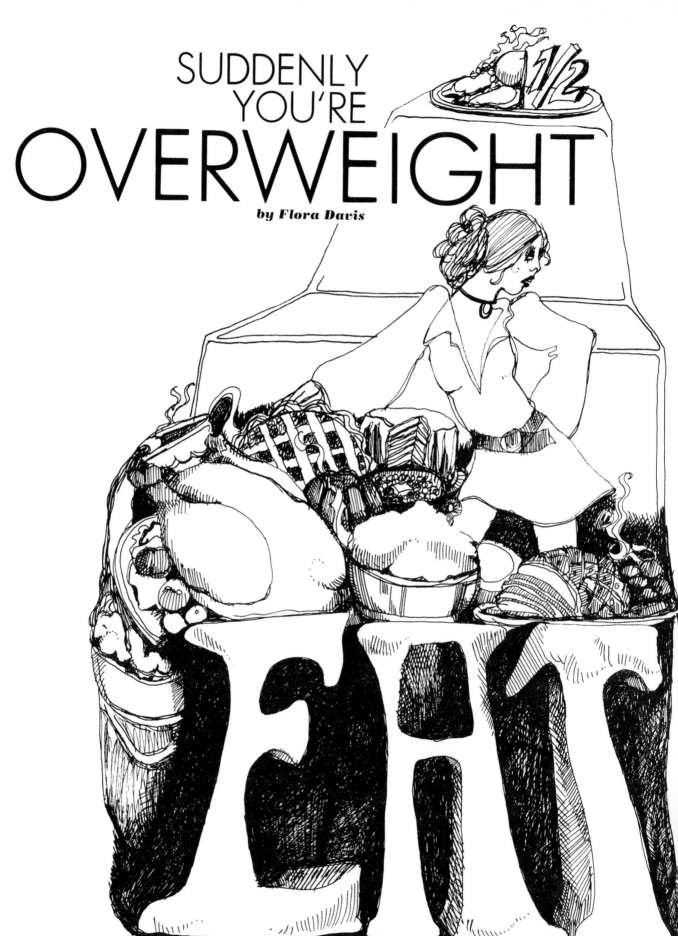

Overweight is something that usually creeps up on you slowly over a period of months or years. It can also happen practically overnight—so suddenly that it's as if the extra pounds are something you've come down with, like measles. A person may gain fifteen, twenty, even thirty, pounds in a month, without the least idea why it happened.

These sudden weight gains are never as mysterious as they seem. Consider these four case histories:

Elaine K. is a college freshman. Her school is miles from home, but she has made new friends easily and in a letter to her parents reported that she'd never felt better and happier. But the term was barely two weeks old when her clothes began to fit too snugly and now she can't get into most of them at all. The scales tell her she has already gained thirteen pounds.

Jane W. is married and has a healthy six-month-old son. She's only in her mid-twenties but Jane thinks of herself as no longer attractive, almost middle-aged. She never got her figure back, she complains, after the baby was born. She had a normal pregnancy and gained a normal amount of weight in the course of it, but she's fifteen pounds heavier now than she was before she became pregnant.

Barbara P. wanted to be an airline stewardess for as long as she could remember. Now, at twenty-two, she's through her training at last. Her life is as exciting as she'd imagined it would be, but she had a shock the other day when one of her supervisors pointed out that she'd recently picked up a lot of weight and suggested that she ask a doctor's advice about getting down to her normal size again.

Patty A. has always thought of herself as down-to-earth. A few months ago she became engaged and almost immediately her fiancé was sent to Vietnam. She tells friends that she doesn't let herself think about the war or the danger he is in because "if I once started worrying, I'd just never stop." She seems her usual calm, sensible self, but in a short time she has gained twenty pounds.

For each of these four young women it's the first weight problem and in each case the overweight can be traced to one of two factors: either to an abrupt change in the life situation or to sudden, acute anxiety.

Going away for the first time to college or boarding school is a life change that can pile on pounds. An overly starchy dormitory diet usually gets the blame, but it can as easily be the unlimited opportunities to snack. In Elaine's case there were other more basic causes: homesickness and tension. It's true she didn't *feel* unhappy, but that was because she was doing such a good job of comforting herself with food. As soon as she tried to diet, she felt strung up and depressed. It wasn't until summer vacation that she managed to stay on a diet long enough to lose weight. Now in her sophomore year, she still has to fight the urge to go on food binges.

Another common time for a weight spurt is at the end of a first pregnancy. Usually, the pregnancy itself gets the blame.

"It must have done something to my metabolism or my glands," Jane explained vaguely.

The real cause was Jane's eating habits and the damage was done not before the baby was born but afterward. Modern obstetricians are weight-conscious and insist that patients watch their diets. But after the baby is born, the new mother is on her own and for many women this is a grueling time. Babies are demanding and Jane, feeling more irritable than loving, became guilty and draggingly depressed. She began to eat indiscriminately because food was such a comfort and was so available now that she was at home all the time. Jane felt fat and nearly forty for months after the baby was born. Finally, she resolved her own mixed feelings about her new life and settled down to a sensible diet.

In Barbara's case what brought on the weight gain was her new job, which changed her eating habits drastically. As a stewardess, she was apt to have lunch in one time zone, dinner in another, and in between there was always free food available aboard the plane. With the help of a doctor's diet, Barbara quickly lost the weight she'd gained.

Patty's problem was pure anxiety. When her fiancé left for Vietnam, she took on more worry and tension than she could handle and learned to lull her problems with food. She stuck to a diet grimly for a month, but at the end of that time felt so irritable and unhappy she gave it up.

"I'll just have to stay unpleasantly plump for now," she said. "I'll do my dieting after Tom is safely home."

There are other situations with a built-in weight hazard. For example, some teenagers after reaching their full growth go on eating as if they still had growing to do—and fatten up accordingly. Most young people, though, instinctively cut down on their food intake at the right time. Getting married is another weight-hazard situation. Many new wives, startled by sudden weight gains, blame them on birth control pills. It's true that The Pill can cause body cells to retain more water and thus may add on a pound or two, but for most women it can't be blamed for a gain any bigger than that. A new life, with a change in eating patterns, is much more likely to be the source of the problem.

Then there are the more bizarre psychological reasons for piling on weight. Some people feel safer, more able to cope with life and social situations, when they're bigger. Others are actually afraid of becoming too thin—they associate thinness with being sick and weak. Eating also has sexual overtones—a well-known fact that was celebrated in the food-orgy scene in the film *Tom Jones*.

Is it always necessary to understand *why* you've suddenly gained weight in order to lose again? When this question was put to two doctors who are authorities on weight problems, both answered "No." Understanding the cause of the gain is a help because defining problems usually puts them into better perspective, but it's more important still that you be willing to put the blame where it ultimately belongs: on your eating habits.

"People gain weight only when they eat too much or significantly cut down on their exercise. And the only way to lose weight is by dieting—there is no easy magic to make the pounds go away," said Dr. Morton Glenn, a New York internist whom GLAMOUR often consults about weight problems.

As for overweight caused by a change in the life situation, Dr. Glenn pointed out that it is very seldom practical or even desirable to go back to an old way of life just to lose weight again.

Psychotherapy is sometimes suggested as a cure for overweight caused by anxiety. Over a period of time, it may relieve the tensions that drive you to overeat, and in helping you to understand yourself it can help you to stay with a diet and to maintain a weight loss once you've achieved one. But Dr. Claude H. Miller, a psychiatrist who was project director of the Weight Control Program of the Karen Horney Clinic, cautioned: "Solving psychological problems does not guarantee normal weight, and it's definitely no substitute for a good, strict diet. Once the emotional problems are out of the way, you still have to settle down to eating less."

Dr. Miller's advice is to start dieting first, to face up to why you're overweight as you go along and to expect a certain amount of tension to develop while you're dieting. Psychotherapy is indicated only if you have other serious problems, though a chance to talk things over with a professional—not necessarily a psychiatrist, possibly a clergyman or doctor—sometimes helps to put things into proper perspective.

As the cases of the four girls show, the urge to eat can be irresistible under the stress of anxiety and change. There are several reasons for this. Food is a convenient oral tranquilizer, and most human beings use oral tranquilizers from time to time. Some people smoke, some overeat, some bite their nails. When the habit begins to interfere with health, it must go, and substituting another oral pacifier—such as gum-chewing—is never a good idea, because if the substitute is later given up for any reason, the original bad habit is likely to return. Another reason eating is so lulling is that when you really pack in food, you draw the blood down to the digestive system and away from the brain. You quickly feel bloated and drowsy rather than alert and on edge. People who feel very edgy when they're too thin—or even a normal weight—usually find that as their weight increases, their tension dwindles. Food is also an excellent sedative, which may be why so many people go in for bedtime snacks.

"Overeating doesn't really solve any problems," said Dr. Glenn, "any more than brushing crumbs under the tablecloth gets rid of them effectively. The crumbs are still there, even if out of sight, just as the anxieties are still there even if they're lulled by overeating."

But Dr. Miller disagreed: "Human beings need some way to cope with tension, and eating is a safer tranquilizer than most," he said. "It's better than drinking or taking drugs, and you'd have to be at least forty pounds overweight to do your system as much damage as you'd do by smoking two packs of cigarettes a day."

To Dr. Miller, the most important thing is to set a realistic goal for yourself. If you can't handle the tension you live under when you weigh what the charts say you should, then perhaps you should allow yourself to put on a few pounds. Dr. Miller said that you can weigh up to 20 percent more than the recommended chart weight without doing your system any real damage. Beyond 20 percent, the fat begins to be stored in dangerous places—the heart muscle, the liver, the pancreas.

A woman whose weight seesaws frequently should think carefully before dieting. The seesaw syndrome works this way: at lower weights, the woman gets anxiety symptoms—tension, insomnia, nightmares. She overeats to relieve the anxiety, then eventually diets to get back down to what she thinks she ought to weigh. But then she feels anxious again, and again turns to food for comfort, and so it goes. There is evidence now that blood vessels can be damaged during periods of weight gain and that this damage, if it's repeated again and again, is much more harmful than any of the consequences of gaining weight and staying heavy. The seesaw weight gainer can, of course, take her anxieties to a psychiatrist for help.

"But for most people," Dr. Miller said, "going to the refrigerator is much simpler than going to a psychiatrist."

Consulted specifically about the problems of Patty, the girl whose fiancé is in Vietnam, the two doctors gave quite different opinions.

"Overeating won't bring back her man any faster," said Dr. Glenn, "and he may not appreciate a fat fiancée when he returns."

"If some kind of tranquilizer is absolutely necessary for the girl, overeating is one of her better alternatives," said Dr. Miller.

Sudden weight gainers are lucky in some ways. The shock of unexpectedly finding themselves pounds and pounds heavier than they want to be may be enough motivation to start them dieting. Also, the prognosis for the truly obese—the long-term fat case with a history of diets abandoned—is not encouraging.

Assuming you opt for willpower and a diet, how do you go about breaking those seductive, bad eating habits? It helps to understand a few things about the mechanics of dieting. The third week, for example, is the one to watch out for. In the first week motivation is high and you see a satisfying weight loss, which is due partly to the fact that the amount of water stored in body cells is reduced. The sense of accomplishment carries you through the second week, but in the third the water balance readjusts itself and the scales show little or no weight loss. This is quitter's week. Millions of people diet again and again and never stick it out past the third week. Women also tend not to show any weight loss in the week immediately before they menstruate, because at that time the body cells store more water. (For more about the effect of water retention on weight, see page 195.) However, the loss is there and will show up dramatically in the week after the period is over.

After the first week, hunger is rarely a problem. Many diets allow you to have certain foods in unlimited quantities—raw carrots, celery, cucumbers, black coffee—and in the first week most people overeat their allowance of these foods. After that, carrot consumption tails off as the system adjusts to the new regimen.

Dieting should be simply an exaggeration of good eating habits. At the end of the diet you drop the exaggeration and the good habits remain. That's why totaling up calories once a day is a poorer way to diet. There's too much temptation to make substitutions. The calorie counts of two foods may be the same, but the chances are the food values won't be. The calorie-juggler doesn't give herself a chance to replace old, bad eating habits with new, sensible ones.

The best way to cope with a real drive to overeat is to get involved in some kind of activity you enjoy. It also helps to have a partner when you diet. Most dieters who come to grief do so because they try to diet alone. You learned your eating habits in company, and it helps to have company when you're trying to change them. That's one reason that consulting a doctor about a weight problem ups your chances of success: along with the diet he prescribes and the medical supervision he provides, he gives you the moral support you need. Anyone trying to lose more than just a few pounds should start with a checkup anyway.

Some diet books suggest that people on long-term diets take occasional, carefully timed vacations from their diets. Most sudden weight gainers can probably afford an occasional holiday once they're safely past the first few weeks. Since the stomach does seem to shrink, they probably won't overeat much anyway. But people with well-established weight problems slip back too easily into their old eating habits if they take a day off. Experiments with the obese have shown that many are totally out of touch with their stomachs and can no longer distinguish between genuine hunger—as indicated by stomach contractions—and appetite, which is simply a desire to eat that's brought on by the thought or sight or smell of food.

Exercise is a good way to prevent overweight but it's never a successful substitute for a diet—unless you're trying to shed just a few pounds. A combination of diet and exercise works nicely for the kind of person who gets a feeling of well-being from using his muscles. The activity releases tension, and in moderate doses won't increase the appetite. But for those who don't have time to exercise or who simply don't enjoy doing it, it's almost simpler just to diet: to give up one slice of bread, worth about seventy calories, rather than to walk an extra mile in order to burn up fifty calories.

But it's partly the decline of exercise along with the abundance of food and tensions in this country that are largely responsible for the fact that obesity is the national problem it is. Experts estimate that one in three Americans is overweight. It's a situation that just a few generations ago would

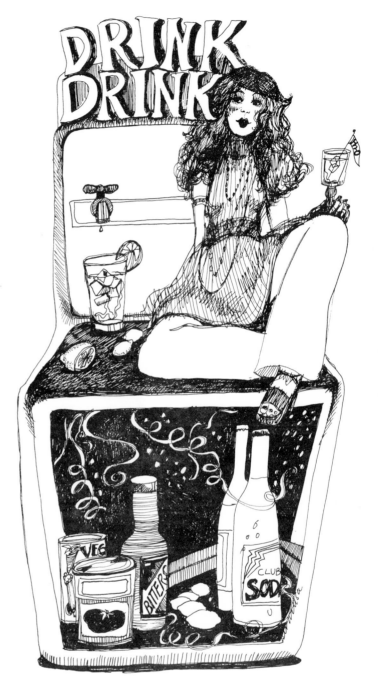

have had a science-fiction ring to it. Americans exercise less and eat more than any other people. High school parking lots are jammed with cars. Refrigerators and freezers packed with food are a constant temptation; in Europe, most people still buy food for only a day or two at a time. The very pace of American life, with all the large and small tensions it sets up, seems designed to produce a nation of overeaters. So, whether you are a victim of creeping fatness or whether your weight gain was the dramatic, overnight kind, you have plenty of company. Unless this country can evolve a new species of human being who can say "no" to food, the United States is well on its way to being, if not a Great Society, certainly a Great Big one.

205

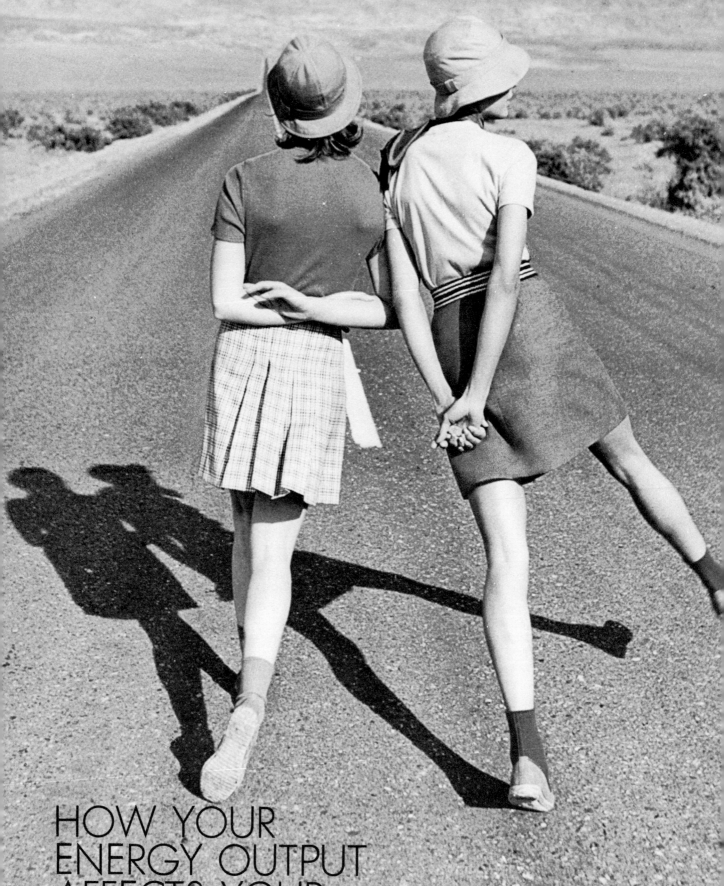

HOW YOUR
ENERGY OUTPUT
AFFECTS YOUR
WEIGHT

In all cases of overweight, food intake exceeds energy expenditure. The food you eat is measured in calories or heat energy units; if you consume more than you expend via metabolism, exercise and routine activities, those calories will add up as extra pounds. 3500 calories equal a pound of body weight. Remember that figure. It is vital to your weight-control problem.

From birth to your early twenties, you are in a period of growth. That is why infants, children and teen-agers often can (and do) consume huge amounts of food without gaining weight. They burn up what they eat in action, of course, and in growing bigger.

The problem of overweight really begins to be important in our early twenties because at that age, significant body changes take place. Usually, you have stopped growing and your metabolism begins to slow down. So your food intake needs to be cut accordingly. Every ten-year period after the age of twenty-five your metabolism loses speed at the rate of about seven percent, and you require steadily decreasing amounts of food to keep your body machinery running smoothly. Even if you eat no more in your late twenties, thirties and forties than you did in your teens, you will actually gain weight. Too, as you grow older you are inclined to be less active.

The American way of life is conducive to gaining weight. We ride instead of walk. To illustrate, an hour of walking expends about 200 calories; if you bicycle to the same place (twenty-six minutes) you will burn about 170; if you drive, you'll get there in six minutes, but at a calorie cost of only 95. The old-fashioned housewife had to cope with inefficient work areas. She walked about six miles a day just to do her chores, and in the process she walked off about 450 calories (75 per mile). In addition, she may have had to walk a quarter of a mile to market. Another 50 calories. Because she relied on hand-manipulated appliances, she used another 180 calories an hour. If she scrubbed the family clothes, she did it at the rate of 250 calories per average load of laundry. Without a dishwasher, she washed and dried dishes by hand, at 130 calories a day. Add up these work calories, and you'll get a total of slightly more than 1,000. Now consider today's housewife whose energy expenditure for work may be cut in half by automatic devices. She burns only about 500 calories a day in housework. In a week, the unused 500 a day add up to a pound.

Here's where exercise can help you. Look at the chart *right above* and you'll get an idea of the number of pounds you can lose simply by walking, doing house or office chores, or your favorite sport. Just for surprise value we included climbing stairs —we're not suggesting an hour of this a week—and sleeping.

	calories consumed		pounds a year
Walking a mile	75	*1 mile 6 days a week consumes 450*	6²/₃
Standing	66	*1 hour a week 462*	7
Ping-Pong, badminton or mopping a floor for 10 minutes	50	*1 hour a week 350*	5+
18 hole golf game	500	*1 game a week*	7+
Tennis	300	*1 hour a week*	4+
Dancing	170	*1 hour a week*	2+
Climbing stairs	1100	*1 hour a week*	16+
Skiing	600	*1 hour a week*	8+
Writing	120	*1 hour a week*	1+
Typing	140	*1 hour a week*	2+
Swimming	500	*1 hour a week*	7+
Knitting	116	*1 hour a week*	1+
Sleeping	65	*1 hour a week*	0
Bicycling	410	*1 hour a week*	6+

Since overweight comes from consuming more calories than we burn, it's logical that a moderate reduction in food and a moderate increase in calories expenditure will help you shed pounds and remain at your proper weight. By looking yourself up on the chart *below* taken from Dr. Herbert Pollack's book *How to Reduce Surely and Safely* you can find out how many calories you burn in a normal day. If you are overweight and want to diet, subtract 1,000 calories. The reduced figure represents the number of calories you can consume and safely lose two pounds a week. Or since 3,500 calories equals one pound of weight, the 7,000 calories you eliminate a week equals a loss of two pounds.

Let's say you are 5 feet 4 inches and you are twenty-two years old. You are a secretary. You will find on the chart that you probably burn 2,220 calories per day. By subtracting 1,000 calories you are left with a quota of 1,220, the number of calories you can eat a day.

The Calories Women Burn per Day
As applied to "light" work (housewives, office workers, clerks, etc.)

Height	Age		
	16-19	20-29	30-49
4'8"	*1960*	*1860*	*1560*
5'0"	*2080*	*1980*	*1680*
5'2"	*2200*	*2100*	*1800*
5'4"	*2320*	*2220*	*1920*
5'6"	*2440*	*2340*	*2040*
5'8"	*2560*	*2460*	*2160*
5'10"	*2680*	*2580*	*2280*
6'0"	*2800*	*2700*	*2400*

For heavier work (dancers, athletes, waitresses, etc.) add 200 calories to all figures except in the 30–49 bracket. Here add 300. Chart from *How to Reduce Surely and Safely* by Herbert Pollack (McGraw-Hill).

HOW TO TAKE CARE OF SPECIFIC TROUBLE SPOTS

SPOT REDUCING EXERCISE CHART

	CHEST/BOSOM	WAISTLINE	STOMACH
SECRET	Sitting in a chair, hold edge of a desk or table firmly with hands shoulder-width apart. Push firmly with hands against desk. Hold six seconds. Repeat three to six times.		Sitting in a chair, hands holding edges, tighten and curve your torso by pushing down with your arms and lifting up slightly from the chair.
BROOMSTICK	Hold broomstick in front of chest, arms slightly bent. Without changing grip or position of hands (keep grip tight) push hands together.		Sit on floor, legs apart, broomstick on shoulders behind head, arms hanging over the broomstick. Twist waistline, trying to touch one knee with the opposite hand—or to touch one foot with opposite end of broomstick. Alternate sides. Do exercise ten times.
YOGA	° Sit cross-legged with hands clasped behind you. Slowly raise arms as high as possible. Keep elbows and spine straight. Hold this position ten seconds. Slowly lower your arms. Relax. Repeat five times.	Stand with feet together, arms overhead, fingers clasped. Inhale. Bend sideways from your waist to left as far as you can. Hold. Exhale and pull arms and body straight and high. Inhale. Bend right. Hold and exhale. Repeat five times.	°Lie on the floor on your back, arms alongside body. Inhale and slowly raise legs up, touch toes to floor over your head. Hold breath. Slowly exhale and bring legs to floor. Repeat six times.

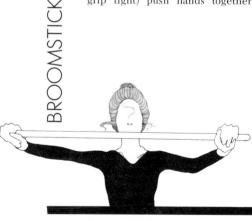

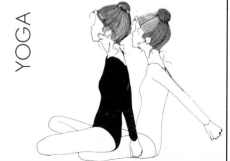

The most effective ways of coping with figure trouble spots that are the result of poor muscle control or body structure—sometimes overweight—are by doing spot reducing exercises and wearing spot reducing clothes. You have to realize at the start though that both these ways are only aides, they can't change the basic bone and muscle structure you were born with. They can however make the difference between a figure fault that no one notices because you have minimized it, and the figure fault that is a needless attention-getter because you have ignored it. Take your pick—here's a whole collection of all kinds of exercises for all parts of the body—for all kinds of girls from those who'd rather exercise in bed to the karate experts. These exercises will not only help firm your muscles but if there is an excess of fat in the area they will make the muscles better able to support it. It is always good to check with your doctor before beginning any exercise program.

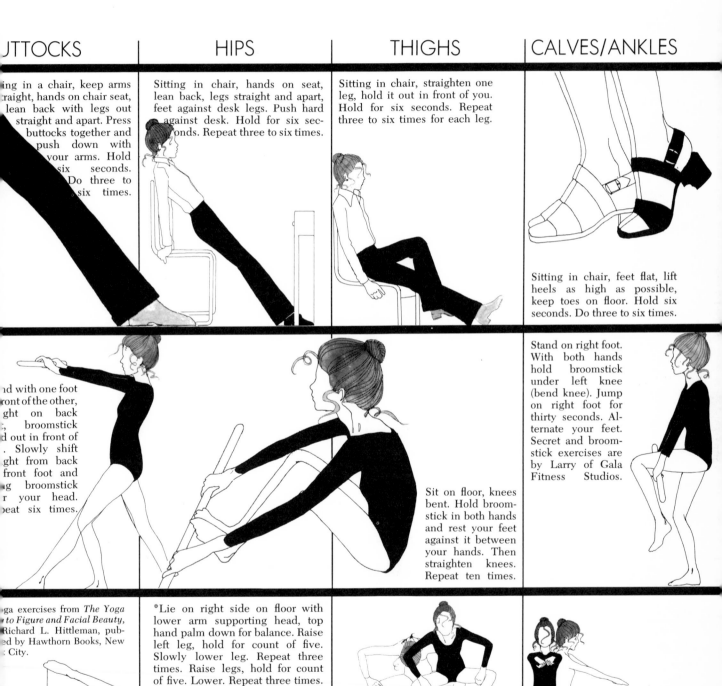

UTTOCKS

ing in a chair, keep arms raight, hands on chair seat, lean back with legs out straight and apart. Press buttocks together and push down with your arms. Hold six seconds. Do three to six times.

nd with one foot ront of the other, ght on back , broomstick d out in front of . Slowly shift ght from back front foot and g broomstick r your head. eat six times.

ga exercises from *The Yoga to Figure and Facial Beauty,* Richard L. Hittleman, pubed by Hawthorn Books, New City.

HIPS

Sitting in chair, hands on seat, lean back, legs straight and apart, feet against desk legs. Push hard against desk. Hold for six seconds. Repeat three to six times.

°Lie on right side on floor with lower arm supporting head, top hand palm down for balance. Raise left leg, hold for count of five. Slowly lower leg. Repeat three times. Raise legs, hold for count of five. Lower. Repeat three times. Relax. Do three on opposite side.

THIGHS

Sitting in chair, straighten one leg, hold it out in front of you. Hold for six seconds. Repeat three to six times for each leg.

Sit on floor, knees bent. Hold broomstick in both hands and rest your feet against it between your hands. Then straighten knees. Repeat ten times.

Sit with knees flexed, soles of feet firmly together, hands pressed against inside of knees. Inhale. Bend toward feet. Hold. Exhale. Inhale. Return to starting position.

CALVES/ANKLES

Sitting in chair, feet flat, lift heels as high as possible, keep toes on floor. Hold six seconds. Do three to six times.

Stand on right foot. With both hands hold broomstick under left knee (bend knee). Jump on right foot for thirty seconds. Alternate your feet. Secret and broomstick exercises are by Larry of Gala Fitness Studios.

°Stand with feet together, arms at sides. Slowly raise arms, come up on tiptoes. Slowly twist body from waist as far right as you can, to left as far as possible, then to front. Rest.

	CHEST/BOSOM	WAISTLINE	STOMACH
IN BED	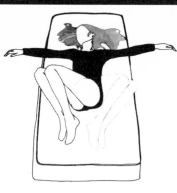 Lie flat on your back in bed. Hold arms out straight at sides. Move them in a fast zigzag motion, each arm crossing the other's path. Keep your arms straight throughout. Repeat the exercise ten times.	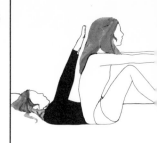 Lie flat on your back in bed. Bend your knees and lift feet off bed. Swing knees together, rocking from left to right ten times without letting your heels touch the bed.	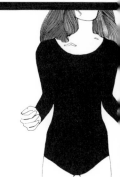 Lie on bed, knees bent planted firmly on bed, arm toward knees. Reach thigh your chest. Lower body s to bed. Repeat exercise six t
KARATE	Stand with feet slightly apart, weight divided, fists at hip. Turn knuckles down, drive fist across body in punching motion, arm slightly extended; snap back. Do five to ten times each arm.	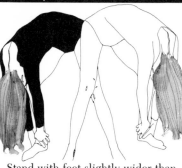 Stand with feet slightly wider than shoulder-width. Bend, grab right ankle with both hands, touch head to right knee. Repeat left. Bend, grab both ankles, tucking head between legs. Do whole procedure three times, work up to more.	Stand with feet shoulder-w apart, arms bent, fists clen elbows tucked. Inhale norm Exhale slowly, pushing i stomach muscles. Five t work to ten, with deeper bre
DANCE	Sit erect with legs wide apart, arms at sides. Swing arms back, bend elbows toward floor. Straighten to position shown here, arching back, chest out, head and shoulders back. Repeat exercise eight times. 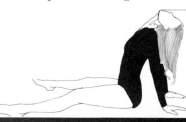	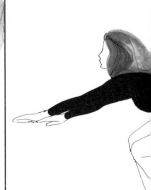 From a standing position, bend forward, knees straight, grasp calves with hands and try to touch head to knees. Straighten up, arms over head, and bend as far backward as you can. Do exercise eight times, slowly.	
TOWEL	Hold arms out, crossed at wrists. With both hands, pull on towel, relax. Pull, relax. Do ten to fifteen times. 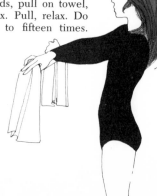	Legs apart, put left foot on side of bathtub. Lift both arms above head, stretch towel. Bend sideways toward left leg, keeping arms and towel stretched. Do ten on each side. 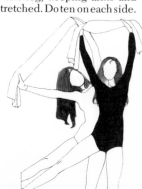	With towel in hand, raise leg forward t level—back knee straight— towel under t hand, stretch arm sideways ten on each

BUTTOCKS	HIPS	THIGHS	CALVES/ANKLES

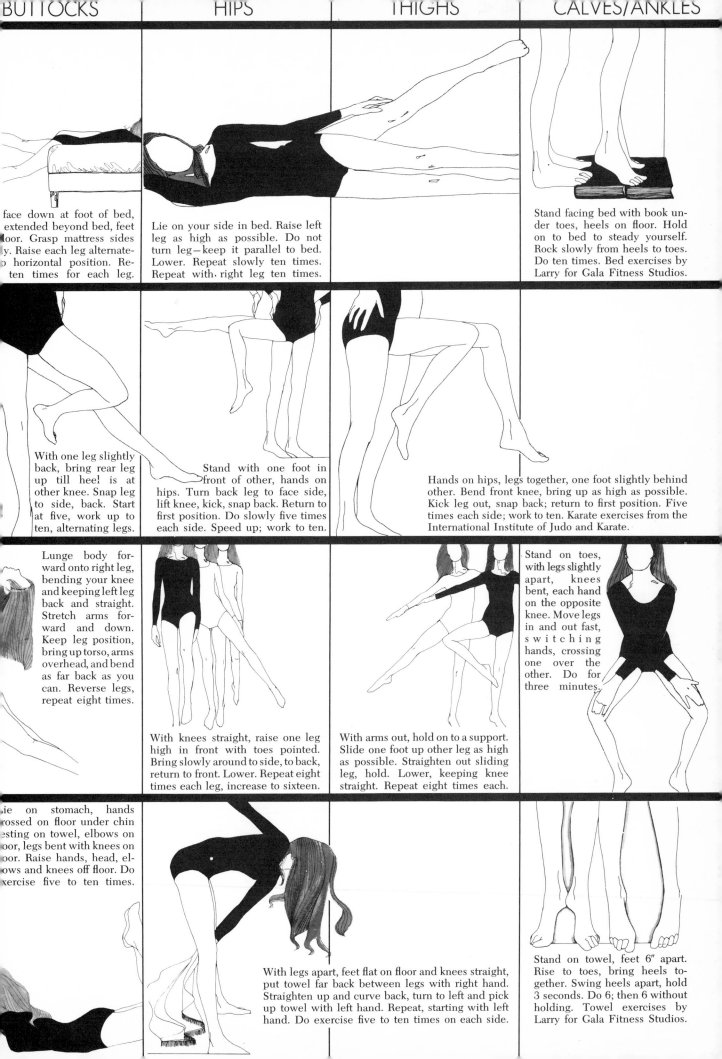

...face down at foot of bed, ...extended beyond bed, feet ...oor. Grasp mattress sides ...y. Raise each leg alternate-...o horizontal position. Re-...ten times for each leg.

Lie on your side in bed. Raise left leg as high as possible. Do not turn leg—keep it parallel to bed. Lower. Repeat slowly ten times. Repeat with right leg ten times.

Stand facing bed with book under toes, heels on floor. Hold on to bed to steady yourself. Rock slowly from heels to toes. Do ten times. Bed exercises by Larry for Gala Fitness Studios.

With one leg slightly back, bring rear leg up till heel is at other knee. Snap leg to side, back. Start at five, work up to ten, alternating legs.

Stand with one foot in front of other, hands on hips. Turn back leg to face side, lift knee, kick, snap back. Return to first position. Do slowly five times each side. Speed up; work to ten.

Hands on hips, legs together, one foot slightly behind other. Bend front knee, bring up as high as possible. Kick leg out, snap back; return to first position. Five times each side; work to ten. Karate exercises from the International Institute of Judo and Karate.

Lunge body forward onto right leg, bending your knee and keeping left leg back and straight. Stretch arms forward and down. Keep leg position, bring up torso, arms overhead, and bend as far back as you can. Reverse legs, repeat eight times.

With knees straight, raise one leg high in front with toes pointed. Bring slowly around to side, to back, return to front. Lower. Repeat eight times each leg, increase to sixteen.

With arms out, hold on to a support. Slide one foot up other leg as high as possible. Straighten out sliding leg, hold. Lower, keeping knee straight. Repeat eight times each.

Stand on toes, with legs slightly apart, knees bent, each hand on the opposite knee. Move legs in and out fast, switching hands, crossing one over the other. Do for three minutes.

...ie on stomach, hands ...rossed on floor under chin ...esting on towel, elbows on ...oor, legs bent with knees on ...oor. Raise hands, head, el-...ows and knees off floor. Do ...xercise five to ten times.

With legs apart, feet flat on floor and knees straight, put towel far back between legs with right hand. Straighten up and curve back, turn to left and pick up towel with left hand. Repeat, starting with left hand. Do exercise five to ten times on each side.

Stand on towel, feet 6″ apart. Rise to toes, bring heels together. Swing heels apart, hold 3 seconds. Do 6; then 6 without holding. Towel exercises by Larry for Gala Fitness Studios.

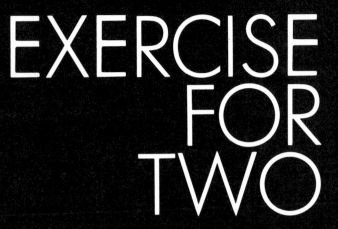

EXERCISE FOR TWO

These are light-hearted exercises. That doesn't mean they won't do you any good. It just means that there's a sense of fun and play about them. They all need to be done with another person, and they're more fun outside, but they can be done indoors, too. Each exercise is for some specific area of your body.

For arms, bust, pectorals

Stand opposite each other, legs slightly apart for balance, legs straight, arms slightly flexed and palms touching, elbows out. Now, fall forward toward each other, hands pressing hard against each other, bending more as you fall. If you can't balance, put one foot slightly forward, but not unless you have to. Keep pushing against each other till one loses balance. Repeat ten times. All exercises by Anne-Marie Bennstrom of The Sanctuary.

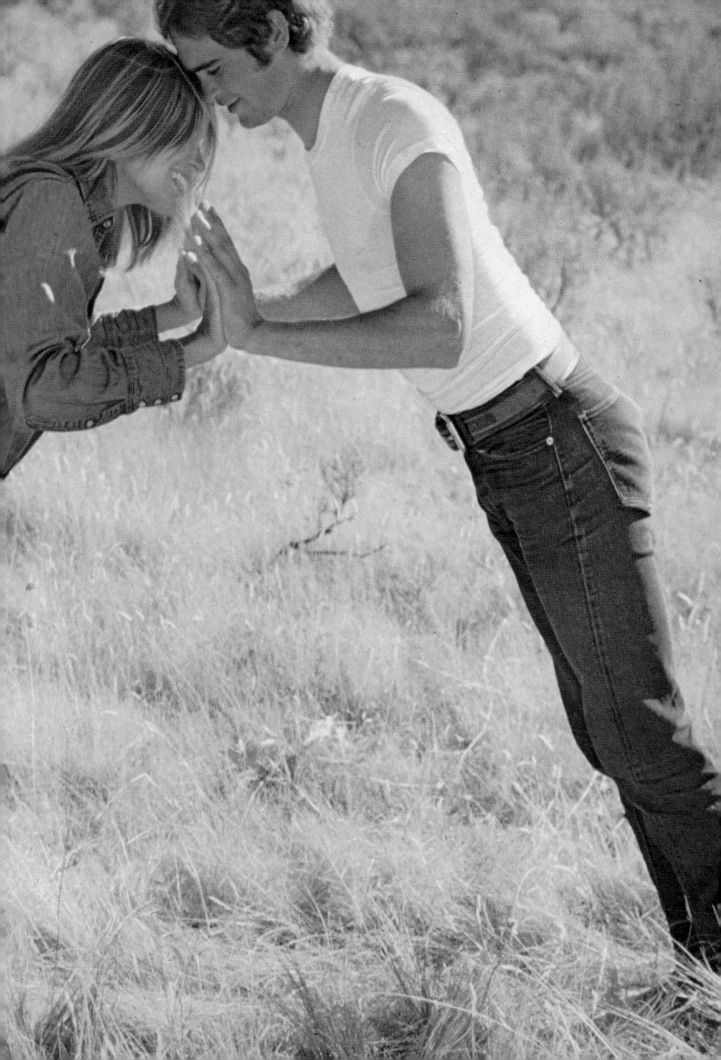

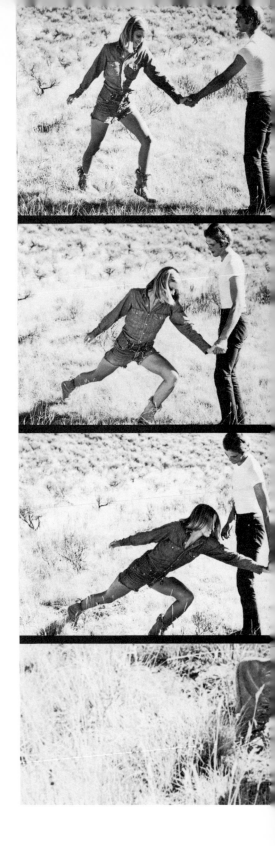

For
stomach

Sit on a large flat rock, mound or bed, something slightly raised, with legs braided. Clasp hands behind neck (if this is too hard at first, fold arms in front). Lie back slowly until both reach a lower than horizontal position, and slowly return to a sitting position. Inhale going down, exhale coming up. Do ten times.

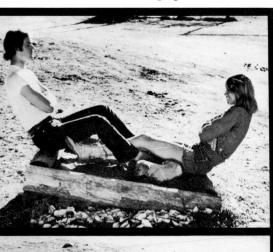

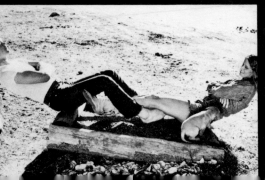

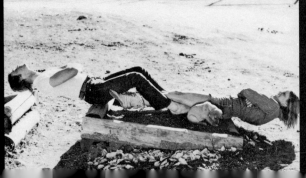

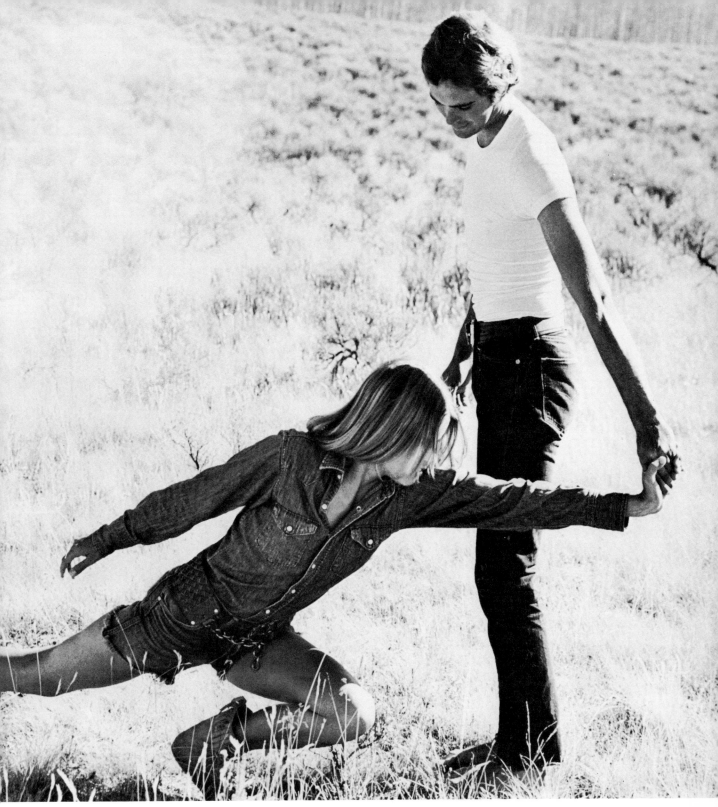

Stand face to face, left hands clasped, see *top left picture*. One partner takes a long lunge forward while the other supports her, holding hand for balance. Keep back leg straight, knee off ground, spine straight. Hold position for a few seconds, then standing person pulls lunging one up to a standing position for a second lunge. Do ten times, turn for other leg. Repeat with lunging partner in the supporting role.

For backs of thighs, bottom

Exercise
for men only

This must be done with one man and one woman. He stands facing tree trunk, door, or something to hold onto for balance, with girl on his shoulders, see *right*. He squats, keeping feet flat on ground, not up on toes. Stand again. Do five to ten times, try working up to using nothing at all for balance.

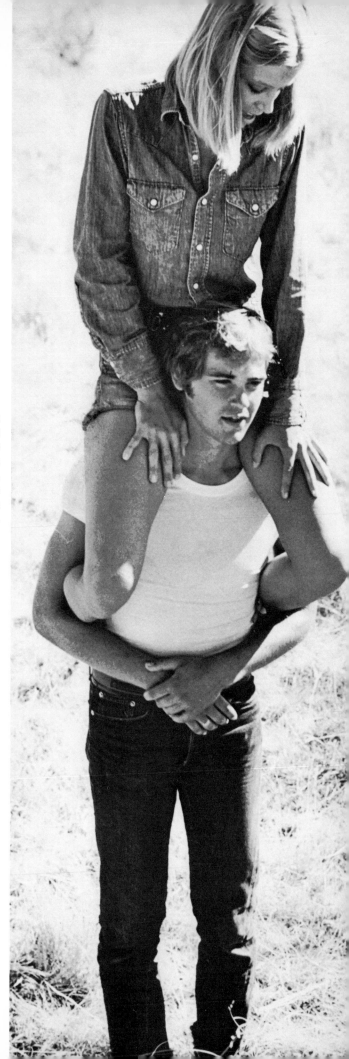

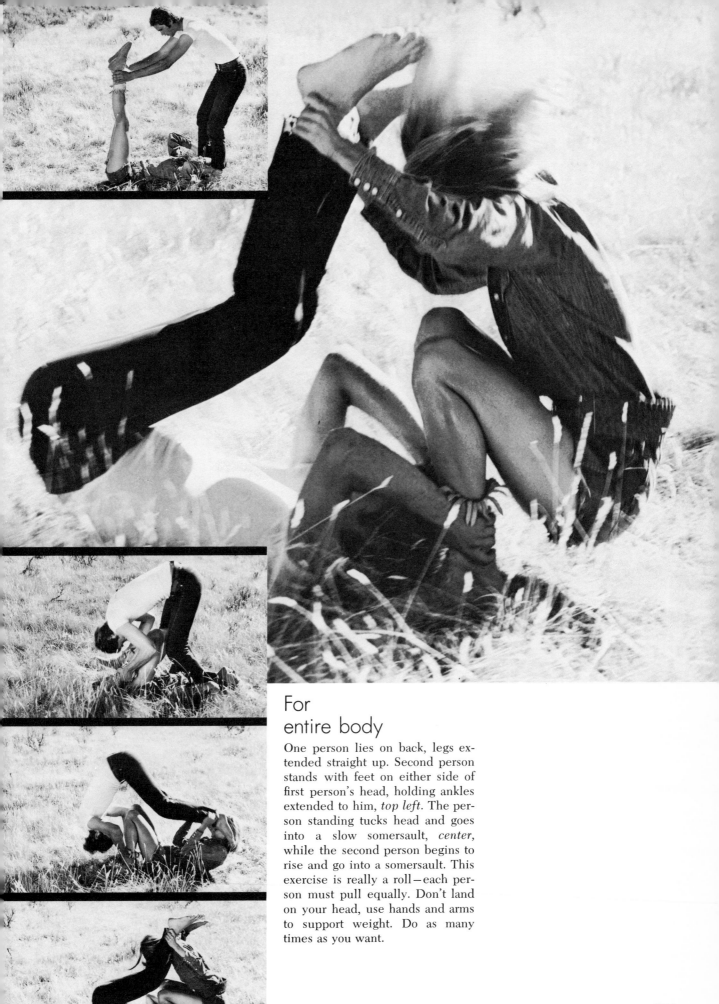

For
entire body

One person lies on back, legs extended straight up. Second person stands with feet on either side of first person's head, holding ankles extended to him, *top left*. The person standing tucks head and goes into a slow somersault, *center*, while the second person begins to rise and go into a somersault. This exercise is really a roll—each person must pull equally. Don't land on your head, use hands and arms to support weight. Do as many times as you want.

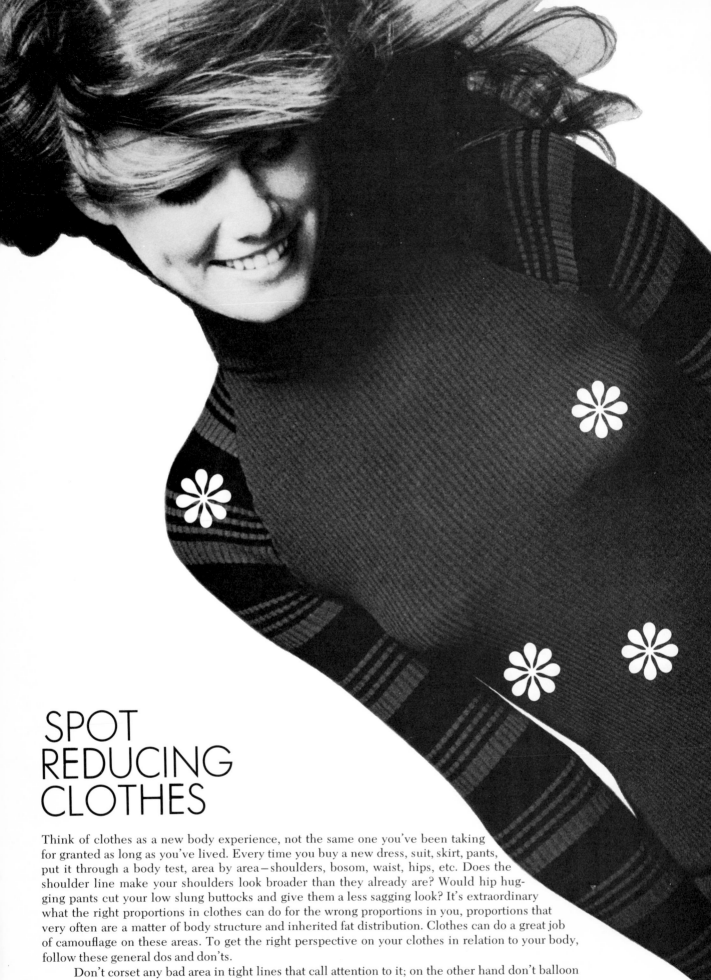

SPOT
REDUCING
CLOTHES

Think of clothes as a new body experience, not the same one you've been taking
for granted as long as you've lived. Every time you buy a new dress, suit, skirt, pants,
put it through a body test, area by area—shoulders, bosom, waist, hips, etc. Does the
shoulder line make your shoulders look broader than they already are? Would hip hug-
ging pants cut your low slung buttocks and give them a less sagging look? It's extraordinary
what the right proportions in clothes can do for the wrong proportions in you, proportions that
very often are a matter of body structure and inherited fat distribution. Clothes can do a great job
of camouflage on these areas. To get the right perspective on your clothes in relation to your body,
follow these general dos and don'ts.

     Don't corset any bad area in tight lines that call attention to it; on the other hand don't balloon
your body in no-shape mu-mu shapes which scream that you're obviously trying to cover something
up. The solution lies in between.

Heavy midriff and waist— Choose dress with long, slightly bloused or loose waistlines, or softly fitted A-shapes, long sweaters and jackets, tunics that don't cinch the waist but follow a shapely line of their own.

Skinny bony midriff and waist— Treat it the same way as the heavy one above.

Broad shoulders— No paddings, no puffed or dolman or leg-of-mutton sleeves, no big broad collars. Choose natural sleeve lines. No exaggeratedly bared necklines, halters or widely curved ones. You need V's or higher covered necks.

Small round shoulders— Nothing with gathers or a too-rounded cut-out back or drawstring neck. If you want to wear back décolletage choose deep V cut-outs or oblongs, never crescents. No puff sleeves, dolmans or leg-of-muttons. You'll look better with wrist-lengths which give an elongated look to the shoulders and arms or simply natural lined short sleeves or no sleeves at all.

Thin narrow shoulders and back— Wear big puffed sleeves, dolmans and leg-of-muttons, wide collars or natural sleeve lines in heavy fabrics to fill you out, wools, linens or their synthetic counterparts. Try to use clothes to fill out this fault.

Big bosoms— Choose lines that don't constrict them but flow softly over them. Don't cinch in your waist or wear tight shirts that make your top heaviness obvious by

contrast. Think in terms of your whole body, filling out the lower portions to match the top with skirts that move out from the figure in an A-shape or flare. No empire lines for the likes of you.

Small bosoms— This is not a real problem. (See section on picking the right bra for you.) Some of the chicest clothes are really made for almost bosomless girls. Don't try to puff yourself out in an exaggerated fashion. If you want a little lift, pick an oval-shaped non-bra bra with a bit of light fiber filling.

Big hips— Again don't constrict in tight-shaped skirts. Choose A's or soft pleats, gathers; sweaters or tunics that slide long and easily over the hips. Don't cinch in the waist. Try clothes that balance the problem by filling out the top half a bit. Always look at whatever you buy in terms of your total body proportions.

Large buttocks— Follow the same rules as those for hips above and pay particular attention to the dos and don'ts for pants and bathing suits that start on page 220.

No hips— No problem at all really, just pick shapes that fill them out, perhaps long-waisted dresses that flare or gather at the hips, or cinch in the waist with a belt over skirts that are gathered, pleated or flared. This way you create the curves you don't have to begin with.

Heavy legs— If the thighs are the problem follow the rules for big hips and see the sections on picking pants and bathing suits for your figure. If calves and ankles are heavy, wear dark-colored stockings, either sheer or opaque and stay away from the heavier textured ones. Be sure the heels of your shoes are thick enough to balance the bulk of your leg —no high, narrow heels.

Skinny legs— Fill them out with heavy or textured stockings, wear pants. Don't wear skirts that billow out so much they call attention to the thinness of your legs by contrast and make them look like two toothpicks trying to support a big potato.

Other leg problems, bow-knees, overall heaviness, thick ankles, etc.— Never take your eye off skirt lengths, develop a seventh sense for the right length and proportion to each piece of clothing you're wearing. You may have to adjust each hemline differently according to the shape of the skirt. Your mirror is your guide.

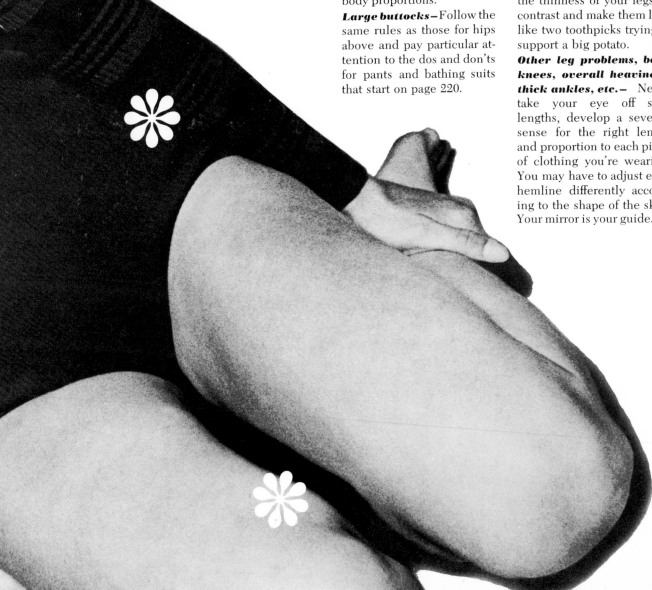

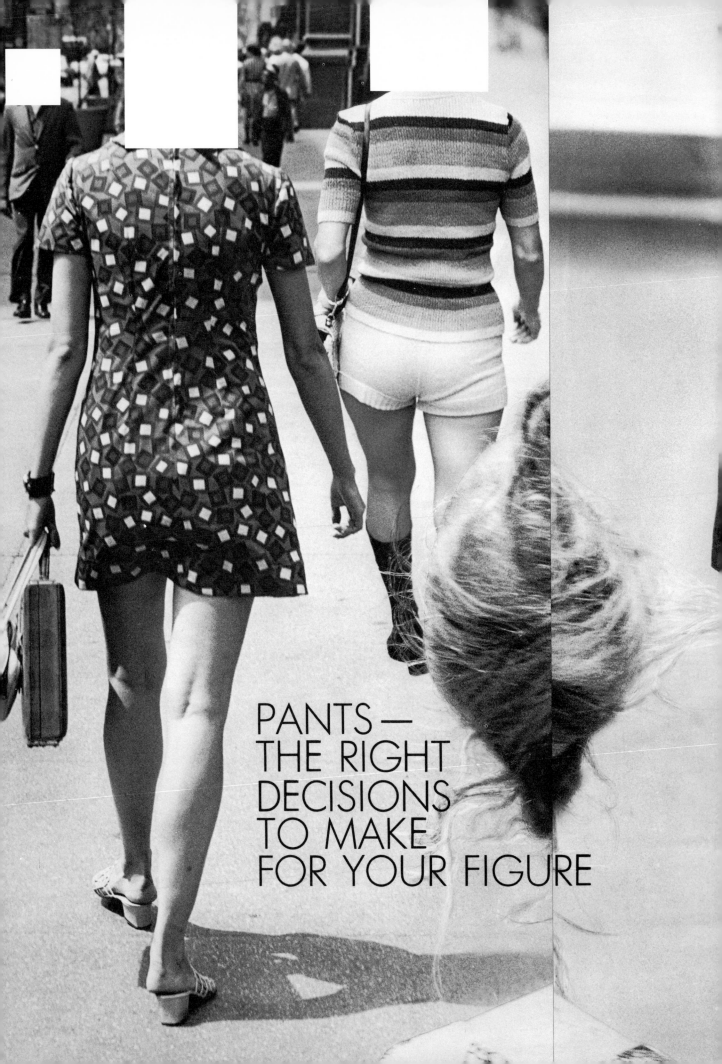

PANTS—
THE RIGHT
DECISIONS
TO MAKE
FOR YOUR FIGURE

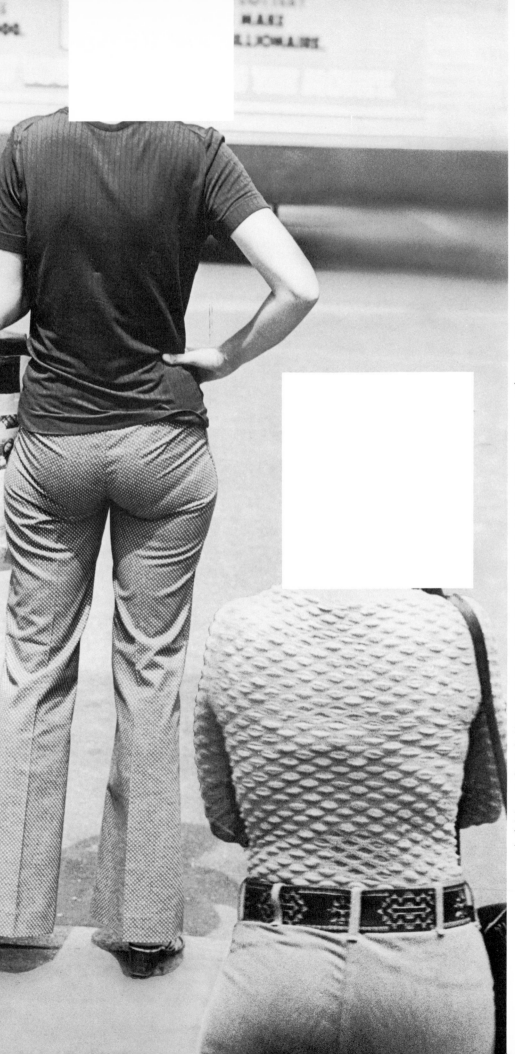

Making the right pants decisions for your figure involves, most of all, knowing the wrong ones. In the case of pants it's clearer to describe what looks don't work for certain figure problems than the ones that do. That's why we give you this list of

Pants don'ts

1. Don't think that a big bottom automatically rules out pants. Provided the size is within reason and not just negligently fat and saggy, you can wear wide-legged pants that fit but don't cup. Their width balances off your bottom's width. Add the help of a long covering jacket. Don't wear snug, tight-legged jeans.

2. If you have very long stilty legs, don't pick high-waisted or wide-waisted pants. The same goes for a figure that's disproportionately long from the waist down. Normal-waisted pants or, better still, hip huggers will cut the long lines. Also cut the length with shirts and sweaters and tunics worn outside of pants instead of tucked in.

3. Don't encase skinny long legs in skinny long pants either, they'll take to wider or pleated pants more appealingly.

4. If you have short legs, don't wear big long tunics and sweaters over your pants—they'll make them appear even shorter by extending the line from the shoulder to the hips or thighs. You're better looking in trim little shirts and sweaters tucked into pants that have a regular waistline.

5. Don't squeeze heavy legs into slim tailored pants, they're more at ease in soft, wide-legged pants.

PICK THE BATHING SUIT THAT'S BEST ON YOU

There's hardly anyone alive who is really uncritical of the way she looks in a bathing suit, but so much of it is do-nothing, depressing criticism. That's why we've grouped together here the usual figure complaints so that you can DO something about them by the cut, the color and pattern, the leg and torso length of the suit you pick. One of the first things to do before you start shopping is to take a good look at your figure in a full-length mirror and decide exactly what body type you are. Do you have a long or short torso, long or short legs? Too many girls really aren't familiar with their bodies. They don't know, for example, whether it's their torso or legs or both that need the illusion of length. Be imaginative about the solution to your figure problems—don't think that a skirt or dressmaker shorts are the only ways to hide heavy thighs or that a suit with a stiff, heavy inner bra is the only answer for a large bosom. And don't be so sure you can't wear a bikini. The right bikini is often a good camouflage for certain faults, like a slightly wide or low-slung bottom. And finally, never walk out of a store without putting the suit through an action test—bend, squat, stretch, sit; test it in front of the mirror on all sides.

If you're very thin, a good maillot with horizontal stripes is your best bet. A girl who is only slightly overweight could wear a suit with vertical stripes. It makes you appear slimmer. If you're really heavy, any pattern will make you look large, so be very careful when you buy.

You have to decide honestly how big you are. If you're not too bad, a bikini could cut the bigness from hip top to bottom. If you really have a problem, a one-piece maillot that fits smoothly down over the seat and well onto the thighs without bulging is the answer.

The girl with short legs should look for a suit that is cut high, like the one below. The higher the suit is cut, the longer your legs will look. Girls with legs that are too long and lanky should wear something with a longer leg, like the trim little shorts below. The slightly longer leg cuts the length.

If your midriff is thick or bulgy with no definable waist, stick to a one-piece suit that isn't fitted close to the body, like the ones below. The darker color helps to slim you; a small print could be flattering, too.

Both figures here are the same height, but the one on the left has a short torso, the other a long one. The left-hand one wants to achieve the longest possible body line: a suit that shows a long midriff. The best suit for the other figure is two-piece to cut the apparent length of the body.

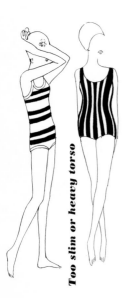

Too slim or heavy torso

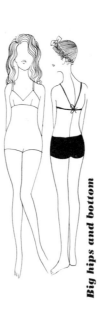

Big hips and bottom

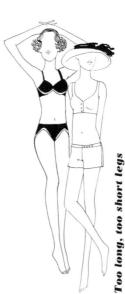

Too long, too short legs

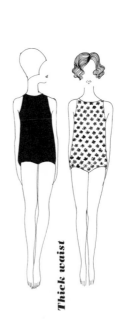

Thick waist

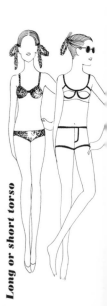

Long or short torso

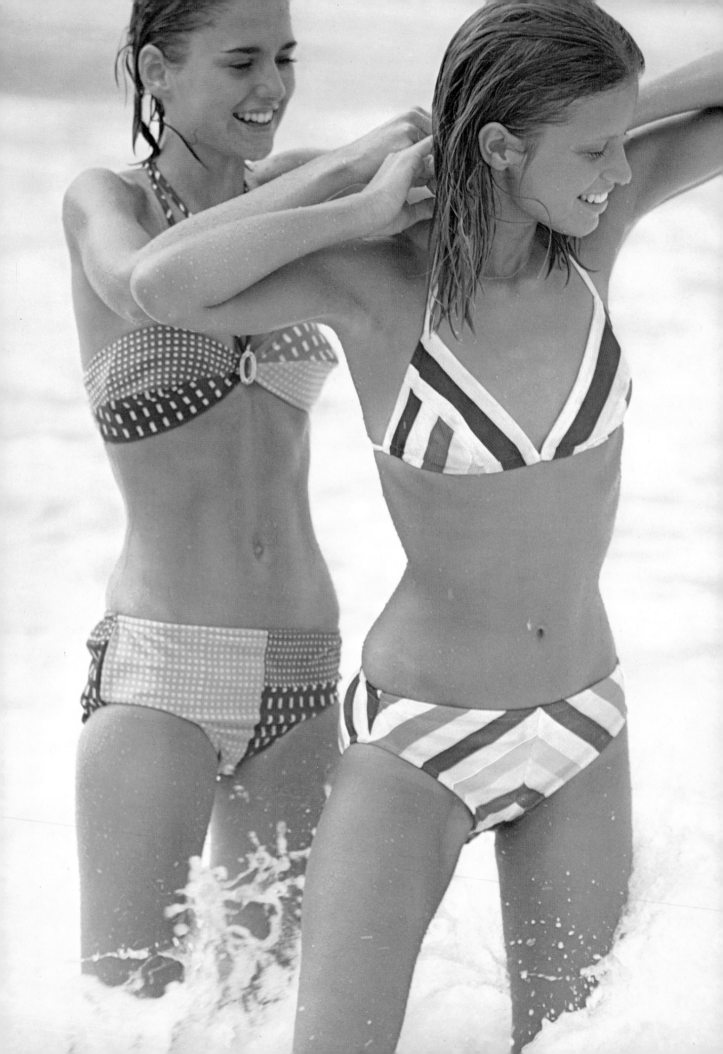

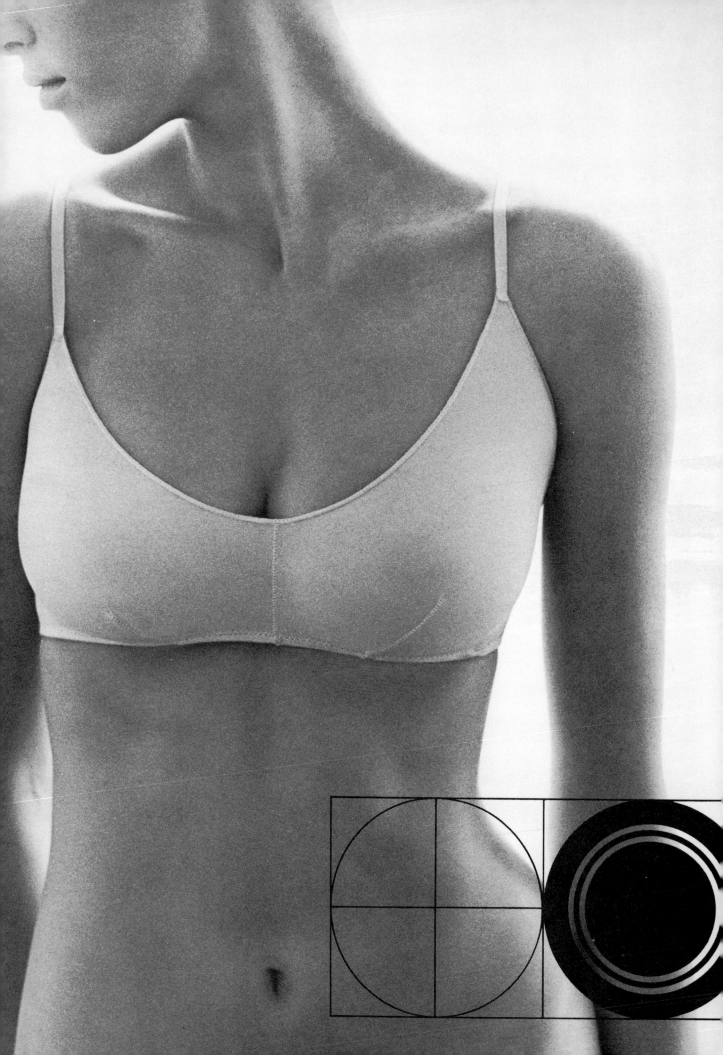

NO-BRA
OR NATURAL BOSOM LOOK

The no-bra or natural bosom look says simply that a woman accepts her body totally, that, liberated by The Pill, it is finally fully her own property, and that she is proud of every part of it *as it is!* The bosom appears now in its natural form, the ideal being neither big nor little but round, firm and proportionate to the individual body. Obviously the girl with a little less rather than more can go totally bra-less now if she is firm enough and wants to. Her luck has shifted after centuries of imbalance and preference (or prejudice) for voluptuousness. Today there's more democracy, but big girls aren't deprived either. There are as many perfectly cut and tailored natural bras for them as there are figures, all designed to look like no-bra and give only as much support as needed for comfort, not a seam or strap more (see the ranges on these pages).

You are bound to hear, though—if you haven't already—all the buts against the no-bra look: it's harmful to go without a bra; it stretches the bosom out of shape; it prevents you from nursing your baby; it gives you cancer—everything from the most reasonable medical doubts to the most outlandish accusations. That's why we asked a number of well-known New York gynecologists for a majority medical opinion. It's summed up in the words of Dr. Martin Stone of the New York Medical College: "There's nothing medically wrong with this fashion."

Even if a woman has large, pendulous breasts, do you still think it is not harmful to go without a bra?

Dr. Stone: "If the size of her breasts causes discomfort without support, she could relieve it with a brassière, but as far as causing any harm or changes in the breasts per se, the lack of support will not."

What about pregnant women?

Dr. Stone: "Again, support is beneficial in terms of comfort because of the pregnancy engorgement, the hyperplasia—that is, overgrowth of tissue—and the presence of milk in the breasts."

Is there any absolutely safe way of making breasts larger?

Dr. Stone: "The oversimplified answer is no. Plastic surgery is now being done with the injection of Silastic and other chemical products, but these all have the same problems. How effective they are, how long the increase lasts, and if there are side complications vary from case to case. There's no chemical means of making the breast larger on a permanent basis. Maybe with the new no-bra look women won't be interested so much in having their breasts made larger. I can't speak for any individual, but surgery is a drastic step and to me not really indicated."

"Pregnancy of course causes a temporary and sometimes permanent enlargement of the breast, but this is obviously not the reason anyone should get pregnant. The same goes for the Pill, which increases the breast size of most women. It's chief function is to prevent pregnancy, not to make women more voluptuous."

Is the enlargement caused by the Pill considerable?

Dr. Stone: "It depends on the woman's own tissue—in some cases there is a significant increase." (Editor's note: We know women who've gone from an A to C cup.)

Is there a decrease when the woman goes off The Pill each month or if she stops taking it altogether?

Dr. Stone: "Yes. When she is off the Pill the bosom regresses, but the regression is only slight during the monthly abstinence, and as soon as she starts back the size will increase again."

What about methods of making breasts smaller?

Dr. Stone: "It can be done by plastic surgery, but again this is a drastic step which I don't think is indicated except in some cases of extreme abnormal size. One type of surgery being done for this definitely deprives the breast of its nursing function, and another promises possible retention of the ability to breast feed but cannot assure it."

Does dieting affect the bosom size?

Dr. Stone: "There is fat tissue in the bosom, too, so that a woman who is generally overweight or underweight and who diets successfully will usually show a reduction or increase in the bosom as well as in the rest of her body."

Does exercise do anything for the size of the breast?

Dr. Stone: "It can develop the muscles underlying the glandular and fat tissue of the bosom to correct sagging and give the bosom a lift, but it can't change the actual size. There are no muscles in the bosom itself to be developed by exercise."

Will exercise do anything for bosoms that are droopy after nursing and pregnancy?

Dr. Stone: "Exercise can be effective but it cannot do a 100 percent job of correction. The degree depends on the woman's body build, muscular structure, whether or not she is a placid or phlegmatic person who has never been active in sports or physical work."

Does breast feeding encourage more sagging than is normal in pregnancy?

225

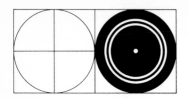

Dr. Stone: "No. In fact, sagging is more apt to be furthered by the more marked breast engorgement seen in non-nursing mothers."

Does breast size have anything to do with the supply of milk for the baby?

Dr. Stone: "No. Oriental women, whose breasts are small by American standards, are among the best nursers in the world."

What do you advise women about the care of their bosoms?

Dr. Stone: "They should visit a gynecologist once a year for checks against breast cancer and learn how to do a self-examination every month or so. Their gynecologist can easily show them how to check for lumps or any sign of abnormal change so that these can be picked up quickly and treated early. The American Cancer Society also has publications and excellent movies for teaching women to do self-examinations, and these are available at local units all over the country. It is a simple procedure and has been very effective. There are, of course, newer techniques, such as mammography, which help detect lesions which are perhaps only questionable or not even palpable. There are doctors who believe that every woman over forty ought to have a mammography regularly."

Aren't there certain times in the menstrual cycle when lumps can be felt in the bosom? Should anything be done?

Dr. Stone: "During the premenstrual phase of the cycle many women experience breast fullness and discomfort, and in some instances areas of multiple cysts are present. These do not feel like distinct lumps, although a woman giving herself an examination might become confused. The hard tissue areas should be diagnosed by a doctor and treated."

What can be done about breast enlargement and soreness during the menstrual period?

Dr. Stone: "The enlargement and the soreness are due to fluid retention that is a result of hormonal changes in the body at that time. Some women can get relief from mild measures such as a diuretic or drug that helps to eliminate some of the fluid."

Is the size and shape of the breast hereditary?

Dr. Stone: "Like all body build, breast structure is related to heredity, influenced by nutrition and other factors."

Is hair on the breast a widespread problem among women?

Dr. Stone: "No. The hair that's sometimes found around the areola of the nipple isn't heavy. It can be cut off with a scissors, or if a woman does not find it uncomfortable, she can pluck out the hairs."

Could we go into a few old wives' tales about the breast and dispel them? Knocking the breast causing cancer, for instance?

Dr. Stone: "More often than not, when a women turns out to have a tumor of the breast, benign or malignant, she can remember knocking her breast and post hoc says that's the fault. It is rare though that such a trauma causes the cancer."

What about sex enlarging the breast? Is that more of an old maid's than an old wives' tale?

Dr. Stone: "Manual stimulation of the breast in sex won't make it larger, neither will intercourse."

Are there any more questions about breasts that you think women should have straight answers on?

Dr. Stone: "No, but I repeat, there's nothing wrong about the no-bra fashion for women's bosoms."

So freed of any medical doubts about the no-bra look's advisability, you can take any attitude you want about its aesthetics.

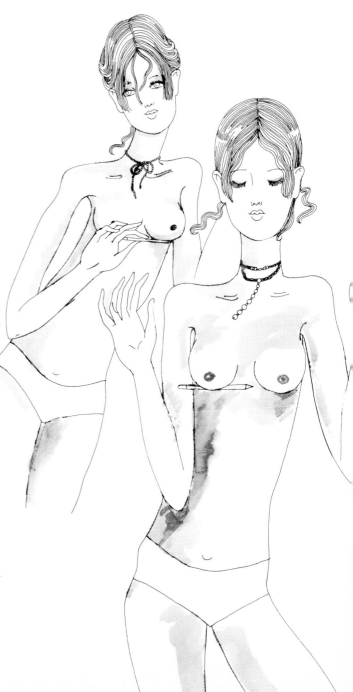

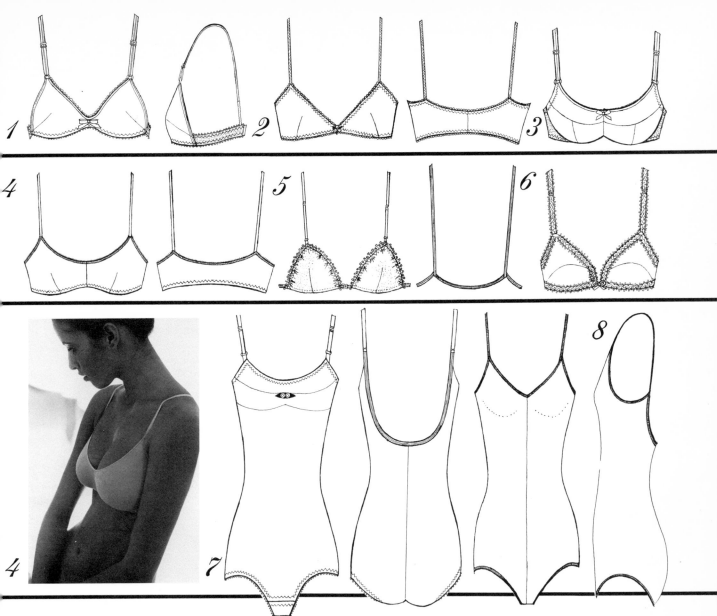

Any of the bras or body-stockings here will give you a soft, natural-line no-bra look. There's one for almost every sort of bosom. The chart at right tells which of them will work best for your figure. Full-bosomed girls can have underwiring in a natural bra; see 3. And for a bra with movable cups spaced exactly the way your bosoms are there is one with sliding cups on an elastic band; see 5. Left: The pencil test is a good indication of whether you'll look good without a bra. Put it at the base of one breast, see sketch. If it falls you can toss away your bra; if it stays put, you'd better wear a bra with most clothes.

BOSOM TYPE	1	2	3	4	5	6	7	8	NO BRA
small and firm (A cup)	✓	✓		✓	✓	✓	✓	✓	yes
medium and firm (B cup)	✓	✓	✓	✓	✓	✓	✓	✓	yes
large and firm (C cup)	✓	✓	✓	✓			✓		?
extra large and firm (D cup)			✓				✓		no
small and unfirm (A cup)	✓	✓		✓		✓	✓		?
medium and unfirm (B cup)	✓	✓	✓			✓	✓		no
large and unfirm (C cup)			✓						no
extra large and unfirm (D cup)			✓						no

Find your figure type in the column, then read across the chart. Wherever you see a check mark, the bra or bodystocking that corresponds to the number checked is a good one for you.

SUPER NAILS
THE PROS TELL YOU HOW

If you were to have the very best manicure money could buy, what would you get? We asked a handful of nail care experts in New York to let us in on what it is that makes a manicure professional. Here's what we got—a whole list of manicure tips in steps from shaping to polishing, a complete how-to on nail buffing, first aid measures for problem nails, plus health-building nail hints. See them on these four pages.

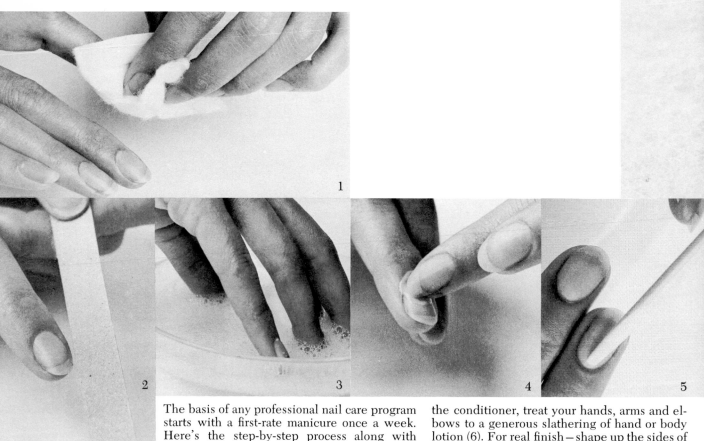

The basis of any professional nail care program starts with a first-rate manicure once a week. Here's the step-by-step process along with some great tips: Start by removing every trace of nail polish. A cotton square or puff saturated with polish remover is best (1). If some polish remains around the edge of the nail, remove it gently with a cotton-tipped stick dipped in remover. Then, with an emery board, file your nails to the rounded oval shape you see in (2). The pros' advice here: Avoid filing to close to the fingertip at the edge of the nail and file gently in one direction from underneath the nail to discourage chips or splits. If you're trimming away a lot of nail, Mimi at The Kenneth Salon suggests soaking in lukewarm water until the nail is softened, then cutting away excess with nail scissors before smoothing the edges with an emery board. When all the nails are shaped, soak in warm sudsy water for two or three minutes until your cuticles are softened (3). Then massage a conditioning cuticle cream or oil into the base of the nail (4). Gently nudge the cuticle back with a fine-tipped orangewood stick (5). While you're letting cuticles soak up the conditioner, treat your hands, arms and elbows to a generous slathering of hand or body lotion (6). For real finish—shape up the sides of your fingertips too. Trim hangnails with small cuticle scissors (7), but never trim the cuticle itself—this causes more hangnails and toughens the cuticle. Then with the fine side of your emery board, smooth any hardened skin at the edges of your fingertips (8). Dip your fingers into the warm soapy water again and gently clean with a soft nail brush to remove every trace of oil or cream (9). Dry your fingers with a terry towel (10). One of the manicurists suggests that whenever you dry your hands, make a point of gently pushing your cuticles back with a towel. After hands have been in water, the skin is more pliable and you'll help discourage overgrown cuticles. If the tips of your nails need whitening, run a white nail pencil under them or use a special undernail paste (11). If you're going to buff your nails, or if you have any nail splits or breaks that need mending (see the next page), this is the time to do it. If you want to polish your nails, here's the pro way: Apply base coat first—it's the foundation

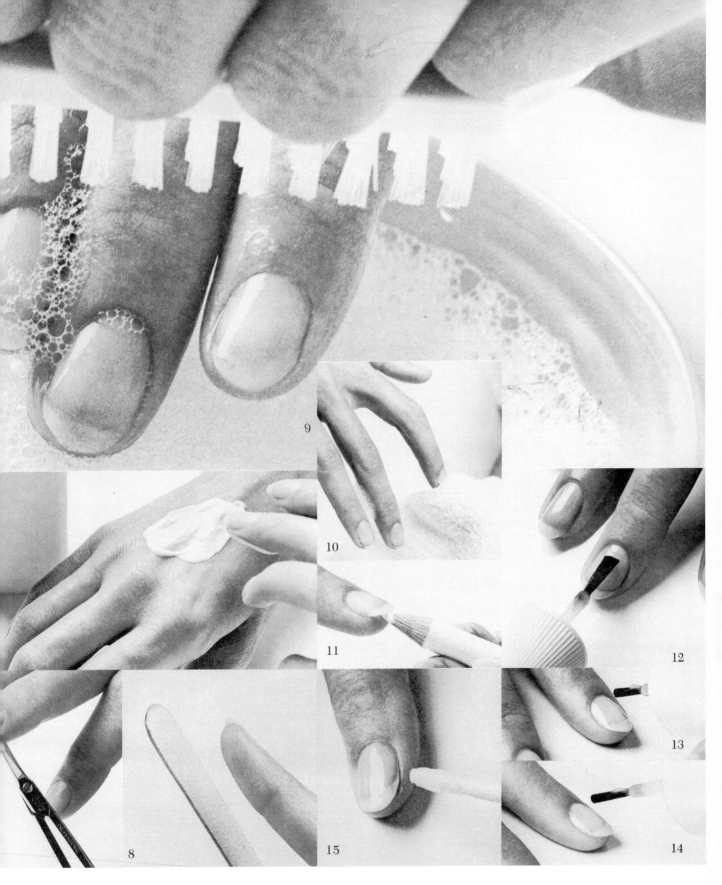

of any good polish job because it gives the polish a surface to stick to and, therefore, lasts longer (12). Then apply two coats of polish (13). To avoid small nicks or smears, let all applications dry at least one minute between coats. And for the smoothest results, apply each coat of polish in as few strokes as possible—our experts say three should do it. Brush from the base of the nail to the tip—the first stroke down the middle of the nail, then one stroke down each side. A top coat or sealer gives polish extra shine, staying power (14). For a neat finish, run an orangewood stick tipped with cotton and dampened with polish remover along the outside of the cuticle and fingertip to clear any smudges of polish (15). Be especially careful with polished nails for an hour or so after polishing.

BUFFING

is one of the best beauty treatments you can give your nails, either as a pre-polish rev-up to stir blood circulation or as a polish in itself. Buffing with a paste gives nails a natural gloss finish. If you've never tried it before, why not start now? You owe it to your nails. But be sure to start at the beginning—with a perfect manicure (follow all the professional steps up to 11 on the preceding pages). Next dab buffing paste over your nails and buff gently in one direction with a nail buffer or soft chamois cloth. If you want a faint pink shine, try a tinted buffing paste. If you want nothing but a clear natural shine, there are colorless pastes too. If you want to buff your nails before putting on polish—simply to promote circulation—then skip the paste. (It would make the surface too glossy for the polish to stick). Buff about a minute on each finger. If your nail feels warm, ease up—you're pressing too hard. You need only the gentlest pressure to bring out the natural shine. This routine suggested by the specialists at Nails by Nena.

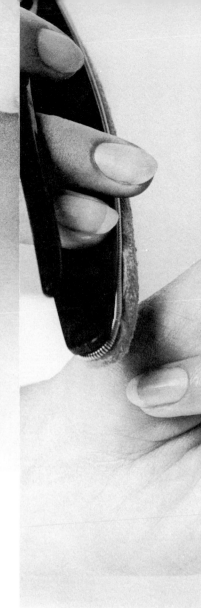

NAIL HEALTH

Softness or brittleness is a sure sign that your nails need help—probably inside and out. Nails are made of protein, so if yours aren't in top condition, it may be because you're not eating enough protein-building foods like meat, eggs, cheese, milk. Yvonne Sergent, corrective nail-care specialist at Saks Fifth Avenue, recommends that you massage a nail cream into your cuticles and nails nightly. A good manicure is another help—shorter, well-shaped nails are generally stronger. Buffing is more than a beauty treat—it's a nail health treatment. It revs up circulation to help build stronger nails. Soft or brittle nails have a tendency to layer, flake and split or crack. If these complications set in, keep your nails short, be especially careful when filing them (see step 2 on the preceding page) and lubricate them with hand cream or a liquid protein conditioner. The problem will be solved when your nails are nourished, conditioned back to health. Be patient. One doctor says it takes about six months to grow a new healthy nail. Meantime, go easy on polishes.

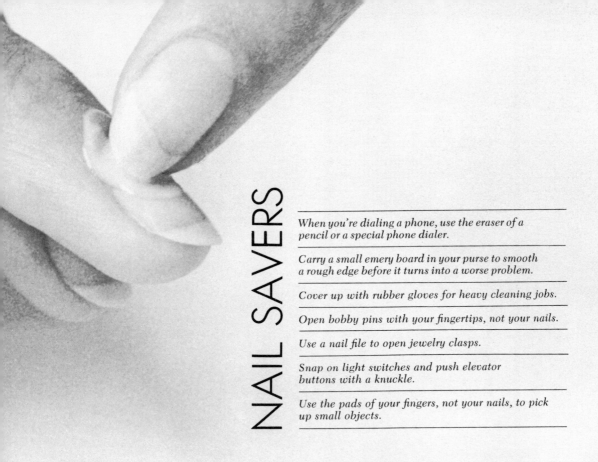

NAIL SAVERS

When you're dialing a phone, use the eraser of a pencil or a special phone dialer.

Carry a small emery board in your purse to smooth a rough edge before it turns into a worse problem.

Cover up with rubber gloves for heavy cleaning jobs.

Open bobby pins with your fingertips, not your nails.

Use a nail file to open jewelry clasps.

Snap on light switches and push elevator buttons with a knuckle.

Use the pads of your fingers, not your nails, to pick up small objects.

MENDING

Don't give up on an otherwise-healthy half-broken or chipped nail. Mend it. There are kits to buy at cosmetic counters with everything you need, but you can do it with things you already have at home too. You can use any fibrous sheer tissue like eyeglass-cleaning tissues or paper facial blotters and regular household cement or glue. First tear off a small piece of tissue large enough to cover the break or chip with a little left over to tuck under your nail (1). Brush the patch evenly with household glue, then put it on your nail, wet side down (2). Smooth the surface lightly with an orangewood stick so there aren't any ripples in the tissue. Trim the tissue lapping over the edge of the nail with cuticle scissors (3), but leave enough to tuck under the nail. If glue gets on the scissors, wipe it off with polish remover. To tuck the edge of the patch under your nail, dab a little glue on the overhang and smooth it under the nail tip with an orangewood stick. Continue smoothing until all the ripples are evened out (4). A little polish remover on the edge of the stick helps in smoothing. Then a little glue under the nail on the patch seals your mending job (5). Polish with a base coat, two coats of nail enamel and a top coat (6). See the rewarding finished patch-up job (7).

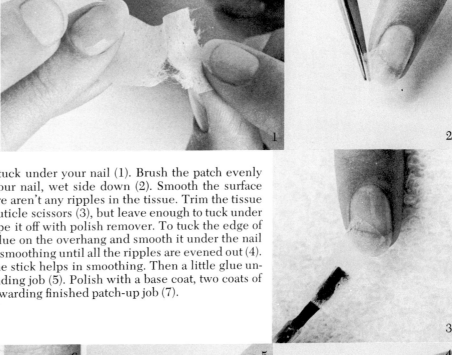

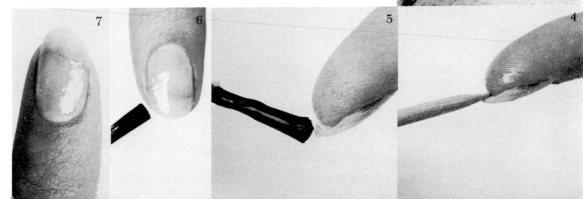

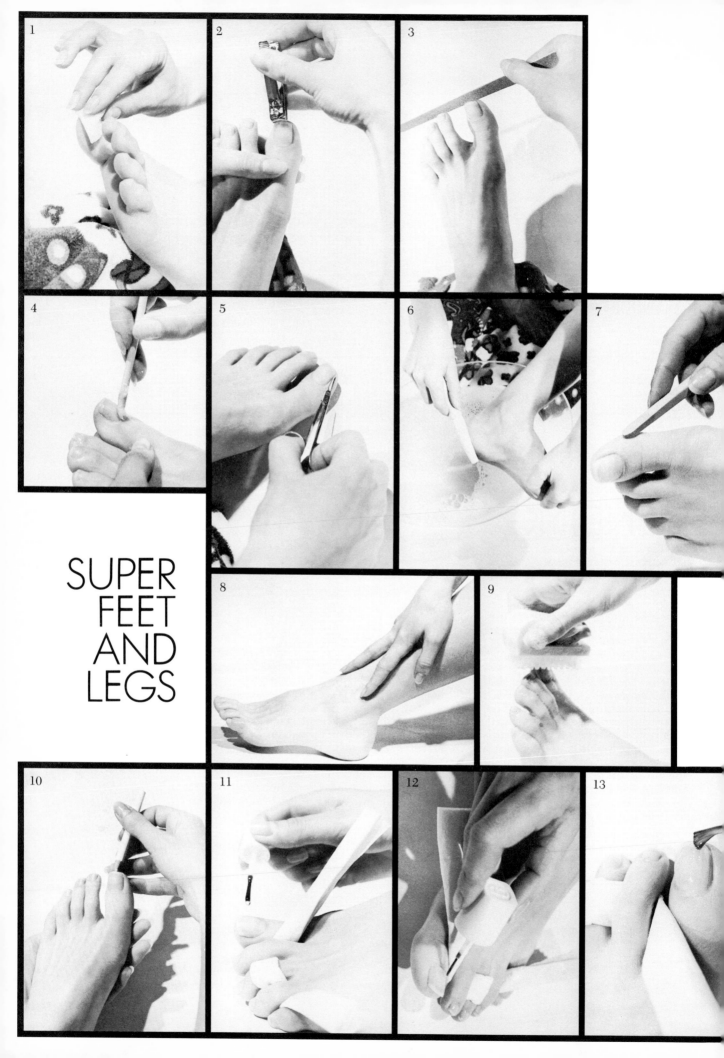

SUPER
FEET
AND
LEGS

POLISHED FEET

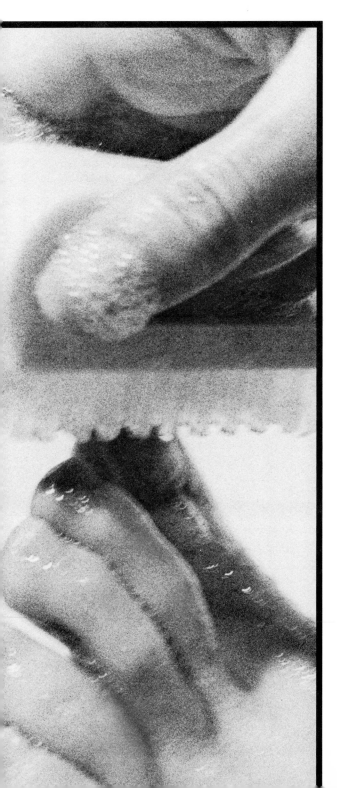

Polished feet are a must if you're going to bare them—and who isn't—in bed, on a furry rug, on the beach or in sandals. All it takes to get that polish is a good pedicure every two or three weeks. Here's how to give yourself one: Start by soaking your feet in warm sudsy water, one foot at a time. Then use a good bristle brush, like the one to the left on this page, to scrub them. Remove any old polish, 1, and trim water-softened toenails with clippers, leaving nail edges squared, 2. File rough edges with an emery board, no closer than one-eighth inch from the sides, 3. This helps discourage ingrown nails. Now put cuticle oil around the cuticles and gently ease them back with an orange-wood stick wrapped with cotton, 4. Trim off any rough or excess cuticle, 5, but be careful to cut *only* the excess or you'll make the area around the nail sore. When both feet are finished, start pumicing your heels with a wet pumice stone, 6. Work pumice around heel and on sole of each foot. (Try to pumice lightly every night as part of your bath routine.) A smaller, finer-grained one is good for toes, 7. After pumicing, cream feet and legs with rich lotion, 8, then scrub *toenails only* with a brush to remove any cream, 9. A nail-whitening pencil used under each nail will give them a pretty finish, 10. Now you're ready for polish. Fold a tissue into a strip and weave it between toes to separate them and to keep polish from smudging, 11. Apply base coat, then two coats of a pretty shell color if you like, 12, 13. While polish is drying, slip into a pair of wide-open sandals, *below*.

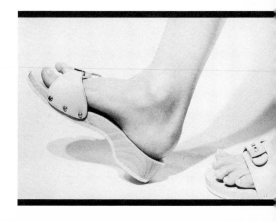

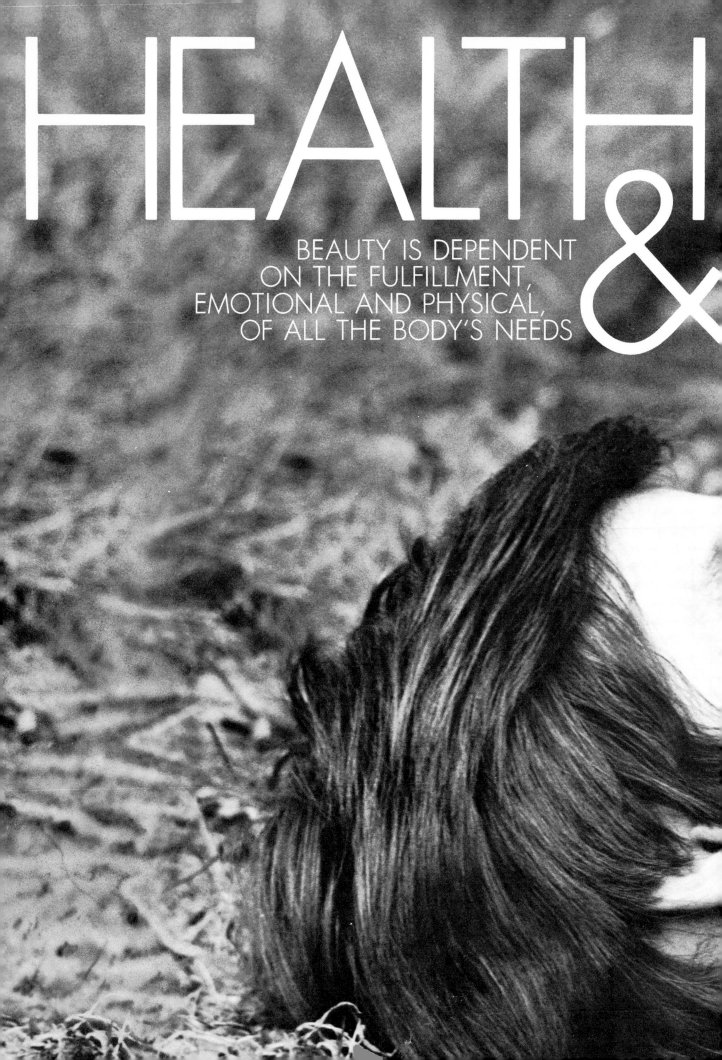

HEALTH &

BEAUTY IS DEPENDENT
ON THE FULFILLMENT,
EMOTIONAL AND PHYSICAL,
OF ALL THE BODY'S NEEDS

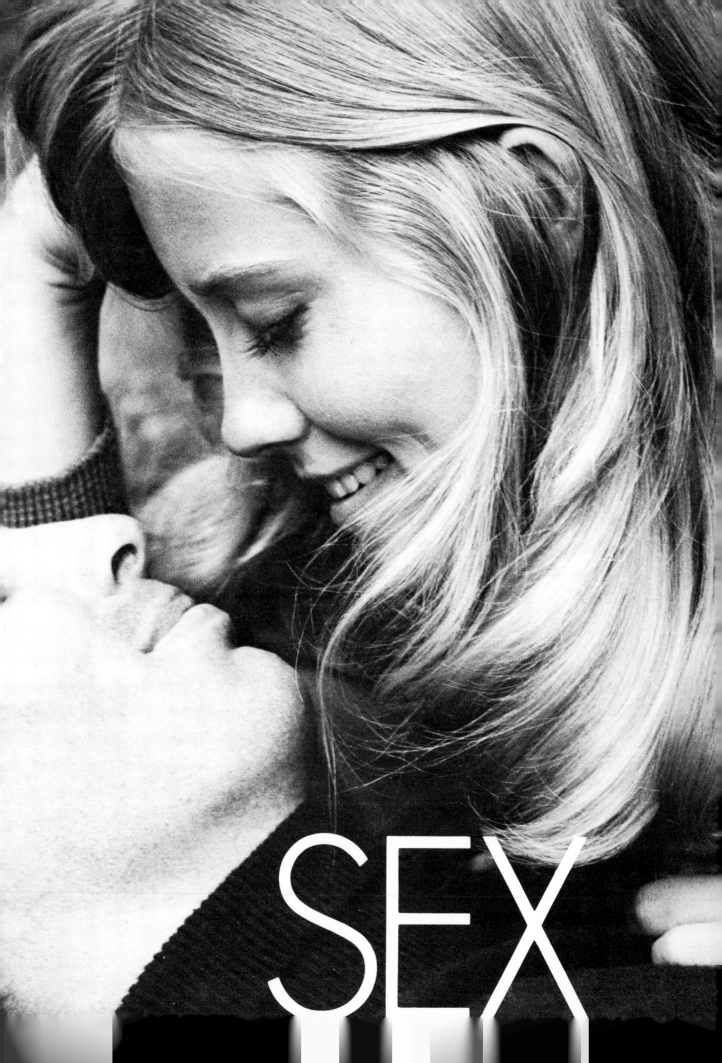

SEX

HEALTH
AND
SEX

There is a freshness and life about the healthiest bodies that add up to a special kind of beauty—even the most perfect features and figure can't compensate for it when it's lacking. Its presence depends on the fulfillment, emotional and physical, of all the body's needs. That is why a woman's sex life eventually becomes a factor in her beauty. As the famous psychiatrist Charles W. Socarides said, "No aspect of women's lives can be untouched by the rewards of fulfilled sexuality, or conversely, impoverished by blighted sexuality."

Until the 70's many young women's sexual lives were shadowed by mystery and misinformation. Many still are. But this is not a healthy situation, and it is not one that has to be. With the present openness about sexuality there is no reason why any young woman should suffer anxiety, fear and ignorance about her sexual desires and functions. Women's magazines discuss these matters frankly in almost every issue. There are any number of excellent and serious books published on sexuality, books that have made or come close to best seller status in the last few years. Here in this chapter of the Glamour Beauty Book you will find a collection of articles that will give you some of the basic information that young women need to know about gynecological problems, menstruation, contraceptives, current sexual misconceptions and attitudes plus a guide for establishing a clear understanding of your requirements from your doctors—the family physician, gynecologist, obstetrician or whatever kind of specialist you may have to consult.

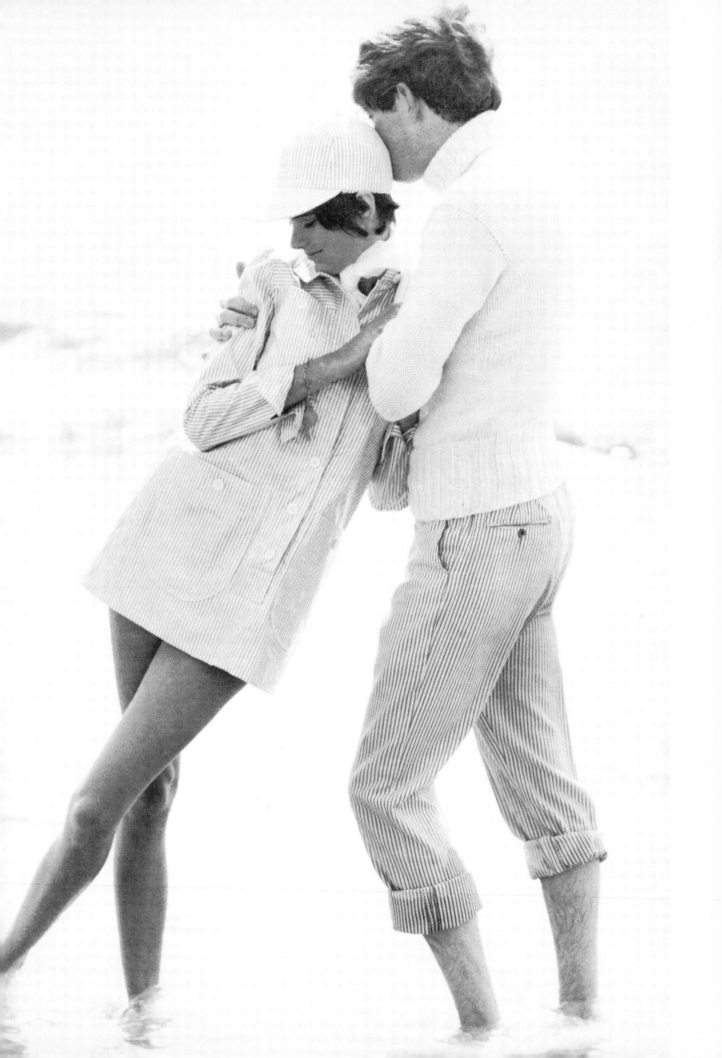

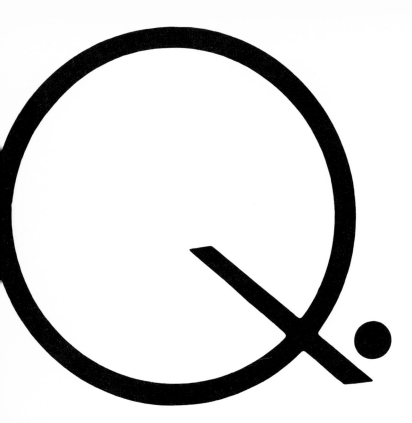

QUESTIONS TO ASK YOUR DOCTOR

About Sex,
Pains, Operations,
Even Imaginary Symptoms
And the Importance
Of Speaking Frankly
With Him,
Even When
It's Embarrassing

by Cyril Solomon, M.D.

You have decided to consult a physician. You have sat in his office, waiting for your turn. You have been asked questions, some of which have seemed irrelevant to your original complaint. You have been poked and prodded, examined; you have had blood and urine taken from you. Finally, you reach the inner sanctum.

You may think, at this point, that the rest is up to the doctor. But it isn't entirely. It is at this point that you can help yourself and him as well.

First, have a pen and paper ready to take notes. In addition, have some questions ready to ask.

I know of no physician who does not welcome questions from patients. You, of course, have no way of knowing which of your questions are pertinent. But it's much better to ask some that may seem silly than to risk omitting something that may be important. I can recall a patient to whom I was about to give a clean bill of health when she asked me if there was anything to be done for a persistent itch. This is a warning symptom of diabetes—and subsequent tests proved that she was an incipient diabetic!

Your doctor does not know how much you really know about yourself. The only clues he has are the questions you ask him. Unfortunately, not many patients think to ask. In one survey of a group of doctors and patients, one third of all the patients involved never asked a single question during repeated visits, even after the doctor had given the diagnosis and prescription.

Your doctor is probably over thirty, but you've got to trust somebody. He may know your mother and father, but he also reads the medical literature that stresses the importance of privacy for you, even though your parents press him to the wall. Doctors and young patients must understand the problems of communication that may exist. One way is for the patient to take the initiative. She must try to make the doctor aware, through the questions she asks, of her own life patterns, which may be quite different from his.

Young women frequently come to doctors because of disturbances that are sex-related. These should be discussed frankly and openly. Although many of your generation are living by a set of values which is different from the mores of the 1940's, this does not mean that all of you are necessarily well-informed about sex. You may think you know, but many of you do not—as evidenced by the number of young girls coming to doctors these days with unwanted pregnancies. (At the present time, about one out of twelve babies is born out of wedlock, and one survey shows that 10 percent of all women in this country have had a pre-marital pregnancy.) Practically all women who visit doctors are curious about the Pill and want to know more about contraception. Most women, especially young women, are woefully ignorant about the norms of sexual adjustment. Ask questions about these things. In today's society, there should be no problems that cannot be discussed in a doctor's office. If your doctor is embarrassed by these questions, that is his problem, not yours. Bring them up anyway. If he feels that he cannot, or doesn't wish to, advise you on matters relating to sex, he will undoubtedly refer you to someone who can be of help to you. It is very important that you be able to communicate fully with your doctor. (In fact, that should be a factor in choosing a doctor in the first place.)

Our present culture is designed for rebellion, if sometimes only symbolic rebellion. It provides support for sexual experimentation, drug usage and hippie behavior. It questions all authority. Many who are in school feel that education is another name for baby sitting. Resentments spring up against parents, school, the law. You may be troubled by emotional conflicts within this framework but feel that there is no one you can ask about them. Ask your doctor about these feelings. He can help you put them in perspective and help advise you on whether they indicate a need for help.

If your doctor feels that psychiatric help is indicated, you should know that psychiatry is going through a revolution. Psychiatrists today deal with patients within their own community, which means a psychiatrist will consider and treat your problems in the context of your values, mores and life-style, not your parents'.

Serious diseases are rare in the eighteen to twenty-four age group. The physical complaints that turn up most frequently are obesity, skin disorders, allergies and diseases related to the female genital tract: Menstrual disorder, painful menstruation, vaginal discharges and cystitis, or related urinary tract disturbances. Some of these and other complaints may be emotional in origin; it has been established in many surveys that about 50 percent of the complaints young women bring to the doctor's office are psychogenic, even though they may be masked by or accompanied by physical symptoms. Doctor and patient must relate to each other in order to discover what the real problem is.

When you are ill and undergoing, or about to undergo, a course of treatment, there are certain general questions that should be asked, regardless of the ailment:

1. The reasons for laboratory and X-ray tests.
2. The test results.
3. The cause of the illness.
4. Why treatment is instituted—what does it consist of and how well does it correct the problem?
5. The prognosis? Can I work, how long may I feel tired or in pain?
6. The complications of the disease.
7. The complications of the treatment itself.
8. The cost of the examination and treatment and the coverage by insurance.

Get the financial questions out of the way early. Don't be afraid to ask your doctor what it's going to cost. In return, be frank with him about your financial resources. Some expenses may be adjusted according to ability to pay. Your doctor or his secretary can explain to you fully what you are entitled to under your insurance coverage, plus provide you with forms and help you fill them out.

If you are to be operated upon, you will want to know the following:

1. What is to be done?
2. What, if anything, is to be taken out of you?
3. What will the removal of an organ or part of an organ do to you?
4. What is the usual length of hospitalization and convalescence?
5. What pain or discomfort can you expect?
6. When can you go back to work?

If you are concerned about the Pill, discuss it thoroughly with your doctor before taking it. Ask what symptoms should make you discontinue the Pill. Ask about abnormal vaginal bleeding, ask about weight gain and swelling of your legs, ask about the incidence of blood clots and other symptoms. Ask about psychological changes, gastrointestinal symptoms. If you have a baby, ask about nursing while on the Pill. What happens if you forget to take one or more?

When you are given a prescription for any medication, ask exactly what it is. It may be a drug you have been sensitive to before. Ask what the drug usually does and ask what the complications of taking it may be. Ask whether you can have alcoholic drinks or whether any food should be avoided while you are taking the drug. Ask whether the new drug can be taken along with some other medication which you might be taking.

If your problems are emotional, try to expose your fears and anxieties. Ask questions. Your problems may turn out to be part of a normal sequence. You may be depressed in the aftermath of some viral infection. If you are given tranquilizers or mood-elevating drugs, ask how soon you can expect relief. You will want to know if, or at what point you might need psychiatric help.

Mutual understanding is essential to a good doctor-patient relationship and is best achieved when the patient takes the initiative by asking questions. And a good continuing relationship with your doctor is vital to your well-being, now and in the future.

In a time when science has taken over and computer language has become the medium of communication, it is especially important to hold onto the humanizing factors in your life. One of the best places for you to start is in your doctor's office.

WHAT WOMEN WON'T ASK AND DOCTORS DON'T TELL THEM ABOUT MENSTRUATION

by Phyllis Starr
with Robert W. Kistner, M.D.

Almost everyone thinks everyone talks openly and unprudishly about everything today. But who does about menstruation? It is one of the last living taboos of our society. Although women menstruate every month of most of their adult lives, it remains to many of them a mysterious problem that they won't discuss with their doctors or that their doctors don't, or won't, talk about sympathetically to them.

More intelligent talk and less callousness and skittishness could do a lot to relieve the situation, which is nearly international. In a study done on accident prevention in Great Britain, 10,000 working women indicated that they were accident-prone a few days before and during menstruation. Certain European countries regard premenstrual tension as "temporary insanity." In the U.S. 70 percent of women experience this tension, and 120 million working days a year are lost because of it and other menstrual disorders. In one British prison, half of 156 newly convicted women committed their crimes just before or during menstruation.

One of the best men to do the talking about menstruation is Dr. Robert Kistner, a leader in gynecological research and a professor at the Harvard Medical School. He speaks clearly, easily and unselfconsciously, as if he were telling you about your sinuses. "Painful periods, premenstrual tension, even gynecological diseases as severe as endometriosis, are suffered and accepted by an unestimatable number of women, when they could be helped by a kind and interested doctor," he said.

Women are full of misconceptions even about the purpose of menstruation, one of the first things Dr. Kistner puts his patients straight about. Menstruation does not cleanse the body of poisons; that's an old wives' tale that hangs on obstinately. Menstruation is the casting off of the lining of the womb, which has been thickened or built up by the two hormones, estrogen and progesterone, secreted by the ovary to make the womb receptive for the implantation of the fertilized egg, in other words, to becoming pregnant. It has no other purpose, Dr. Kistner said. It is good for only one thing.

Most women have roughly a twenty-eight day cycle, during which estrogen builds up the womb-lining tissue for fourteen days. Then ovulation, or the shedding of eggs from the ovary, occurs, and for the next fourteen days a combination of estrogen and progesterone continues the building process. At the end of this time a woman menstruates unless an egg has become fertilized and she is pregnant. Since the cycle is frequently not exact, doctors advise that anyone who wants to become pregnant is most likely to do so between the twelfth day after menstruation and the sixteenth. That gives two days before and after the fourteenth day when ovulation should occur. But Dr. Kistner quotes a colleague: "There is nothing so regular about

1 2 3 4 5 6 7 8

a woman's menstrual cycle as its irregularity." Some women have a twenty-one to twenty-three-day cycle, and for them this is perfectly normal; others, a thirty-two- to thirty-five-day cycle. A woman who has a twenty-eight-day cycle might in one cycle, for an unknown reason, ovulate on day nine. If she does and has intercourse without using a contraceptive, she'll get pregnant. It is possible, too, for a woman who observes certain practices of the Jewish faith which forbid her intercourse during and for a time after menstruation and who ovulates close to the last day of her period to be infertile. Such a patient may be given estrogen to hold off ovulation until the fourteenth day. There have been cases of conception with intercourse occurring seven days prior to ovulation and no other intercourse intervening, even though the human egg is capable of being fertilized for only about twenty-four hours. The sperm, however, can live as many as seven days, although forty-eight to seventy-two hours is generally regarded as maximum survival time.

Of course, ovulation cannot be detected in advance, only retrospectively by charting a basal body temperature. If a menstrual period (sometimes even two or three) is missed, this is not cause for serious concern, particularly if a woman has been under emotional strain, or moving from one town or college to another, or traveling or has gone on a strict diet. If she is on the Pill, she can expect to miss periods. But if she is not and is worried after missing a period that she is pregnant, it is helpful to know that pregnancy can now be diagnosed by the new types of tests—not the old rabbit or frog—as early as seven to ten days, definitely two weeks, after the expected first day of the missed period, i.e., about twenty-one to twenty-eight days from ovulation.

In treating menstrual disorders, the contraceptive pill has been of enormous value to girls and women of all ages—from ten to fourteen, when most girls in the United States and the United Kingdom begin to menstruate, up to age fifty or fifty-two, when menstrual periods cease completely because of menopause. (Menopause will not be included in this article since it is outside of GLAMOUR'S average readership age.) Certain problems are actually more prevalent in one age group than another and can be talked about with the same chronological regularity that Gesel & Ilg talk about the growth symptoms of children.

Excessive and irregular bleeding in early teen-age girls

Frequently when a girl first starts to bleed, her periods tend to be rather irregular and profuse because she is not ovulating, and ovulation is what brings about the pattern of rhythm in menstruation. If her intervals of bleeding are, for instance, between sixty to ninety days, she is building up an excessive lining of the womb, and her flow, when she menstruates after all that time, is apt to be profuse, even occasionally resulting in severe hemorrhaging. This can be treated very simply now by giving the girl the Pill for twenty-one days, which induces an artificially normal cycle and usually a light flow. The giver should be a doctor, not a well-intentioned mother prescribing her own birth control pill for her daughter. Sometimes such bleeding can be caused by a disorder of the blood clotting, leukemia, a cyst on the ovary, rarely an ovarian tumor, and other diseases that only a physician could detect. A doctor will usually continue the girl on the Pill for six to eight months, after which she will be taken off it and usually begins to ovulate and menstruate regularly.

It might seem silly to use a contraceptive pill to control abnormal bleeding due to lack of ovulation when the Pill actually is effective in preventing ovulation and subsequently pregnancy. But it really isn't. The abnormal bleeding in some teen-agers is due to the constant release of estrogen from the ovary without the beneficial effects of the second hormone secreted after ovulation, progesterone. Without it, the womb lining gets thicker and thicker, overflows, and profuse bleeding results. So the Pill simply replaces progesterone and produces an artificial menstrual cycle until the teen-ager's menstrual pattern is established.

9 10 11 12 13 14

Painful periods, problem for many sixteen to twenty-odd year olds

Once ovulation begins to occur regularly, with a certain amount of rhythm, in a twenty-eight- to thirty-two-day cycle, the next disorder that annoys many young women is painful periods, medically named *dysmenorrhea*. There are two kinds: primary and secondary. Primary means that when a doctor examines a patient he can find no disease that would account for the pain—she simply has pain. Secondary *dysmenorrhea* is due to an infectious process or disease in the pelvis and is not usual in this age group (it will be taken up in an older division). Girls with primary *dysmenorrhea* may have pains—cramps located just above the pubic bone—that come on about a day or so before menstruation, along with a variety of other symptoms—back-, leg- and headaches, depression, nausea, vomiting. The cause of the pain can't be pinned down exactly. Some gynecologists, strongly influenced by psychiatry, believe it is merely a release mechanism for basic insecurity or conflict within a woman. It is, in fact, more usual and severe in highstrung nervous women and girls whose mothers have had painful periods, so that obviously they grow up associating menstruation with being "sick," "unwell," or even "cursed." Marked differences of pain thresholds in menstruation, as well as in childbirth, have been observed among different individuals and ethnic groups. Dr. Kistner has noticed that painful periods are more frequent among girls of Italian or Spanish descent that he has treated; they are a rarity in those of Nordic extraction and hardly ever seen among Negroes. He believes the pain has only a possible psychological overlay and is definitely a physiological mechanism—caused by hormonal changes, chiefly secretion of progesterone, and the degeneration of the tissues of the lining of the womb. A tightly closed cervix, through which the tissue must pass, may aggravate the process in this way: the muscles of the uterus have to work harder to slough off the tissue, so a true muscle cramp, like a charley horse, can occur.

The best treatment for primary *dysmenorrhea*, Dr. Kistner finds, is a sympathetic, factual explanation of what menstruation is all about. This may involve some superstition-breaking or undoing of resentful attitudes that menstruation is a curse or sickness rather than a natural process that happens to all women. He tries to persuade patients that there's no reason for curtailing any of their activities—sports or sex—during the period. Sex is purely a matter of taste at this time, in no way harmful physically. Some women's sexual desires are actually increased in the immediate premenstrual and menstrual phase, just as they sometimes are during pregnancy, possibly related to the elevated hormonal level. To relieve menstrual pain many women need only reassurance and understanding from their doctor that nothing is really wrong with them. For mild menstrual cramps, Dr. Kistner suggests taking an aspirin compound, possibly with the admixture of an antispasmodic, and a warm bath.

If this approach doesn't work, Dr. Kistner usually has success with suppressing ovulation by the use of the Pill or just plain estrogen. For some reason the second hormone, progesterone, together with estrogen, is responsible for the symptoms. Women who don't ovulate don't have painful periods. Even women with severe *dysmenorrhea* placed on an ordinary oral-contraceptive pill do not suffer after they've been on it for several months. If, however, after preventing ovulation with the Pill, a patient still has pain or it shifts from the pelvic region to other parts of the body, head or back maybe, it is possible that she needs this pain for some psychological reason to get sympathy or attention. Another alternative, if the pain is not improved and actually gets worse during the period after taking the Pill, is a disease known as *endometriosis*. This disease occurs when the lining of the womb is expelled through the Fallopian tubes and is implanted in the abdominal cavity on the ovaries, bladder, colon and other ligaments that support the uterus. These expelled cells grow and bleed, causing painful periods, irregular bleeding and eventually infertility. Until 1955, pregnancy

15 16 17 18 19

or hysterectomy were the only effective treatments, neither very satisfactory for young unmarried women. Estrogens and male hormones had been successful, but the prolonged treatment and the side effects were disturbing to patients. Besides, these hormones lacked the comprehensiveness of pregnancy as a treatment. Dr. Kistner's own search for an improved therapy led him to the discovery that a false pregnancy could be induced by the medication which finally became the Pill. On a combination of estrogen and progesterone, not given in the same cycles now used for the Pill, these patients did not menstruate, their breasts increased in size, nipples became larger and darker, sometimes the line along the abdomen, the *linea alba*, darkened, they gained weight, felt nauseated when they first started, had changes of appetite, and some even complained that their martinis tasted differently—a rather usual complaint in real pregnancy. As the dosage was built up, the pseudopregnancy shredded and disintegrated the diseased tissues, just as natural pregnancy does. Today any contraceptive pill can be used, and 80 percent of patients show improvement. This disease, once a major cause of the hysterectomies so dreaded by young women, is now effectively controlled.

The child-bearing period, roughly eighteen to thirty-five

After a woman has had a baby, she usually doesn't have to worry about painful periods; they disappear. That doesn't necessarily mean the end of menstrual problems. The most usual complaints in the eighteen to thirty-five group are failure to ovulate, which, of course, prevents pregnancy, and profuse and irregular bleeding, like the fourteen-year-old teen-ager. All are signals to see a doctor because they could be evidence of endocrine disorders involving the pituitary, thyroid and adrenal glands, or diseases of the ovary.

If a woman who wants a baby has not become pregnant after one year of trying, she should ask her gynecologist to find out why, especially if her periods are irregular. Warnings that should send her to him even sooner: staining before or after the menstrual period, frequently caused by a fibroid tumor or polyp; bleeding or particularly a watery-pink staining after intercourse or douching may indicate a disease of the cervix, often cancer. (In fact any woman of any age who has these symptoms should have a pelvic examination and "Pap" smear.) After excluding these diseases, the doctor may give her the drug called Clomid to induce ovulation. This drug produces ovulation in about 70 percent of properly selected patients, and almost 50 percent of these eventually become pregnant. The incidence of multiple pregnancy after Clomid is one in ten as compared to one in eighty in non-Clomid pregnancies, but almost all of these were twins. This, in Dr. Kistner's judgment, is the most successful treatment of infertility due to irregular ovulation. And there is, he added, no substantiation of evidence that placing a nonovulating woman on the Pill for three to six months and then taking her off will increase her fertility potential, as was suspected at one time.

Unmarried women in this age group who have irregular periods should see a doctor for an additional reason. If the lining of the womb continues to be stimulated month after month, year after year, by estrogen without regular menstruation, a process known as *hyperplasia,* or overgrowth, occurs. If untreated for prolonged periods of time, it may, in roughly 10 percent of the cases, develop into cancer. *Hyperplasia* can be successfully treated by inducing ovulation and subsequent pregnancy, but in the case of a single woman this is hardly desirable. The lack of progesterone caused by nonovulation can be substituted for by providing artificial cycles with the Pill. This gets rid of the *hyperplasia,* brings about perfectly normal bleeding every month and provides adequate hormonal replacement.

In this age group Dr. Kistner has noticed a recent increase in the number of girls with another problem that reveals some of the conflicts of young women in our time. These are all exceptionally intelligent girls who were usually at the top of their high school classes before going to college. Once on campus, and perhaps living away from home for the first time, they find they not only have to compete rather fiercely with boys and girls for high academic standing but with other girls for

20 21 22 23 24

dates, perhaps even for their own female identity. They begin to overeat or undereat to ease their conflicts, then either gain some twenty pounds or lose twenty to thirty, and the pituitary gland becomes affected. It may shut off completely its hormones which stimulate the ovaries. The ovaries are thus unable to produce estrogen and progesterone, ovulation ceases and eventually all bleeding stops. The breasts gradually diminish in size, since they are no longer stimulated by estrogen, and the female body contour begins to disappear. Aside from the seriousness of their psychological state, these girls are living in a state of estrogen insufficiency which could eventually, if not treated, predispose them to certain metabolic diseases: *osteoporosis*, an increase in the brittleness of bones; *arteriosclerosis*, hardening of the arteries.

Treatment from even a physical point of view is not easy. These girls are unmarried, in college and uninterested in having babies (pregnancy, as in so many other gynecological disorders, could help). First they should be examined thoroughly to exclude the possibility of a brain tumor that might cause these same symptoms. When that is ruled out they can be given estrogen for the first fifteen to sixteen days of an induced cycle, then estrogen and progesterone for the last five days, and a normal withdrawal flow will begin. In addition, an attempt is made to solve the basic psychosomatic problem that is causing the pituitary gland to function abnormally. Sometimes just the mere fact that bleeding begins again, along with the reassurance of the gynecologist, will improve these girls' eating habits and get them on the way to solving their psychological problems.

Premenstrual tension, no respecter of age but fixes usually on the late-thirties to early-forties

It may be all right to trust a woman over thirty, but not during the five or more days before her period if she is subject to premenstrual tension. Her irritability and depression, along with a score of other symptoms that may include weight gains of up to nine pounds, are two of the enigmas of gynecology. The symptoms of premenstrual tension vary enormously—some women are plagued for two days to two weeks before each period. One or two or more symptoms may attack at the same time or at different intervals before and during menstruation: headache, fullness and/or tenderness of the breasts and nipples, swelling of the ankles and feet, numbness and tingling in the fingers, weight gain, abdominal pain, backache, migraine, aggravation of acne, nervousness, insomnia, irritability, change in sexual desire, poor concentration. "At this time, women complain of feeling bloated," Dr. Kistner said. "They are and they act bloated too." He has had husbands beg him to do something to relieve their wives of these symptoms because they cannot live with their periodical bitchiness.

For the most part these symptoms seem to be related to salt and water retention, which is caused by elevated estrogen levels in the body. Doctors don't know why premenstrual tension occurs chiefly after thirty. The current feeling is that the syndrome or disorder is caused by a change in the metabolism of estrogen and progesterone or the effect of these hormones on sensitive end organs or tissues. It is possible that water retention may occur also in tissues of the brain. Some women have a fantastic ability to retain salt and water and can, after one cocktail party where they've had a few drinks, hors d'oeuvres or salted nuts, gain six to nine pounds in a matter of twenty-four to forty-eight hours.

Controlling water retention depends to a certain extent on a woman's willpower. She has to stay on a low-salt (sodium chloride) diet eight to ten days prior to the menstrual period. Any condiment used in cooking that has sodium chloride on the label should be rejected. Anything that reads sodium, in fact, particularly common salt, increases the tendency to swelling. Taking a diuretic pill will help because it increases the outpouring of salt and water through the kidneys, and the swelling is relieved. Actually, if you look in the *Physicians' Desk Reference* under premenstrual tension, there are about sixty different remedies. Dr. Kistner de-

25 26 27 28 29

scribed one as a sort of shotgun type—combining a diuretic to get rid of fluid, a little progesterone because there has been some evidence that if more were around at this time, it would be a good thing, and a mild tranquilizer as well.

If an oral contraceptive is being used, the incidence of premenstrual tension markedly diminishes. But a woman has to be careful that the Pill she is taking does not contain excessive estrogens. Estrogen causes the retention of salt and water. For this reason, and others, various pharmaceutical companies reduced the amount of estrogen in the Pill from 125 micrograms to 100, then to 80, and now have it down to a minidose of 50. After it was noted that women using oral contraceptives for conception control had less premenstrual tension, physicians began to use these combinations to treat the disorder.

The selection of the proper Pill for the proper woman will have excellent results. Even a woman with the multiple complaints of all age groups—premenstrual tension, irregular flowing and painful periods—is relieved, and conception control is added as a bonus. She will not have pain, her premenstrual tension will diminish, her flow will become regular and she won't get pregnant. It sounds too good to be true, which may be, in part, why some people, including doctors, mistrust it.

The Pill scare

Claims that the Pill may cause cancer of the breast, the most common cancer among women, and of the cervix, the second, Dr. Kistner considers rigamarole and not based on statistical evidence. The Pill, however, he said, may aggravate an already existing breast cancer. This is why a doctor who is giving the Pill for contraception or menstrual disorders should examine the breasts and female organs every six months and should do a Papanicolaou smear test for cancer of the cervix at least once a year. In Dr. Kistner's estimation, if this is done, a woman will never develop cancer of the cervix, on or off the Pill, because detection and treatment at an early stage, called *anaplasia,* or at a little later stage, cancer *in situ,* will prevent the disease.

Answering another claim, that fibrocystic disease, or breast cysts, another common plague of

women, is caused or aggravated by the Pill, Dr. Kistner said that he actually used a certain type of Pill successfully in the treatment of the disease. Fibrocystic disease is related to the repeated stimulation of the breast every month by a woman's own estrogen and progesterone hormones. According to him, the best treatment is again pregnancy because it provides a constant level of hormones plus the benefits of nursing—the purpose for which the breast was designed. Menopause, too, is effective in lowering the estrogen level. For years, the breast pain and also the spread or development of this disease was treated with a male hormone that negated the estrogen effect on the breast. Now Dr. Kistner uses one of the oral contraceptives with a progestin that is slightly androgenic, i.e., has male hormone characteristics, with a very low amount of estrogen. When a pill of this type is given, he said, the amount of estrogen and progestin is much less than the woman is making herself each month in her own ovary. It is, incidentally, a mistake to think that women taking the Pill are consuming tremendous amounts of hormones which are going to do all sorts of serious damage. The amount taken is constant in contrast to the cyclical ups and downs of estrogen and progesterone that take place naturally in her body. The newest treatment for patients who have extensive and painful fibrocystic disease is an injectable synthetic progestin called Depo-Provera, now being used as a contraceptive. This preparation, given at intervals of two to three months, prevents ovulation and reduces the amount of estrogen and progestin produced each month. The breasts soften, masses disappear and pain is forgotten.

The value of the Pill in treating disorders of menstruation has been greatly overshadowed by its reputation as a contraceptive. Women still suffer everything from minor cramps and premenstrual tension to more severe symptoms privately and unnecessarily because they are unaware of the therapeutic values of the Pill—a situation that Dr. Kistner speculates might be due to the predominance of men among medical news writers who can't perceive this widespread distress which women themselves hide in fear of being indelicate. It is up to women to stop being embarrassed, to ask and insist on relief from their doctors, and if it is not given, to change doctors. It is just as important to find a doctor who keeps up with advances in medicine so that he can give his patients maximum medical care.

30 31

GUIDE

TO GYNECOLOGICAL PROBLEMS

by Ellen Switzer

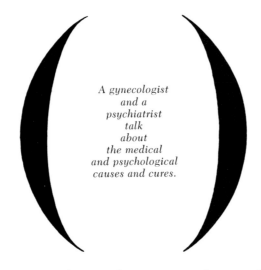

*A gynecologist
and a
psychiatrist
talk
about
the medical
and psychological
causes and cures.*

Most gynecologists, physicians specializing in the diseases of women, agree that too many patients wait entirely too long before reporting even the most distressing symptoms. This is particularly true of young, unmarried women who don't know a specialist and who somehow can't bring themselves to discuss intimate physical details with their family doctor. The shyness is particularly unfortunate because most gynecological conditions found in young women respond readily to simple treatment *if they are diagnosed early.* On the other hand, the same conditions hardly ever clear up without treatment, as the patient hopes they will. Usually, after the condition has persisted for a while, therapy will be more complicated, costly and time-consuming. Often, surgery is needed for a long-standing problem which earlier might have been cured through medication.

Why are women so hesitant to consult a doctor for such conditions as abnormal vaginal bleeding, vaginal discharge, menstrual irregularities and severe menstrual cramps? Psychological reasons are among the basic causes.

Many women are afraid that there is something terribly wrong with them. By "something terrible" they usually mean cancer. It might be comforting for them to realize that cancer of the reproductive organs in young women is most unusual. It occurs even more rarely in a woman under thirty who has never been pregnant. There are two types of uterine and cervical malignancies: carcinoma, representing 95 percent of all cases of diagnosed cancer, and sarcoma, representing somewhat less than 5 percent. Carcinoma doesn't occur often in women under thirty—none of the physicians interviewed for this article could remember even one single case in a woman that young. Sarcoma can and does, but it is such a rare form of lesion that most experienced physicians see only a very few cases in their entire careers. And, although cancer is highly unlikely, it might be well to remember that by far the best chance for a complete cure is the earliest possible diagnosis and treatment.

But in spite of the fact that cancer is so unusual, young women will suffer for months, trying to find enough courage to see their doctor, because they suspect that they are afflicted by some terminal illness.

Another common worry is the fear that they might have some abnormality which will make it impossible for them to have children. Again, this is exceedingly rare, although some conditions, if untreated, may in the long run produce sterility. An occasional woman will become so worried and upset by the gynecological symptom that she turns up at a psychiatric clinic in a state of panic or depression. Often it takes only one or two visits to the gynecologist to cure the simple infection or slight hormonal imbalance that caused the original symptom. It may take much longer to deal with the emotional problems the symptoms have brought on or aggravated.

Another quite opposite reason for not calling the doctor is the patient's conviction that there is really nothing at all wrong with her. Dr. Stephen Fleck, professor of psychiatry at the Yale University School of Medicine who has worked on several joint studies with professors in the Department of Obstetrics and Gynecology, says that "such a young woman is afraid that the doctor will tell her that it's all in her head. There is now a great deal of sophistication about psychosomatic illness and still very little about the basic facts of life," Dr. Fleck said. "The patient who doesn't want to bother the doctor, because in her inexpert opinion it's all nerves anyhow, should remember that her physician is better equipped than she to decide whether the problem is in her head or in that part of her anatomy which hurts."

Another physician told about a psychiatrically oriented actress who had recently been his patient. She was rehearsing a new play and started to have severe pains in her right side almost from the day rehearsals started. She was convinced that she was suffering from a large case of hostility towards the play's director, who reminded her of her brother. So she took a few tranquilizers and decided to talk herself out of her pain. On opening night she collapsed on the stage, and it soon became obvious that she was suffering from a large ovarian cyst. She had to undergo emergency surgery and was incapacitated for several months.

Probably the most frequent reason for not consulting a physician is plain embarrassment. In spite of all the new openness about sex in the media, many women today are just as shy about discussing intimate physical problems as their mid-Victorian great-grandmothers were. Very few women have had an opportunity to discuss specific sexual functions and malfunctions. Their sex education, if any, is usually sketchy and euphemistic.

A recent report on sex and the college student by the Group for the Advancement of Psychiatry (GAP) states that sex-education courses in American colleges "explain the anatomy and physiology of reproduction, often avoiding explicit sexual references by using examples from the plant and animal world." In addition, "As a consequence of emotional conflicts, students with access to the full range of sexual information often fail to master or make use of it."

It is not astonishing that a woman who is inhibited about sexual matters cannot absorb factual information about her reproductive system and finds it almost impossible to discuss, even with her doctor, problems that are related to her own sexuality. She *knows* that her doctor will not be shocked by what she tells him, but somehow she can't bring herself to make that appointment in spite of her knowledge. However, if she realizes that she has these inhibitions, she may find it easier to cope with them. Most doctors will understand a patient's embarrassment and make the consultation as easy as possible for her.

The number of common gynecological symptoms that young patients have is fairly simple and limited, but the conditions which can cause them are varied. The usual signs of trouble are excessive vaginal bleeding during periods, bleeding and spotting between periods, irregular menstrual periods (or no periods at all) after the menstrual cycle has become definitely established, premenstrual tension, painful, disabling periods and vaginal discharge. These are *symptoms*, not diseases in themselves, and medical advice should be sought as soon as possible to establish the cause and begin treatment.

According to Dr. C. Lee Buxton, professor of obstetrics and gynecology at the Yale University School of Medicine, some of the most common gynecological conditions encountered by young women have very similar symptoms. So self-diagnosis is no good. Only a physician can tell what the cause of the symptoms is after a thorough internal examination of the patient.

One frequently seen condition is endometriosis. The principal symptom is incapacitating pain during periods, especially after a girl has had a history of relatively pain-free menstruation. There may also be some bleeding between periods or heavy bleeding during periods. This seems to be a twentieth-century disease. It was first recognized at the turn of the century, but now has become one of the most frequently diagnosed gynecological problems of young women. The condition occurs when cells which ordinarily line the uterus (the endometrium) attach themselves to sites outside the uterus. These cells continue to function as if they were still part of the uterine lining: i.e. they swell and grow during the menstrual cycle and bleed during the menstrual period. Some physicians believe that the condition is congenital, that girls are born with the rudimentary cells already in their abdominal cavities. Others believe that the cells somehow escape from the uterus and attach themselves to various inappropriate sites. Every once in a while a really wild theory hits the newspapers. For instance, several years ago someone proposed that since, in his opinion, airline stewardesses got the disease frequently, changes in air pressure might have something to do with it. Recently, someone in England blamed water-skiing. But physicians are convinced that such simple explanations, unfortunately, won't do. Non-water-skiers and girls who have never set foot in an airplane turn up at their offices fairly regularly with endometriosis.

Women who marry late and who postpone pregnancy seem to get it more frequently than those who have babies when they are young. Also, pregnancy is considered a good treatment for early endometriosis. Since menstruation stops, so do the unpleasant symptoms. And sometimes the symptoms don't come back after the baby is born.

If endometriosis is diagnosed and treated early, the condition can usually be arrested by simple hormone therapy. If allowed to persist and spread, surgery may be needed. Advanced endometriosis can cause sterility. This is just one more reason why it is important to report any symptoms early.

Another condition which laymen often confuse with endometriosis is endometritis. This is an inflammation of the lining of the uterine cavity. It causes similar symptoms, particularly excessive bleeding, pain and fever. Again, if detected and treated early, it is fairly simple to cure. If left untreated, it can cause all kinds of serious complications.

Fibroid tumors also can lead to very similar symptoms. This is one condition which the physician often just watches carefully. Some fibroids just stop growing and cause no problems. If they grow, surgery is usually necessary. If fibroids are too large or spread over too extensive an area in the uterus, they can cause infertility or miscarriages. An operation called a myomectomy can be performed to remove the tumors and leave the uterus in workable condition.

Neither endometriosis, nor endometritis, nor fibroid tumors are premalignant or malignant. In other words, they don't indicate that the patient is more susceptible to developing any cancer than other women who have never suffered from any of these conditions.

Excessive menstrual bleeding, (see page 241 for menstrual information), however, does not always indicate something wrong with the reproductive system. For instance, a hemorrhage may well be a sign of *anemia*, and insufficiency of red blood cells. The bleeding, in turn, makes the anemia

GUIDE

worse and creates a vicious cycle. It could be happening because the girl has been getting a diet that's insufficient in iron and may be helped by a change in food habits (lots of liver, lots of eggs), plus some iron-supplement capsules. But, again, self-medication is a bad idea. The condition may also be caused by a malfunction of the body's blood-clotting mechanism. This, too, can be treated with appropriate oral medication, but only under the careful supervision of a physician.

Malfunctioning of various glands can cause excessive bleeding and is usually corrected with hormone therapy. It certainly should be treated before the patient is weak, tired and miserable from excessive loss of blood every month.

There is also a whole series of complaints that are caused by infections. The most frequently mentioned are the venereal diseases, *syphilis* and *gonorrhea.* For the past ten years or so there has been a lessening of concern about these diseases because it was assumed that they could be easily eliminated through the use of antibiotics. Unfortunately, this has not turned out to be true. Rather than declining, the rates of both diseases have grown tremendously, particularly among young people. Public health officials feel that people are less apt to seek medical attention after they have been exposed because they think that these infections are no longer dangerous. However, gonorrhea still causes acute infections of the entire reproductive tract, often requiring surgery. It is one of the most frequently encountered causes of infertility in women. Syphilis is even more dangerous. In its later stages it can attack the heart, the brain and the spinal cord. Eventually, it can kill. It can also be passed on to an unborn child by a syphilitic mother. Even the slightest suspicion of exposure to either of these diseases should be immediately reported to a doctor. In most cities, the local department of public health conducts clinics where patients are diagnosed and treated, often free of charge.

Both gonorrhea and syphilis can be caught— through sex relations or close body contact—only from persons who are infected. They are not spread by water, food or air. They are not caught from toilet seats, drinking fountains or eating utensils.

The first sign of syphilis is a painless sore. Unfortunately, it will go away by itself with no treatment. That does not mean that the disease has gone, however. It just lies dormant for from three to six weeks. The next symptom is a rash that may look like a food rash, a heat rash or hives. The patient may also suffer from a sore throat. These symptoms also go away without treatment. But by this time the disease germs have spread throughout the body. The patient may feel fine . . . until much later, when the germs have attacked vital organs. Also, the disease remains infectious and can be spread to other people. The time to cure syphilis most effectively is as soon as symptoms appear. Treatment consists of antibiotics. It is important that these be given by a doctor. Many people are tempted (by embarrassment and false economy) to get an old prescription refilled or to take pills that are left over from an earlier prescription. Nothing could be more unsafe. Since the symptoms disappear even without a treatment while the disease remains, only a doctor will be able to tell when the patient is cured and how long the treatment must be continued.

The symptoms of gonorrhea are different from those of syphilis. The first indication is usually a slight vaginal discharge, burning and itching. This too can go away without treatment. However, the disease then spreads through the Fallopian tubes and ovaries, causing infections and infertility. It can also cause blindness in newborn babies. Again, early treatment with antibiotics is essential, and only a doctor will be able to tell what antibiotic to use, what dosage is needed and for how long a period the treatment must be continued to effect a complete cure.

Symptoms similar to early gonorrhea can be caused by other kinds of infections which are very common and uncomfortable but relatively harmless. The most frequently diagnosed is *Trichomonas vaginitis,* which is caused by a germ and is often seen in group-living situations, for instance dormitories or hotels for women. Doctors are not entirely sure how it is spread, but unlike the venereal diseases it can be caught without having physical contact with an infected person. Symptoms are vaginal discharge, itching and burning. It is cured through local treatment, and if persistent, with oral medication.

Although the condition is neither dangerous nor debilitating, it can become chronic. Therefore early attention is important. Dr. Buxton estimates that 20 to 25 percent of all women have this condition sometime during their lives. He emphasizes that it is nothing to be ashamed of, that it is easily treated. He also points out that a great many girls, fearing that they may have gonorrhea, start self-medication with powerful antibiotics which may be dangerous. "This would be extremely foolhardy if they really had a venereal disease, and it's unnecessary and just plain stupid when they have a condition for which a simple local treatment would be effective," he added.

A girl who has never had any gynecological problems and has therefore not had any occasion to consult a specialist should have a complete physical examination, including an internal check, before marriage. Most states require a blood test for syphilis, but that is not nearly enough. The best time to have such an examination is about eight weeks before the wedding date. This will give the doctor enough time to take care of any conditions which might interfere with normal childbearing and to prescribe an appropriate contraceptive method if this is what the couple desires. Birth control pills, for instance, may have some side effects. The time to discover these problems is well before the excitement of pre-wedding festivities. Dr. Buxton pointed out that some types of pills which cause all kinds of problems for one patient (i.e. nausea, weight gain, excessive bleeding) work very well for another. Usually, the doctor can find the right pill for his patient, given enough time. Incidentally, no one should take birth control pills without medical supervision. They are very easy to obtain. Most prescriptions are indefinitely refillable, and girls have been known to get their own prescriptions refilled for their friends. But, although these pills are usually considered effective and relatively harmless, there are some conditions under which they can be harmful. For instance, if the blood-clotting mechanism of the patient is not functioning properly (i.e., women with infected veins) the pills can be downright dangerous. This has been recognized by the Federal Food and Drug Administration, which makes the labeling on birth-control pills indicate this danger.

There is one other important reason for seeing a doctor before the wedding. Surprisingly large numbers of girls come to see their doctors in a state of panic weeks and sometimes months after they have been married because they find that intercourse is extremely painful or impossible. Sometimes gynecologists don't see these women until they show up at infertility clinics—they are too embarrassed to discuss their problem in any other context. Often this particular problem is psychological. "Girls who have spent years fending off male advances suddenly find that they can't stop when they are married," Dr. Fleck said. "Also, they have read and heard so much about the great sexual partners they are supposed to be all of a sudden that they get a simple case of stage fright. In that case, often reassurance of both bride and groom is all that is needed. Sometimes, when the girl is so inhibited and frightened that her frigidity continues, psychotherapy may be indicated."

In some cases, there is also a very simple physical reason for problems early in marriage: a very thick, inelastic hymen. This can be spotted during the premarital examination. In some cases the hymen can be stretched. When this does not work, the hymen can be cut under local anesthetic. Most doctors will not perform this operation without discussing it with both bride and the groom because of the psychological implications. However, physically, it is a very minor procedure, and can be done in the doctor's office. It should be done about six weeks before the wedding.

Obvious problems to conception and childbearing will probably be spotted in the premarital examination. However, more subtle problems may turn up later. It might be reassuring to a couple anxious to have a baby to note that *infertility* is not even considered a serious possibility until the couple has tried for one year to have a baby with no success. Among normal and ultimately fertile couples, approximately 65 percent will conceive within six months, an additional 15 percent within a year, and the remaining 20 percent within two years. There are many reasons for infertility, and both husband and wife should have a thorough checkup if the wife fails to conceive after a reasonable period of time. Many teaching hospitals have infertility clinics which are especially well-equipped to find out what is causing the problem and to try to remedy it.

In cases of pregnancy almost all women know enough to see a physician. However, even relatively sophisticated and well-informed women sometimes wait too long before their first prenatal appointment. A woman should certainly see a doctor after she has missed two periods; earlier if she has any reason to feel that anything may be wrong. Most doctors include prenatal care in their bill for the delivery of the baby, so there is not even any saving in money if a woman waits until her fourth or fifth month. And she may be causing all kinds of serious problems for herself and her unborn baby by not having regular checkups much earlier.

Both Dr. Buxton and Dr. Fleck had some advice on how to pick a gynecologist. In her own home town, a woman might want to ask her family doctor for a recommendation. If she is living in a strange town, the local medical society will give her the names of three board-certified gynecologists. She can then decide which one she wishes to consult. It's particularly important to find a gynecologist with whom she can talk easily and comfortably. If she finds that she simply cannot relate to the doctor, the best thing might be to change doctors. However, as Dr. Buxton put it: "Doctors are human just like everybody else. We get tired, upset and sometimes discouraged. There may be days when we seem abrupt or impatient or too busy. But we want to help our patient, we want to answer her questions, to reassure her if that is what she needs, to help her over the rough spots. In return, we hope that we can gain her confidence so that she will tell us what is really bothering her. It won't embarrass us and we don't make moral judgments. We just want to be able to help."

CONTRACEPTIVES

WHAT MANY WOMEN STILL DON'T KNOW ABOUT THEM

by Roberta Brandes Gratz

This is the Age of the Pill. And in the dozen years since it was introduced on the open market a strange phenomenon has developed. A whole generation has grown up believing that the pill is almost the *only* birth control method to use.

Before, a girl about to be married or involved in her first affair would go to her doctor to be fitted for a diaphragm or would depend on her partner's use of contraceptives. Now she immediately thinks of the Pill.

That the Pill has provided a new freedom for women—new control over their bodies and their destinies—is not questioned. The traditional moral codes on premarital sex are challenged. The threat of becoming pregnant, which once worked even if the stricter morality didn't, is now minimized.

But with this new freedom and with the dominance of the Pill has come a whole new problem, an increase in ignorance or misinformation about the larger concepts of birth control and the complexities of the Pill.

Many doctors renege on *their* responsibility, too. They hand out the little packets, rarely even mentioning which kind of Pill they contain—combination or sequential—and fail to fill their patient in on any pertinent information. They certainly don't encourage any further inquiries, which leads to confusion, if not fear.

Several doctors report scores of women, old and young, flatly refusing to consider one kind of contraceptive or another because their friends have had a bad experience with it. Or they have been completely scared off by reports questioning the safety of the Pill *for some women*. They have often not read those reports themselves. Their fear is secondhand, and they refuse to investigate on their own to let it be determined if their own medical history warrants this concern.

Doctors are alarmed, too, at the lack of information about contraception in general. Dr. Selig Neubardt, a young suburban obstetrician, observes in his book, *A Concept of Contraception:* "The choice for too many women is the Pill or nothing. The idea should be that there is contraception and one form is the Pill but it's not that great. There are others, too. Women have to understand the whole picture and know about all techniques before deciding on one for themselves."

Birth control education, many doctors argue, should begin in the early teens. "What would make a young college girl have sex without using a

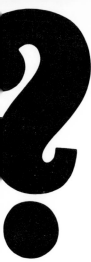

contraceptive?" Dr. Neubardt asks rhetorically, "The fact that we have failed her in education, failed her in the beginning. She has learned about creation and conception but never about how *not* to create."

Not too long ago I had the occasion to interview many women who for an assortment of reasons had undergone one or more abortions. The assumption that women with unwanted pregnancies usually have failed to use a contraceptive is not always the case. More often than not they "misused" their particular form of contraception. Several had carelessly forgotten to take one or sometimes two pills in a row. One had not been refitted for her diaphragm since before the birth of her last child five years earlier. An unmarried girl, who in spite of the use of a diaphragm, has had two unplanned pregnancies (and two subsequent abortions), still believes "It's probably physically, emotionally and morally better to have two abortions than to use birth control pills."

Doctors of course differ on which methods they prefer to prescribe, all emphasizing that each woman is a highly individual case with a lot depending on her attitude. One may loathe the idea of inserting a diaphragm, another have a general antipathy toward taking *any* pill other than aspirin, another fear the idea of having a foreign object, like a coil, remain inside her.

Dr. Alan F. Guttmacher, president of Planned Parenthood-World Population, likes to tell his medical students: "Sex is not below the waist but above the neck." A prime exponent of oral contraceptives, Dr. Guttmacher said, however: "The tendency to shift methods is unnecessary. If the diaphragm is being used satisfactorily with a satisfactory sex life, that's fine."

The doctors interviewed here were asked to outline the most basic misunderstandings they encounter about the more common birth control techniques—the condom, diaphragm, Pill and coil. (An in-depth discussion of potential Pill side effects was avoided.) All agreed that women should of course follow the latest reports on the subject and stressed the need for comprehending the basics of the methods to help them with their doctors to choose the most appropriate for each individual woman.

The diminishing interest in use of the condom, one doctor observed, reveals the shifting responsibility of birth control. "It used to be," he pointed out, "that the man was expected to handle the contraception. Today most women are almost ashamed not to be the ones. I still consider the condom the best technique for unmarried couples. It is also the only method that also protects against venereal disease. Now any American-made condom is electronically tested and quite reliable. I would still recommend that the woman use a vaginal foam along with his use of a condom. This gives two techniques that together are 90 percent effective, and each partner has some responsibility."

Another doctor cited the additional advantage that some young and inexperienced men do better reaching orgasm with a condom. Ironically, the condom is still the most widely used technique but, in his opinion, by the wrong age group, i.e., middle-age people. With this age group it may actually be a sexual imposition, because the ability to reach orgasm has probably diminished. A couple may have started with condoms and never switched.

The diaphragm, doctors frequently argue, is the most misused and least appreciated contraceptive technique. "The drawback is not because of the times it failed," said Dr. Neubardt, "but more because it is a nuisance. Some women seem more disturbed about removing it than inserting it. One should be quite sophisticated to use it. It is not suitable for borderline motivation.

"It doesn't provide protection against disease and it is difficult for a nonmarried couple because they don't know when and if. Inserted ahead of time, in anticipation, too much time can go by for it to still be effective. Actually, though, I can't think of any technique suitable for most of the time. Most unplanned pregnancies result from just one time without protection. Those sperm don't know it's the first time."

Dr. Sherwin Kaufman, medical director of Planned Parenthood of New York City, asserts that people are "misinformed that the diaphragm is not as effective as the Pill or the coil. There is a half-truth in the statistics, but there should be a distinction between patient failure and method failure. If a diaphragm is properly fitted and the woman is taught exactly how to use it, it can be as effective as the Pill and probably more so than the coil.

"Contrary to belief, the diaphragm is not physically airtight. It's not meant to be. That's why it must be used with a jelly-outside, around the rim and inside against the cervix through which sperm must pass. So the jelly does the important work."

Dr. Kaufman adds these three firm instructions for maximum security: First, the jelly must be applied to three places—both sides and the rim. Second, the diaphragm should be inserted anytime within three hours before intercourse. If more time elapses, fresh jelly must be applied into the vagina. Third, it should be left in six hours or more after intercourse because there may still be mobile sperm. If it's left in longer, there's no need to worry.

These instructions, necessary as they are, are enough to turn some women away from the diaphragm. Yet, two main features make it worthwhile. It is not felt during intercourse and it has no side effects. A diaphragm should be checked for size once a year and after each childbirth.

One little-known fact was raised by several doctors. At the moment of orgasm, the diaphragm can be displaced by the physical changes occurring during heightened sexual activity. This is particularly true if one has borne a child or is on top of the man.

Another doctor who strongly believes the diaphragm is underrated offers this general rule. If you are after spontaneity above all, use the Pill or the coil; if protection, then the Pill or diaphragm; if abolition of side effects, use the diaphragm.

In any discussion of the merits of birth control pills, the question of side effects is inevitable. The continuing exploration is, of course, legitimate. Some women cannot tolerate the Pill, and others, for reasons of their specific medical history, should not use it. However, certain information should be understood before jumping to conclusions. Much fear is based on a lack of understanding.

When the Pill was first approved for sale on the open market almost ten years ago, the Food and Drug Administration restricted usage to a two-year period. That limitation was subsequently changed to four years, then removed entirely. The impression still lingers that more than a steady two years on the Pill is potentially dangerous.

Doctors now are inclined to set their own limitation, but the reasoning for it is quite different. Dr. Kaufman, for example, gives only six-month prescriptions so that his patients return after that period for a checkup before renewal. Other doctors have similar policies—the time varies—but it is simply to insure regular surveillance which cannot be imposed with certain other methods.

Being able to require more frequent medical visits is one of the many positive dividends of the Pill. Dr. Harold Tovell, clinical professor of obstetrics and gynecology at Columbia University, makes this point: "Deaths from cancer of the uterus are preventable provided regular annual, or more frequent, checkups are obtained and the cancer detected early. Statistics show that the death rate is down about 50 percent from forty years ago."

Dr. Neubardt encourages his patients to occasionally stop taking the Pill for two cycles. "Sometimes," he says, "a woman discovers she feels much better off it though she never had any bad symptoms while taking the Pill. Suddenly there are little differences she never noticed before—she feels peppier, reaches orgasm easier, doesn't scream at the kids."

There are more than a dozen different birth control pills on the market, and what a lot of women are unaware of is that if they try one which causes uncomfortable side effects, another one might not.

There are two basic kinds of pills—sequential and combination. All those on the market are varieties of these two. The combination uses both estrogen and progestin for each pill. The sequential includes only estrogen for the first fifteen to sixteen days and a combination of the two for the remaining pills. The sequential is not as popular with doctors as the combination because, they say, it is not as effective. However, some prescribe it for women who have been having undesirable side effects with the combination pill. It apparently causes fewer side effects. The sequential permits a little less latitude in forgetting. If you miss one combination pill, the danger is not significant. If you miss one sequential, vulnerability is greater, especially during the estrogen-only period.

Doctors suggest that if one misses a pill, conventional contraception should be used for the rest of the cycle. Although uncommon, pregnancies have resulted from missing one pill.

The significance of the wide pill variety is summed up by Dr. Kaufman. "The ingredients are not identical and they are all different in possible side effects and bonuses. Some are good for painful periods, some for heavy periods and still others for regular but scanty periods. Then there are some that are good for premenstrual tension and others that won't aggravate acne. Careful consideration must be given to the complete individual medical history including all these factors. Bonuses can accrue by using a pill to normalize other functions related to hormones. If a patient complains of side effects like nausea, staining, swelling or tenderness of the breasts, bloating or something else, I often encourage her to try a different type."

If a woman's medical history shows any trace of diabetes, cancer, varicose veins, migraine headaches, etc., most doctors would not recommend the Pill.

A misunderstanding that persists is that the Pill causes increased fertility when stopped. It is often confused with a pill that stimulates fertility. And, as Dr. Tovell points out: "There was at one time the rebound-phenomenon theory of Dr. John Rock, retired Harvard professor of gynecology, which held that after the ovary is suppressed for a while, it rebounds more forcefully. That is no longer considered credible, and most doctors say the Pill causes no fertility change."

The idea is currently circulating that the Pill can be taken continuously—i.e., without taking the required break to allow for a menstrual period. The doctors interviewed here did not favor this. Dr. Tovell said: "Biologically, I think it is better to break off. Sooner or later you will get breakthrough bleeding. Actually, the continuous taking of the pills can be used therapeutically, but the occasions calling for it are not common. Under normal medical circumstances I think there are two reasons against the idea. One, we don't know what permanent effect it would have on the pituitary gland, and two, in time a woman will have emotional problems not knowing if she is pregnant or not."

Ovulation, it is commonly thought, occurs in the middle of the cycle. More accurately, it occurs roughly two weeks before a period. This may for some women be the same as two weeks after a period but not for those whose cycles are not the assumed twenty-eight days. Orgasm can stimulate some women to ovulate, which accounts for the rare conceptions during a period.

The first pill in a cycle is supposed to be taken the fifth day after the onset of bleeding, whether or not that bleeding has stopped. Doctors report considerable confusion in deciding actually when that fifth day is. One doctor offers this rule of thumb: "The first day you see blood is the first day of the cycle. If it is five minutes to midnight, it is still that day. The bleeding started six to eight hours earlier but it takes that long for blood to emerge. Protection starts immediately because the suppressive process is initiated with the first pill."

The failure rate of the Pill is quite small but it is there and the cause of some concern. Doctors minimize it. Dr. Neubardt argued: "It is a disservice to stress the failure rate."

"The pregnancy possibility is so remote, one is not entitled to think about it. After a woman selects a contraceptive, she should not worry about failure rates. It robs sexual pleasure. She's doing all she can do. Nothing in life is guaranteed."

Then, somewhat philosophically, Dr. Neubardt added: "With the diaphragm, there's the price of the nuisance. With the condom, there is feeling it. But with the Pill, there's no price but the worry. Yet it's not even dangerous to children. Women are so attuned to paying a price for sex, they can't accept none, so the worry becomes the price of the Pill."

The coil or IUD is a contraceptive method limited in its usage. Until recently it was recommended only for women who had borne at least one child because the plastic loops, coils, or spirals didn't fit comfortably inside a uterus unstretched by childbirth. Now new models—smaller, lighter, more ingenious in shape—are available. "But even with some mothers," Dr. Kaufman reported, "one out of three or four will not be happy with it because of continuous pain, bleeding or expulsion. For some women there are no complications and for them it's great."

Asked why some women reject the coil, Dr. Kaufman echoed the responses of others: "We don't know why it doesn't work because we don't really yet know why it does work."

There is also the problem that the coil can be expelled without the woman being aware of this. Thus doctors urge constant checking by the woman. "If you can't feel the threads," says Dr. Trovell, "kick your husband out of bed."

Among contraceptives the IUD is rated by some authorities as second in effectiveness to the Pill, but it's a poor second. The Pill's no-pregnancy batting average is close to 100 percent, but among every hundred women who use a loop or shield for a year, two or four become pregnant. In addition, about ten in a hundred women who haven't had babies are still likely to expel the device, risking pregnancy until they realize it is missing.

Within a few years the IUD may be running neck and neck with the Pill in contraceptive effectiveness. At least that's what the proponents of a device with a thin copper coating, still in the testing stage, claim. They say that the copper adds an extra anti-fertility effect.

Dr. Guttmacher, however, believes "the future of birth control is in the hypodermic syringe— i.e., monthly shots—"and that in several years it will probably displace the Pill too."

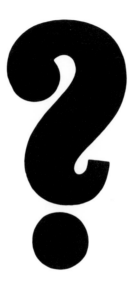

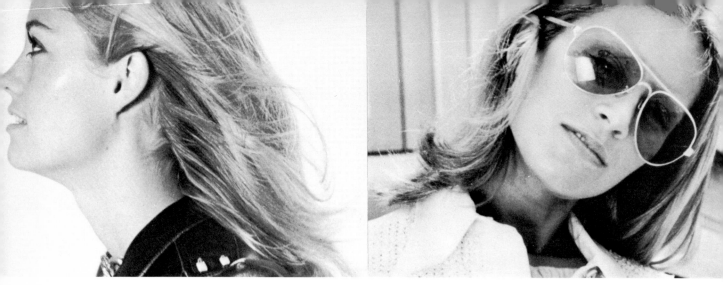

WHICH CONTRACEPTIVE

by Ellen Switzer

Robert and Joanne Adams are in graduate school. They are in their early twenties and have been married for six months. In another year, when Joanne finishes her course work toward a doctorate in English, they plan to start a family. Joanne feels that she will be able to manage writing her dissertation during pregnancy. She'd like to get her degree and have her baby at just about the same time. Since six months before her wedding, she has been taking birth control pills with no apparent ill effects. But recently she has read some of the more alarming testimony given by various medical experts before a U.S. Senate subcommittee investigating Pill safety. She is having second thoughts about her chosen method of birth control. A premature pregnancy would seriously disrupt her plans for a college teaching career. However, she doesn't want to take any unnecessary chances with her health either. Should she stop taking the Pill? If so, what are her alternatives?

William and Susan Peters have been married for five years and have two children. Susan is twenty-five, William, twenty-eight. Early in their marriage Susan started taking birth control pills. She stopped when she wanted to become pregnant. During her first pregnancy, she developed varicose veins. Her physician suggested that after the birth she consider another method of birth control, and when she agreed, he inserted an IUD (intrauterine device). Six months later she was pregnant again . . . and this time the baby was not planned. Apparently she had expelled the IUD without realizing it. After her second child, she tried using a diaphragm and now a year later, she is pregnant again. The thought of three young children, two in diapers, depresses her. She had con-sidered an abortion, but decided against it. However, both she and her husband want to be sure that this will be their last baby. They asked their physician, is there a completely safe, 100 percent certain method of birth control?

Barbara Taylor is not married. She is twenty years old, going to college, and has been dating Jim Allen, a law student. Quite recently they started having sexual intercourse. Barbara is almost sure that if she gets pregnant, Jim will agree to marry her. But she's not happy about the idea of being forced into marriage by an unplanned pregnancy, particularly since this would mean that Jim would have to quit law school and take a job. She knows that their attempts at contraception have been haphazard at best, but she doesn't know how to solve her problem. She doesn't feel that she can go to the old family doctor who, she insists, is "quite puritanical and old-fashioned." Her college health service has a policy of not giving birth control information to unmarried girls. Where can she go for the best medical advice?

These three situations are typical, based on over one hundred interviews with young people. Names and other identifying data have, of course, been changed. The interviews show that many young couples, in spite of their apparent sophistication about sex, are puzzled about which contraception is right for them. Much of the publicity about the real and alleged dangers of birth control pills has added to the confusion. Polls indicate that many women have stopped taking the Pill as a result of the 1970 Senate hearings alone. Also, immediately following the hearings, birth control clinics reported a decrease in the number of women using oral contraceptives.

Many family planning experts are very concerned about this. They point out that the hearings did not produce any new evidence about the real and alleged side effects of oral contraceptives. They

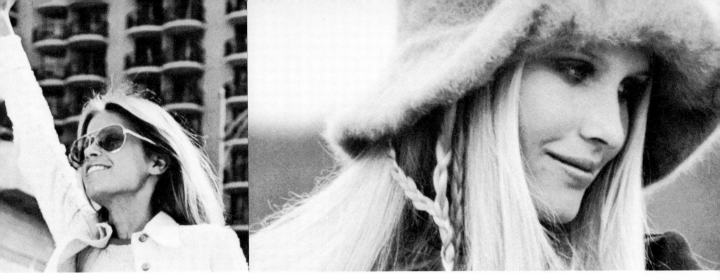

S RIGHT FOR YOU? . . .

know that the Pill is by far the most effective method of birth control and expected more than 100,000 unplanned pregnancies just within the first few months after the hearings, according to testimony by Dr. Alan F. Guttmacher, president of Planned Parenthood-World Population and an internationally known specialist in obstetrics and gynecology. When one of the senators on the committee interrupted him to voice the hope that the resulting babies wouldn't be named after members of the subcommittee, Dr. Guttmacher didn't think that the remark was very funny. He pointed out that many of those unwanted pregnancies would probably be terminated by abortions, most of them illegal and really dangerous to the women's health, if not their lives. Even the most anti-Pill faction of the medical community concedes, when pressed, that the number of legal and illegal abortions will probably rise as women abandon oral contraceptives for less failure-proof forms of birth control. And statistically, even the most expertly performed surgical abortion presents a higher risk than oral contraceptives in terms of possible side effects including permanent injuries and deaths.

But even when the pregnancy is not terminated, an unwanted baby can mean a serious interruption of life plans or even a major psychological disaster. Certainly the Adamses, the Peterses and Barbara Taylor were not willing to take this chance. How were their questions answered, and what are the implications of these answers for other young couples with birth control problems?

Joanne went to see a gynecologist who is a faculty member at one of the major medical schools in the Northeast to ask whether she should stop using the Pill. He told her that he could see no medical reason why she should change her form of contraception and a great many why she shouldn't. Joanne had received a thorough medical check-up before she was given the Pill prescription. The doctor had her entire medical history, plus considerable information about the medical history of her parents. Joanne had never suffered from varicose veins, headaches, chest pains or shortage of breath. During the time she had taken the Pill, her physician had seen her every six months, taken her blood pressure, checked on liver function, measured urine sugar, took a Pap smear once, and inquired carefully about any possible side effects. Joanne had reported none. There was no history of diabetes or vein disease in her family. In short, her doctor could see no evidence that the Pill was harming her health now, nor that it might be potentially damaging.

Could he promise Joanne that there might not be some as yet unknown future damage? The answer to that question, unfortunately, had to be a qualified "no." He told her that, according to British studies published last year, three in every 100,000 women taking the Pill had died from unexplained blood clots. After the studies were reviewed by the U.S. Food and Drug Administration, a warning that the principal ingredient in the oral contraceptive, estrogen, might cause overclotting of blood in some users, was stated in a leaflet that now accompanies the drug. If this fact worried Joanne sufficiently to want to change her birth control method, her doctor pointed out that should she get pregnant, her chances of death in childbirth would be *eight times higher*. In her age group, twenty-five of every 100,000 women die in childbirth each year. If she decided to obtain a legal abortion early, her chances of injury or death would be about the same as if she had the baby. In illegal abortions, about one hundred in 100,000 die, a totally unacceptable risk.

Her physician also pointed out that blood clots were the *only* well-established lethal hazard associated with oral contraceptives. Some researchers have noted an increase in blood sugar in

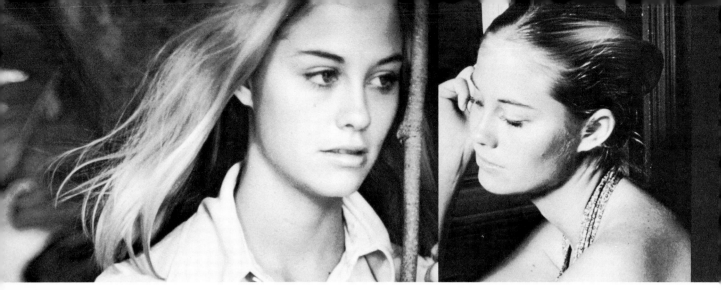

HOW TO FIND THE RIGHT

women taking the Pill. However, while the vast majority of physicians feel that this side effect should be watched, they do not consider it sufficiently alarming to take their patients, except those with a history of diabetes, off the Pill. "You'll be reading a lot about side effects of birth control pills during the next few months," the doctor told Joanne. "You'll hear that everything from frigidity to nymphomania, from baldness to cancer, may be caused by birth control pills. There is little scientific evidence for any of these allegations. But I can tell you one important side effect of *not* taking the Pill: pregnancy."

Joanne's physician agreed with every doctor interviewed for this article. Oral contraceptives are by far the most failure-proof form of birth control short of sterilization. Among one thousand women who take their medication regularly as prescribed, only between one and seven a year will become pregnant. The next most secure method is the IUD. But many physicians, including Joanne's, prefer not to use it for women who have never had a child. Insertion into a tight cervix is more difficult, and the chance of expulsion is higher. All other methods of birth control are considerably less effective than the Pill or the IUD.

Susan Peter's physician is also a faculty member at a well-known medical school. He did not advise her to start using oral contraceptives again. She had the one condition that almost all doctors feel can make the use of birth control pills dangerous: varicose veins. She had already expelled one IUD. But the physician suggested that he might try inserting another one after the third baby was born, possibly trying a larger size or a different shape. He told her that she would have to check herself carefully to make sure that the device remained in place, especially during and right after her menstrual periods. He would give her a vaginal foam to use for at least six months after the IUD

was inserted, as a form of extra insurance. "IUD's that remain in place for six months usually stay there," he added. However, he warned that even an IUD securely anchored in the uterus is no absolute guarantee against pregnancy. "We don't really know how and why IUD's work," he said, "or why they seem to work better in some women than in others." The failure rate with IUD's is about two to four times higher than the Pill; about fourteen to twenty-eight women per thousand per year get pregnant using this form of birth control, as opposed to between one and seven per thousand per year on the Pill. That the diaphragm had not worked well for Susan didn't surprise the doctor as much as it did her. Even when consistently used and correctly inserted, the diaphragm is still somewhat less safe than the IUD. The Masters-Johnson studies of the physiology of sexual intercourse have shown that many diaphragms, even those that are well fitted, don't stay in place during lovemaking. Also, apparently a great many women are tempted to take a chance "just this once," particularly when they feel that they have reached the "safe period" during their menstrual cycle. How often this turns out to be a mistake is shown by recent studies of contraception failures in clinic patients using the diaphragm; pregnancy figures have gone as high as three hundred women in a thousand in one year.

The completely safe, absolutely failure-proof contraceptive that the Peterses had requested was unfortunately not available. However, in view of Susan's previous contraceptive failure, plus the fact that in her case the Pill was not indicated, he suggested that a tubal ligation might be performed right after the birth of her third child.

"Normally, I would consider you too young for such an operation," he said. "I usually don't recommend it for a woman under thirty. But you have had three children fairly close together al-

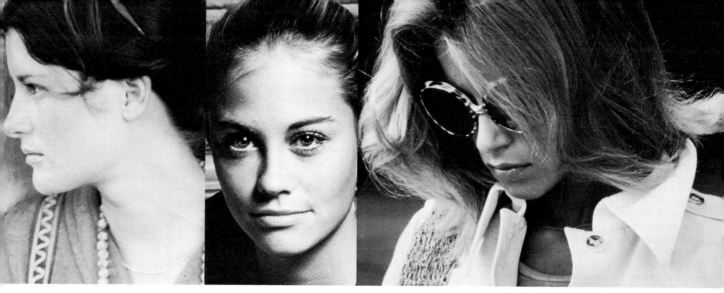

CONTRACEPTIVE FOR YOU . . .

ready. Pregnancy, with your vein condition, is even more dangerous than birth control pills, and I can't advise those. Besides, you were quite depressed for several months after your last delivery, and you look pretty unhappy to me right now. I agree with you that you probably shouldn't have any more children after this one. If you and Bill agree, I will plan to tie off your Fallopian tubes right after I finish delivering your next child. It's a very minor procedure. You will only have to stay in the hospital one or two extra days. Then you won't have to worry about either pregnancy or birth control again. But you must realize that, should you change your mind about wanting more children later on, the chances are only between fifty and sixty-five percent that we will be able to restore your fertility with surgery."

If Susan accepts her doctor's suggestion, she will be one of well over 100,000 persons who had sterilization operations during the past year. The number of such requests is rising, according to the Association for Voluntary Sterilization, which provides information for individuals and couples with questions about this form of birth control. The most frequently performed procedure is the one suggested by Susan's doctor: a cutting and tying-off of the tubes which carry the ovum to the uterus. If the ovum can't reach the sperm to be fertilized, no pregnancy is possible. The operation has no other effect on the woman. She continues to ovulate and to menstruate. Her glandular secretions and her sexual impulses should not be affected. For any woman who has had all the children she wants and who would prefer to dispense with all forms of contraception for the rest of her reproductive life, this procedure may seem like the ideal solution. There will be no interference from the law except in two states, Connecticut and Utah, which still limit sterilization operations to cases of medical necessity. All other states leave the decision up to the woman and her doctor. Most physicians also insist on the husband's permission. The operation is simple, especially when performed right after the birth of a child, when the uterus is still enlarged and the incision to reach the Fallopian tubes will be tiny.

In the past few years sterilization operations done on men have become increasingly popular. The procedure is known as a vasectomy. It consists of making a small incision in each side of the scrotum so that the ducts carrying the sperm can be lifted out, cut and tied off. Usually this is such a minor operation that it is performed in the doctor's office, under local anesthesia. The operation in no way interferes with the husband's sexual potency or enjoyment. There is no change in the production of male hormones. However, some men, particularly those who feel somewhat insecure about their masculinity, may become consciously or subconsciously upset by the idea that they are no longer able to impregnate a woman. Therefore, most physicians would advise any man thinking about a vasectomy to look closely at his own feelings about his sexuality. There's one additional problem: vasectomies are often performed by urologists. These specialists don't often see the consequences of unwanted pregnancies; such problems simply don't come to their attention. Like most physicians, they may be medically conservative and find it difficult to understand why any patient would want a surgical procedure that is not made necessary by his own health. So, in the past, some urologists have refused to perform vasectomies, and those who agreed to do them had long waiting lists. For more information on the subject of tubal ligations or vasectomies, contact the Association for Voluntary Sterilization, at 14 W. 40th Street in New York, which provides literature and acts as a referral agency to help people find a physician who will do the operation.

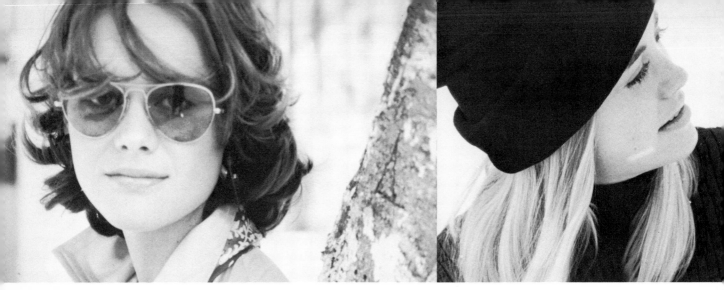

WHERE TO GET THE RIGHT

Barbara Taylor was in a completely different situation from the Adamses and the Peterses. Married couples no longer have a problem obtaining birth control information and advice no matter where they live in the United States. However, an unmarried girl sometimes still finds it hard to get help. Barbara, after spending a thoroughly terrifying week thinking she was pregnant (and looking up all possible sources for legal and illegal abortions in her area), found to her great relief that she was not, and immediately went to see the social worker in her student health service for advice. The counselor confirmed, regretfully, that the college, as a matter of policy, did not provide birth control services to unmarried students unless they could prove that they were engaged to be married and had their parents' permission. "Many other colleges don't have that policy anymore, and we will be changing, too, in the near future, but that doesn't help you right now, does it?" she said. She referred Barbara to the clinic run by the local Planned Parenthood Association. At the clinic Barbara saw a gynecologist who told her that Planned Parenthood, as a matter of national policy, provides birth control service to *all* young women, including minors, who are in danger of becoming pregnant unless they use an appropriate form of contraception. When Barbara anxiously asked whether her family would be notified of her visit, the doctor told her that no discussion with her parents would be necessary. Her consultation with the doctor would be completely confidential. "You are, after all, twenty years old," the doctor said. "If you were much younger, we would probably suggest that you talk the matter over with your family and try to get their permission to come here. But we wouldn't insist, even then. Planned Parenthood policy calls for helping all young women, regardless of age or marital status, who are worried about unwanted pregnancy." At the clinic Barbara had a thorough medical check-up. The physician and other professional staff members explained all the advantages and disadvantages of the various methods of contraception available through the clinic, including the rhythm system, in case she wanted that.

Barbara chose to be fitted with a diaphragm. She realized that the Pill was more failure-proof. But she was seeing Jim only once a week and "we're not having sex all that often," she told the doctor. Actually, Barbara was probably the best candidate for a diaphragm. Because she had never been pregnant, her vaginal walls were not yet stretched, and the chances of the diaphragm staying in place securely were very good. She told the doctor that if she and Jim got engaged, and she decided to transfer to the same college he attended in another town, she would probably be back for a Pill prescription. "I don't see any point in taking any kind of medication unless it's really necessary," she said. "And the way our sex life is at the moment, the Pill doesn't really seem necessary." The doctor agreed. Although she had no objections to prescribing birth control pills to sexually active young women, married or unmarried, she felt that the number of years that any young woman remains on hormones should be watched very carefully. "Technically, someone your age could be on the Pill for twenty-five years or more," she said. "But we prefer not to put anyone on continuous medication for that long. Of course, in actual practice, hardly anyone takes birth control pills in an uninterrupted fashion for more than a few years. Women stop and get pregnant. They switch to some other method for a while. And, increasingly, they have tubal ligations in their thirties."

Should Barbara forget to put in her diaphragm during a part of the month when she is particularly susceptible to pregnancy, the physician had one thought as back-up insurance: the morning-after

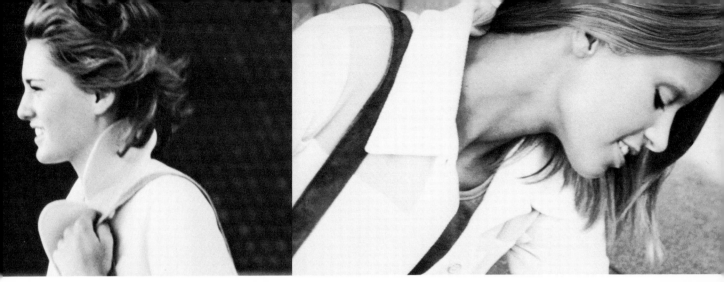

CONTRACEPTIVE FOR YOU . . .

pill. Planned Parenthood clinics often are not equipped to use this method, but many hospital clinics are. It involves giving the woman a huge dose of estrogen, divided over a period of two to three days, preferably beginning within twenty-four hours after possible impregnation (and not longer than seventy-two hours after). Experiments at Yale-New Haven Hospital on a very large sample caseload have shown this method to be highly effective. The estrogen seems to work to keep the fertilized egg from being implanted in the uterine wall. (This, incidentally, may also be the way the IUD works.) In any case, although the girl may technically be pregnant, the pregnancy never has a chance to develop. The morning-after pill method can be used only under the careful supervision of a physician experienced with the technique. "If you feel that you have taken a chance and might be pregnant, for heaven's sake don't swallow a friend's two-month supply of birth control pills. Call *us* and we'll make an appointment for you to see the right physician," the doctor told Barbara.

The Adamses, the Peterses and Barbara Taylor had completely different birth control requirements. With more and better methods available, researchers are working on many different kinds of programs to try to determine which birth control program is best for whom. Dr. George Langmyhr, medical director of the Planned Parenthood Federation of America, is a young gynecologist with great faith in the intelligence of most women to make appropriate choices once they have all the facts. "One of the great new developments in contraception is that we can offer a woman a choice of how she wants to conduct her reproductive life," he said. "We have any number of ways and combinations of ways to help her have only as many children as she wants. We'll tell her the advantages and disadvantages of each . . . and then let her make up her own mind."

To help women decide what's right for them and to allow for more and better alternatives, medical schools continue to investigate the safety, acceptibility and effectiveness of existing birth control methods and to work on discovering new and better ones. A particularly interesting program is under way at the University of Pennsylvania School of Medicine. There the Department of Obstetrics and Gynecology combines theoretical research in reproduction with clinical research and practice in birth control. The department's outpatient clinic serves thousands of women from all walks of life. Data from the clinic are carefully analyzed, and procedures are constantly revised. Have the hearings on the Pill changed the department's attitudes about prescribing the medication in any way? Dr. Luigi Mastroianni, Jr., the department's chairman, answers that question with an emphatic "no." "Those hearings didn't tell us a thing we didn't know before," he said. "We have always told patients that there are certain minimal risks associated with the Pill. We still do. We have always advised some women that they should use an alternate method of birth control. We still do. We have always encouraged anyone experiencing side effects from whatever method of birth control to report the problem to us immediately. We still do. We have always offered a wide selection of methods, including rhythm, with a complete explanation of their advantages and disadvantages. We still do."

Because clinic personnel has found, however, that some women find it difficult to express their fears and concerns to the physician, group discussions have been organized, usually led by a well-trained female health educator. The discussions are scheduled *before* the patient sees the physician so that she already has some idea of available methods and can make a more intelligent choice. Of course, the health educator does not prescribe or even suggest what method might be best for any

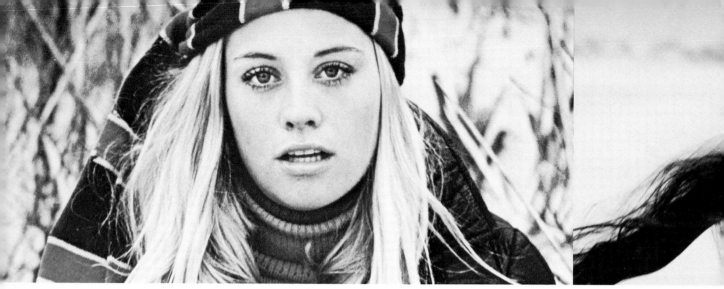

WHAT'S IN THE FUTURE O

would-be patient. She only explains what is available and answers questions.

An especially interesting study is being conducted jointly by the Department of Obstetrics and Gynecology and the Department of Psychiatry. Dr. Karl Rickels, professor of psychiatry, explained that the two departments are investigating cooperatively some of the psychological and psychosomatic effects of *all* forms of birth control. "For instance, we have been told that for some women, birth control pills produce anxiety and depression. Private physicians often hear this, and they don't have the time to go into the background of the situation. We are trying to pinpoint whether the chemical in the Pill or the patient's own feelings about taking it are causing the reaction. We now suspect that if a patient goes into a deep depression after taking birth control pills, she may have been a candidate for this particular form of psychiatric illness all along. The estrogen in the Pill might not be the culprit at all. Almost any new development in her life might have triggered her condition. But the medication is such an obvious, concrete object on which to blame her unhappiness."

Additional research reported by Dr. Celso-Ramon Garcia, professor of obstetrics and gynecology, seems to bear out these conclusions. Dr. Garcia, in a paper on emotional factors in oral contraception, tells of a comparative study done on reported side effects of birth control pills between a group of middle-class private patients and women on an Indian reservation. "In the former, nausea, breakthrough bleeding, headache and breast tenderness were more prevalent," he said. The middle-class women also showed much greater weight gain than the women on the reservation, an observable fact that unlike the other effects could not have been influenced or suggested by the questions of the interviewer.

The two departments are also planning a study on why an IUD may seem unbearably uncomfortable to one woman, while hardly noticed by another. They are interested in the whole field of contraceptive failure. Why do some couples have so many "accidents," while other couples seem to be able to control the size of their families effectively, regardless of what method of birth control they select?

While investigating the relationship between female psychology and the reproductive process, the department is also looking into other aspects of birth control. For instance, clinic physicians have found that many women who have never had children can use an IUD. "We have tried it with women who specifically asked for this method and we have found that retention is much better and side effects fewer than we had originally believed," one clinic physician said.

Sometimes patients have to switch from one method to another several times before finding something that is just right for them. Many physicians, at the University of Pennsylvania and in other clinics, recommend that a backup method be made available even to patients who have already found a method that seems right for them. "We give our patients containers of spermicidal foam, whether they are on the Pill, or use an IUD," said Dr. Virginia M. Stuermer, medical director of Planned Parenthood in Connecticut and associate clinical professor of obstetrics and gynecology at the Yale School of Medicine. "It's always possible to forget to take the Pill . . . and even one slip during the menstrual cycle increases the chances of pregnancy. An IUD might be expelled days or weeks before a patient can get back to the clinic. A diaphragm might be punctured or mislaid. In such cases, the foam is there as extra insurance." Other physicians and clinics provide a package of condoms for the patient's sexual partner.

Like all physicians interviewed for this arti-

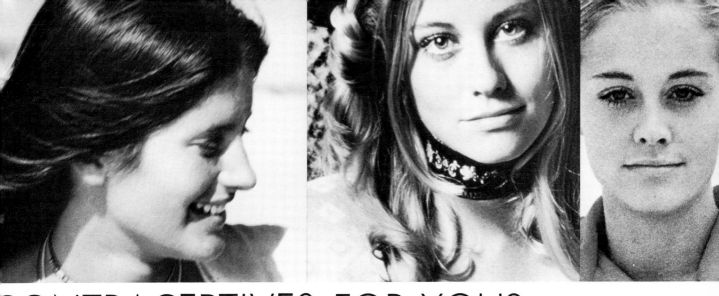

CONTRACEPTIVES FOR YOU?

cle, Dr. Stuermer believes that effective contraception is better than abortion. But she agrees with the majority of physicians that abortion laws should be changed as rapidly as possible. "The best time to terminate an unwanted pregnancy is very early," she said. The danger is minimal then. But even in states where abortion laws are fairly liberal or where hospital administrators interpret laws permissively, administrative procedures often take valuable time. Dr. Stuermer advocates that statutes relating to abortion be removed entirely from the books. "This should be a matter between the woman and her physician," she said. Physicians who prescribe the morning-after pill now are obviously taking the problem into their own hands. In almost all states they are technically breaking the law when they use this method to terminate a pregnancy. However, the most frequently used procedure, dilation of the cervix and curettage of the uterus, should be done only in a hospital operating room, which means the physician has to go through the proper channels. "Something can always go wrong even in the simplest operation," Dr. Stuermer said. "Women who don't want to be pregnant will find ways to get abortions. We should make it as safe for them as any other medical procedure."

In England and Sweden a new form of abortion without surgery has been used experimentally and apparently successfully. The patient is injected with a hormone-like substance, which produces a prompt abortion as late in pregnancy as five months. However, European doctors recommend that the injection be given much earlier. According to medical reports, hospitalization of the patient is not necessary if the pregnancy has not progressed beyond eight weeks. This method is not yet available anywhere in the United States and is used only experimentally in Europe. If it is really perfected, however, it might make changes in abortion laws unnecessary, since the procedure will take place usually in the privacy of the physician's office. Meanwhile, abortion laws are changing too.

New York State has passed a bill to remove all legal restrictions on abortions, leaving the decision up to the physician and his patient. Hawaii has passed a similar law. However, there is a residence requirement there. The patient must have lived in Hawaii for three months prior to the operation. This bars many out-of-town women from taking advantage of the law's liberal provisions, since physicians consider an abortion after three months medically hazardous. Several other state legislatures are considering bills modifying or eliminating legal restrictions on abortion. Alaska recently passed a liberalized abortion bill. But even if all these laws pass, the necessity for effective contraception remains. Any form of surgical abortion is more hazardous, in terms of possible side effects, than any form of contraception.

Dr. Stuermer indicated that an excellent form of birth control might be a chemically harmless pill that is taken routinely immediately after intercourse which would thus prevent the implantation of the fertilized ovum in the womb and thus cause an instant abortion. Actually, this may be the way the IUD works. Such a new, and as yet undiscovered, form of medication would eliminate the mechanical difficulties of the IUD as well as the day-after-day, month-after-month introduction of chemicals into the patient's system.

At this time, however, few researchers have any firm expectations that a new form of birth control that is mistake-proof, completely safe, unrelated in its applications to the time of intercourse, and acceptable to all couples will soon be discovered. "Anyone who is waiting for medical science to perform this miracle in the near future, while having a baby every year, had better settle for something less perfect," Dr. Mastroianni said.

MIS-CONCEP-TIONS ABOUT SEX

by *Phyllis Starr*

In sex everybody has to be finally his or her own expert, and few people are. Misconceptions, fears, guilt and incredible to humorous ignorance run right down the line of sexual experience from teenagers to octogenarians, from graduate students in the greatest medical schools of America to underprivileged young mothers in the ghettos. Everyone talks about the new openness that surrounds sex—clergymen, psychiatrists, novelists, anthropologists, actresses, editors—everybody discusses it on TV. Nudity is commonplace in the movies. Many publishers would rather publish books and articles on sex than on any other subject. But the actual facts of anatomy, sexual response, psychological development, male and female relationships, abortion, contraception, pregnancy, childbirth and masturbation remain as unavailable to many people as if they had never been let out of the nineteenth century.

Even the young, who have probably had more sex more openly than any generation in American history, are far from competent or knowledgeable on the subject or in the act. To find out some of their problems and misconceptions a good source is Dr. Philip Sarrel and his wife, Lorna, who offer a sex counseling service for students at Yale. They have helped organize and conduct courses in human sexuality at Yale as well as Brown, Mount Holyoke, Smith and Amherst. Dr. Sarrel is an assistant professor in the Department of Gynecology and Obstetrics at the Yale University School of Medicine, and Mrs. Sarrel is a social worker. The noncredit, elective, co-ed courses are jammed, but the Sarrels wonder if the students who don't sign up aren't the ones who need them most. "That's not to say," explained Dr. Sarrel, "that the students who do take the courses don't need them. But we have the feeling that many students with hang-ups and problems about sex who should be there attempting to straighten them out, aren't."

The crucial thing about sexual ignorance is that it can, in some cases, lead to serious problems that could have been relieved or prevented if brought into the open. Some people still consider masturbation an abnormality. Some actually think masturbation can lead to insanity. Some students who masturbate often think "I am the only one in the world committing this sin." Then a lot of energy and concern goes into worrying about it. When you have a mode of behavior that is anxiety-provoking it doesn't just stop; in fact, it usually increases if it is allowed to go unresolved. The person who is suffering anxiety and guilt because of masturbating may masturbate more. This really leads to the core of why sex needs to be taught. Mrs. Elise Ottesen-Jensen, the founder of the Swedish system of sex education, said that she spent her whole life teaching sex so that people could be free to use their energies in other ways. She was president of International Planned Parenthood Federation from 1959 to 1963, and in her eighties she is still a much demanded lecturer about sex education.

In order to really teach sex, Dr. Sarrel believes, you have to have "some outlet for peer sharing," peer instruction and experience, which is why the sexuality courses divide into small question-and-answer groups directed by student leaders. "This experience is probably much more important than anything we can do in the lectures. An authority can turn students off when he starts to moralize, but he can hold them if he talks honestly and tells the facts without implying that 'this is what I think you ought to do.' I always keep in mind when I'm talking to a group that there are as many students in that group who are going to be as potentially relieved by what I am saying as there are those who are going to be threatened. I try to let the students make their own decision."

One of the real crises in what we call the sexual revolution is that sex today is being used as an entity in itself and not as part of a broader relationship. What used to be the problem of petting has now become intercourse; and the questions are, Where is the more meaningful relationship? Where is the deep commitment and how do you express it? How do you communicate it?

Students now think in a very freewheeling way. They define systems of their own. And some of the things a few of them are defining, or redefining, are virginity and intercourse. Some of the more sophisticated students think virginity is an ancient concept. They are essentially saying "What is a millimeter of tissue? It's insignificant and the important thing is the commitment in the relationship."

One girl described her petting relationship this way: "This is ridiculous. This is mutual masturbation." She had come to the conclusion that this was more immoral than having intercourse.

Then there are students who define sex as something different from intercourse. "I had one girl tell me she had sex with some boys and intercourse with others," said Dr. Sarrel. "When I asked her what the difference was she said, 'Well, intercourse is when a guy comes inside me, sex is when he doesn't.' I've had students say to me, too, 'I'm a virgin, the boy never came inside me.' He ejacu-

Can a virgin become pregnant?
Can sperm fertilize an egg as long as one week after intercourse?
Can you become pregnant during your period?
Can orgasm last for minutes?
Can you answer these questions?

lates only in the area of the vagina. They think this cannot impregnate them, but if the sperm works its way up into the uterus, which is possible, it can."

Conception is one of the areas in which students have the grossest misconceptions. "They are always surprised when we tell them that sperm can live as long as a week," said Lorna Sarrel, "and impregnate at any time during that week if the girl is ovulating."

"The male students," said Dr. Sarrel, "often have no idea when pregnancy occurs." Dr. Haskell Coplin, the professor of psychology at Amherst who has been responsible for the sexuality courses along with the Sarrels, has been studying students over the last eighteen years and has found that 95 percent of the Amherst men had only a vague and somewhat inaccurate understanding of when conception occurs.

The Sarrels once came across a couple who had been together for about a year. They only had intercourse when she was menstruating as a way of birth control, which may not be much of a control. If a girl ovulates on say the second day after her period, which is possible, and she has had intercourse at the end of her period, sperm still can be alive and fertilize her egg. "Another factor in the occurrence of pregnancy," Dr. Sarrell said, "is the feeling some girls have that you have intercourse for awhile before you can become pregnant. Or, as one girl put it, 'You have to do something else in order to get pregnant.' In the last two years I have seen close to a dozen girls who became pregnant the first time they had intercourse. In addition, a number of pregnant girls seemed to have had intercourse at a 'safe time.' Either the factor in their pregnancy was a prolonged sperm survival or, perhaps as in animals, there are some women who are 'reflex ovulators' responding to intercourse by releasing an egg. Such cases have been reported in medical literature."

There's another category who get pregnant because they manage to deceive themselves into thinking that they just couldn't, that nothing could possibly happen to them. It's the invulnerability syndrome. They don't use contraceptives, "like the girl in Good-bye Columbus," Mrs. Sarrel pointed out. "You remember the boy is furious when he finds out she wasn't using anything. Contraception has become a female responsibility. He says in effect, 'What's the matter, are you so spoiled you think nothing bad can happen to you?'" Other risk takers that the Sarrels have observed among students are those who are having intercourse without contraception, but feel "we aren't going to do this again." Particularly if they're a little hung up about it, guilty. They're going to try not to have intercourse the next time they're together. They refuse to face up to the fact that intercourse has become a regular thing for them, and going to a doctor to get birth control is really facing up to exactly what it is you're doing. That's a big step for most girls.

Students who do face up and who are on the Pill sometimes fall into another error. The Pill can cause a discharge and increase susceptibility to vaginitis. When they get a discharge or irritation some of them think it means they have a venereal disease. Some get terrified and think it is instant punishment for having intercourse. "Actually," said Dr. Sarrel, "venereal disease in college students, at least the ones on the campuses where I have been, is rare. These students are for the most part in a one-to-one relationship. There is something I admire tremendously about these college students. It's not that they're freer to have sex than other generations. To be suddenly faced with so much freedom can be very threatening. But it's that they can be open, honest, and develop relationships that are not based on a lot of superficialities. The fact that so few male college students today have a prostitute experience is great and accounts partly for the rareness of V.D. among them."

As might be suspected, another big misconception area is orgasm. Mrs. Sarrel had one student tell her, "My orgasms just aren't like my friends'. They're not as good and my friends' last for minutes and minutes." "Either your friends are lying," said Mrs. Sarrel, "or they have overactive imaginations, because a single orgasm lasts only a few seconds." Another difficulty is that in many instances first intercourse is painful and a little traumatic. Often it's a disappointing experience. Girls build up great expectations and then find a kind of lukewarm situation. They don't understand that a process of learning is involved. But the amount of physical discomfort is insignificant compared to the disillusion, the so-that's-all-it-is attitude; it's not like D. H. Lawrence. There are some realistic students who say, "I expected it would be a little uncomfortable, I didn't hear bells or see stars, but it was a good experience as a beginning." And others who say, "Sure, I didn't have an orgasm the first time and I didn't expect to, but in the course of time it's now built up to where I do have an orgasm, and it's a wonderful, meaningful experience." But it's necessary to realize the problems of students who have become depressed as a result of their first intercourse experience and to offer them counseling that can help put that experience in the perspective of their own backgrounds and individual lifestyles.

There's a great need among girls to have orgasm, and some worry about it. They want to know, have they or haven't they? What is it? That's a very hard question to answer. "Some girls who have been orgasmic have not realized they were," said Dr. Sarrel. "The chapter in Masters and Johnson's Human Sexual Response in which women describe orgasm is a resource I refer to. However, it still isn't very easy to imagine an orgasm if you have never been orgasmic."

This, of course, gets at an important issue of sex education—what you can and can't teach. You

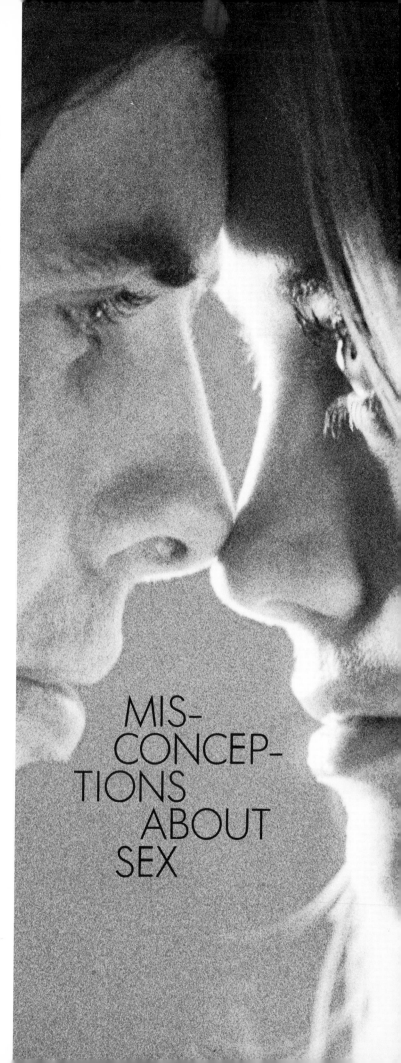

can't get on a platform and didactically teach feelings and attitudes; you can only explore them. You can't say to Martha, "Look, your orgasm is going to be just like Peggy's," because everyone's is different.

The misconception that there is just one way to feel, one way to do things and that if you don't, then something is wrong, abnormal, psychologically inferior, causes all kinds of trouble. Oral-genital sex, for example, seems to have become more common. Students see it in movies very clearly. It can be harder in many ways for some to assimilate and handle than intercourse. Positions in intercourse come under this heading too. "Take a girl who has a climax only if she is on top,' said Dr. Sarrel. "That's not so unusual, but her boyfriend considers it to be emasculating and has responded by not being able to maintain an erection. He is depressed and tells her she is oversexed. They both need to understand the culturization they have brought into the bedroom, in order to avoid turning their relationship into a hassle instead of a learning and maturing experience in intimacy."

The pressure to be like everyone else causes problems in sex too. Male students do an awful lot of bragging about intercourse with girls, and if a boy doesn't have it, he begins to wonder if he is normal. Mrs. Sarrel said, "We had one boy who was very upset about the kind of bragging that was going on in his dorm. He found himself doing it, being hypocritical, and he couldn't stand it. He wanted to know what would happen if he were honest with them? We told him to try, maybe the others would be honest too, and everybody would be better off."

"Many students regard sexual relationships as an important part of the maturing process," Dr. Sarrel said. "Although they appreciate the importance of respect for each other and for the commitment that sex means between two individuals, they do not equate sex with love. This attitude can work in many ways. On the one hand, there are students who separate sex and love and are especially active sexually because, as one student put it, 'I just couldn't think of any reason not to be.' On the other hand, there are those who are not so victimized by the sex revolution and who are able to develop relationships based on feelings in addition to purely sexual ones. Many are not ready to 'fall in love,' for they feel they have not yet developed an individuality they can share in the way that the intimacy of a love relationship demands. That is an important difference between many teen-agers and college students. The teen-agers are absolutely sure they are in love. They get pregnant, married and have babies, then get divorced. Immaturity is the most common reason for marriage dissolution today. The college students are more skeptical about love. They want to enter the continuum of the love relationship from a more meaningful starting place."

MIS-CONCEP-TIONS ABOUT SEX

CHILDBIRTH

ADVAN

MORE IN THE LAST FIVE YEARS THAN IN THE PREVIOUS HUNDRED!

by Ellen Switzer

In a labor room at Yale-New Haven Hospital a young woman lies on her bed, reading a magazine. Occasionally, as she feels a contraction, she winces slightly. Otherwise she is the picture of relaxation, although she knows that the obstetrical and pediatric staff have classified her as a "high-risk mother." Two years ago, in another hospital, she delivered a dead infant. This time a similar tragedy will be avoided. Next to her bed, on a rolling table, stands a small electronic device that looks a little like a tape recorder. The machine is a fetal monitor, now used almost routinely at the Yale Medical School when trouble might be expected during labor and delivery. The machine keeps the mother and her unborn child under close electronic vigil from the start of labor until her baby is safely born. She can feel easier and assured, because she knows that the monitor will instantly pick up the slightest abnormality in her baby's heartbeat. A team of obstetrician, pediatrician and anesthesiologist will be notified at the central nursing station by a flashing yellow light and will be at her bedside in less than a minute to do what is necessary to eliminate the cause of fetal distress.

In another labor room down the hall, a twenty-three-year-old girl and her husband are playing chess. She wins. A few minutes later a doctor and a nurse enter to examine the patient. As they leave, the husband, who is waiting outside the door, is told that his wife will be going to the delivery room shortly. Within half an hour he will be a father. Fastened to his wife's hospital gown is a small glass tube that looks like a hypodermic without the needle. Attached to the tube is a slender plastic catheter, which in turn is taped into the patient's back. For the past four hours an anesthesiologist has been occasionally injecting a small amount of a Novocain-like solution through the tube into her back. The procedure, called peridural continuous lumbar anesthesia, has eliminated pain, although it has not made the mother sleepy (sleepy girls don't win chess games, even when their husbands are not competing very strenuously), nor has it paralyzed her. She is also able to move her legs and to feel her contractions as pressure. This means she can cooperate in the baby's birth by bearing down and pushing when she is told to do so by her doctor. When the baby is born, she will be able to hear its first cry, even before the cord is cut. As a pediatrician examines the baby carefully and a nurse cleans it, the obstetrician finishes the necessary repairs on the mother and leaves to tell the husband that he is the father of a healthy girl. Only then is the catheter taken out. She is moved from the delivery table to her bed and is rolled into the corridor. "Was it bad?" her husband asks. "The only trouble with peridural anesthesia is that it may increase the birthrate. It's so easy to have a baby!" she says.

In a conference room on another floor of the same hospital, a group of young doctors is meeting. They are discussing babies—babies that have not yet been born. The first case involves a mother with diabetes in her eighth month of pregnancy. The baby looks and feels large. However, is it really as mature as it seems? The results of various chemical tests made on the mother and the fetus are brought into the discussion. The physicians decide that labor should be induced. "The uterine environment is probably no longer right for the fetus," one pediatrician says. "We can do better with the infant in our new-born intensive care unit."

Only recently have doctors been able to be sure that they could not only simulate the uterine environment for some babies, but they could improve on it. One member of the medical team is a new kind of specialist. He combines training and experience in obstetrics and pediatrics with another medical specialty: computer science. The computer can record an enormous volume of data about the mother and the fetus, correlate the information in various combinations and help the physician to make the best-informed and most carefully considered decisions possible.

What is happening at the Yale University School of Medicine, Dr. Nathan Kase, the recently appointed thirty-nine-year-old chairman of the Department of Obstetrics and Gynecology, calls "The New Obstetrics." For several days last month I had an opportunity to talk with Dr. Kase and his staff, to observe recently developed electronic devices at work and to watch in the labor and delivery rooms as babies were born and cared for by some of the new methods.

"More has happened in obstetrics in the last five years than in the previous hundred years," Dr. Kase said. "We have probably made more progress faster in obstetrics than in almost any other branch of medicine. Daily, in our clinical practice, we are helping mothers and babies with new tools that were not even in the research stage ten years ago."

Basic to Dr. Kase's approach to the new obstetrics is the fact that each pregnancy involves *two* patients: the mother and her unborn child. This means that pregnancy, labor and delivery are now the concern of a number of different specialists. Obstetrician and pediatrician work together almost from the beginning of the pregnancy, assisted—as

needed—by other kinds of physicians (internists, blood specialists, psychiatrists). Increasingly, the computer specialist and the electronics engineer are also involved.

This, of course, does not mean that every pregnant woman who has her baby at Yale-New Haven Hospital sees all these scientists. She may see just her obstetrician (although Dr. Kase, for one, likes to have a pediatrician involved early and certainly prefers to have him in the delivery room during and right after the birth of the baby). However, if any complications should arise, a team of specialists stands ready to help as a matter of routine in all pregnancies and deliveries under the supervision of the Yale Medical School staff. They are also available to private physicians in the community for consultation as needed. Most of the young mothers with whom I talked found that fact alone immensely reassuring.

I spent over a week in the Yale Department of Obstetrics and Gynecology. During that week I talked to the women in labor, stood beside several of them while their babies were being delivered, then accompanied the babies to the nursery where the fast but expert checkup they receive in the delivery room is followed up by a complete physical and neurological examination. I spoke with obstetricians, pediatricians, blood specialists, several anesthesiologists and the director of Yale's new medical computer department. Most illuminating, perhaps, were my conversations with young women who were about to have babies, who were in the process of having babies and who just had babies.

The labor and delivery suite is the quietest and by far the pleasantest part of the hospital. During the two days I spent there I did not hear one scream, or even a groan. Some of the women were having unmedicated labor. Some were using the breathing methods advocated by Dr. Grantley Dick-Read; others, those recommended by Dr. Fernand Lamaze. Dr. Dick-Read recommends abdominal breathing with complete relaxation and sleep between contractions. Dr. Lamaze is against abdominal breathing; he recommends chest breathing. Both methods also have their own set of exercises, which are practiced during pregnancy and are considered by some as useful in combating pain in childbirth.

The physicians at Yale, like most of today's obstetrical specialists, avoid the term "natural childbirth." ("What's unnatural about having a baby, regardless of *how* you do it?" one doctor asked.) They feel that the breathing exercises are chiefly of psychological value in that they distract some women from concentrating on their own fears and apprehensions. These doctors do, however, feel strongly that a woman should know what is happening to her own body and to the fetus during pregnancy, labor and delivery. The term they use is "prepared" or "educated" childbirth.

Most of the women with whom I talked had attended prenatal classes and had read several books for expectant mothers (two of the obstetricians recommended *Pregnancy and Birth* by Dr. Alan F. Guttmacher as "a reassuring, accurate and informative book." It is available in paperback). In spite of the "education," however, most of the first-time mothers were frightened when they arrived at the hospital. All felt their fears had been needless by the time their babies were being delivered.

The calm atmosphere on the floor helped. So did the fact that nurses and doctors were constantly available to answer questions and provide reassurance. The medical staff encourages husbands to remain with their wives in the labor room until the actual delivery of the baby. If, for some reason, a husband cannot remain with his wife, there's usually a succession of student nurses who remain in the room once contractions are firmly established.

No one tells anyone that childbirth is supposed to be painless. "I never tell a woman in labor that her contractions don't or shouldn't hurt," said Dr. Robert Hook, maternity floor anesthesiologist and professor of anesthesiology. He has specialized in obstetrical anesthesia, which he considers a fascinating, fast-changing and challenging field. "When a patient tells me she is in pain, I grant her the simple human dignity of believing her."

The most frequently used method of relief from labor and birth pain at Yale-New Haven Hospital is continuous lumbar peridural conduction anesthesia. This can be applied continuously from the time the cervix is about half-dilated, long before the most painful contractions start.

"Labor and delivery are divided into two stages, with a brief transition in between," said Dr. Gerald G. Anderson, assistant professor of obstetrics and gynecology. "During the first stage, the cervix dilates about ten centimeters. Then there is a brief transition while the baby gets itself into the right position for delivery. During the second stage, the baby is pushed out through the cervix and the birth canal. Early in labor, while the cervix is dilating to about four centimeters, there is probably not much discomfort. A woman will experience her contractions as a hardening of the uterus, with possibly some relatively mild cramps or a pulling sensation. We don't like to start the peridural anesthesia until dilation is nearing five centimeters, so for a period (between four and five centimeters) she may be uncomfortable. If she's really unhappy, we can, at that point, give Demerol (a synthetic morphine-like drug) or tranquilizers. But, frequently, just reassurance and the husband's presence are enough. It is during this relatively brief time when we prefer not to give medication that the relaxation techniques she has taught herself may be helpful. But in my opinion, a good detective story or an interesting crossword puzzle would do as well. For the vast majority of women, after we have put in the peridural, pain is just no longer a problem."

Dr. Hook agrees. There are some exceptions. For instance, a few women are allergic to one or all of the local anesthetics used in peridural anesthesia. "If a woman tells us that her face blows up to twice its normal size after a Novacain injection by her dentist, we feel that she's probably not a good candidate for peridural . . . so we work out something else," he says. There are a small number of women who, after the peridural has been injected, still have a "window" of pain. For some unknown reason a section of their lower abdomen is not affected by the anesthetic. In that case it may be supplemented with a few whiffs of gas.

As I talked to women who were having their babies with peridural anesthesia, Dr. Hook's point became obvious. One nineteen year-old first-time mother (let's call her Sally, although that is not her real name) had had mild labor pains for several days. She was not in great discomfort, but just uncomfortable enough to have had her sleep interrupted for two nights. When she came into the delivery suite, she was discouraged, exhausted and close to tears. Her physician introduced me as a medical writer (this was done with all patients to whom I talked), told her that I was doing an article on the new obstetrics, and asked her if she minded talking to me. Sally wasn't too enthusiastic about this prospect at first. As a matter of fact, at that point she wasn't too enthusiastic about having the baby. But at least I was a distraction, so, along with the floor nurse, I went into her labor room. Sally was badly frightened. When Dr. Hook dropped in to see her and asked whether she was in severe pain, she said, "No." But she knew it would get so much worse. Her mother had told her so much about the horrors of childbirth, and how could she forget those awful scenes she had read in *Farewell to Arms* and what she had seen in a recent British movie?

Dr. Hook conferred briefly with Sally's obstetrician and then assured her that not only were things not going to get worse, they were going to get better almost immediately. The obstetrician had decided to reinforce Sally's slow contractions by dripping a hormone into bloodstream. But before starting the drip, she would be given peridural anesthesia.

"Roll up like an angry cat," Dr. Hook said. "I'm going to give you a little local anesthetic before I start the peridural. It may sting a little . . . but nothing more." He injected the drug. Sally didn't even wince; she just looked interested. "Now I'm going to put the needle in place between your spinal vertebrae and your spinal canal . . . that's what we call the peridural space," Dr. Hook continued. "As I put in the needle you may feel a little pressure. But we won't get into your spinal canal. The drug won't mix with your spinal fluid, so you won't be paralyzed and you won't get any headache later." By that time he had inserted the needle, threaded with the plastic catheter, removed the needle, and the nurse had taped the slender plastic tube to Sally's back. "Now roll over and relax," he said. A few minutes later, the nurse commented, "I think Sally's having a contraction." Sally agreed . . . a strong one, judging from the hardness of her uterus. But there was no pain . . . not even any discomfort.

I visited Sally off and on for the next two hours. She was still tired (after all, she hadn't slept much for two nights), but by now her enthusiasm for becoming a mother had returned. She was also delighted to talk to me, partly because she wanted to share her exciting experience with another woman.

As she was rolled off into the delivery room, she noted that I was wearing the green operating room gown used at Yale-New Haven Hospital, plus head-covering, mask and all the other delivery room gear. She asked me if I wanted to come along and watch the delivery. I had watched several others (with the patients' express permission) and was interested in how Sally would do. So, along with the floor nurse, I helped push her bed into the delivery room and stood next to her there.

It turned out that the baby was well down in the birth canal. "Push, Sally," the doctor and nurse encouraged in unison. She did, several times, eagerly and enthusiastically. Between contractions she turned to me and kept repeating, "When I tell this to my mother tomorrow, she just won't believe me." The baby uttered its first cry before it was even completely born. It turned out to be a healthy squalling eight-pound girl. Sally looked over the baby carefully, counted toes and fingers, and the infant was turned over to the pediatrician who did a fast, careful, preliminary check. "Apgar score 9," he announced. The Apgar scoring system is the standard method of checking a newborn infant's responses. Ten points is tops; 8 or 9, normal. Low Apgar scores may mean that the baby is either sleepy (from too many drugs that have crossed into its bloodstream through the mother's placenta) or that it has some other problems. Sally's baby was obviously in great shape, in spite of her relatively long early labor. After some brief necessary work on Sally and a clean-up job on the baby, they were both transferred to her bed, and I helped roll them to the room where Sally's husband was waiting to meet the new addition.

Peridural conduction anesthesia is the new obstetric technique of interest to the vast majority of mothers whose only foreseeable childbirth problem is that of physical pain. However, the new obstetrics includes as well equally dramatic and revolutionary techniques that apply in the minority, but very important minority, of births in which there may be complications.

Amniocentesis is a key new diagnostic tool that keeps track of the progress of the fetus. A local anesthetic is injected into the mother's abdomen. Then a needle is inserted through her abdominal wall into the uterus and a small amount of amniotic fluid is withdrawn. Its composition is incredibly complex. The amniotic fluid can tell the physician whether the fetus is male or female, sick or healthy, mature or immature. Amniocentesis, before the second month of pregnancy, will reveal whether the fetus has certain inborn genetic abnormalities, whether it has been affected by German measles contracted by the mother, or by drugs she may have taken. If known abnormality is present, a therapeutic abortion can be performed at that time if this is what the patient and her doctor wish. Although few states specifically permit abortions when the fetus is badly damaged, many hospitals interpret existing abortion laws liberally enough to allow operations in such cases. Amniocentesis also makes it possible to treat the mother and/or the fetus to improve the baby's chances.

There are other new techniques of observing the unborn child. Up till now, the only method for observing the skeletal structure and the head size of the fetus has been X-rays. Physicians have known that repeated X-rays, particularly early in pregnancy, could be harmful and have been searching for a safer, better technique. A new method, called ultra-sound, is based on the principle that was used for submarine detection during World War II. A very sensitive microphone is placed on the mother's abdomen that picks up the signals from the fetus. They are recorded on a sort of radar screen. When correctly interpreted, they can give accurate data on the fetal position, head size, skeletal structure and other information invaluable in anticipating possible birth complications.

The *fetal monitoring system,* developed by Dr. Edward H. Hon, until last year professor of obstetrics at Yale, now at the University of Southern California, may well be the most exciting development in the new obstetrics. Dr. Hon studied electronics before changing his field to medicine. He felt that the most serious threat to the baby's safety during labor and delivery was the interruption of its blood supply to the brain. Oxygen deprivation has long been associated with stillbirths, cerebral palsy and other types of brain damage in infants. Until the development of the fetal-monitoring machine, the only tool the physician had for diagnosing fetal distress was the stethoscope, an inaccurate measure at best. Fetal heartbeats are measured by the stethoscope about once every twenty minutes (less on a busy delivery floor). Fetal distress, however, can occur in seconds, and damage can be serious before the stethoscope has even picked up a clue. Also, according to Dr. Hon, the stethoscope can pick up signals only *between* contractions. However, the baby is in most danger *during* contractions. So, by the time the physician realizes that something has gone wrong, it is frequently too late to save the baby from harm, even with an emergency caesarean section. Dr. Hon's little machine picks up signs of difficulty long before they become apparent through the stethoscope. The remedy is frequently exceedingly simple. The mother may just be asked to change her position, because she is pressing down on the cord and interfering with the fetal blood supply. Or medication may be changed or stopped.

The monitor can be used without any medical hazard and without discomfort to the patient. It is applied by clipping a small electrode to the infant's scalp when the cervix is sufficiently dilated (usually as soon as labor is firmly established). At the same time a small plastic tube is passed into the mother's uterus. The graph on the monitor records fetal heartbeats and maternal contractions. At the slightest indication of abnormality, a yellow light flashes, and remedial action can be taken instantly. According to Dr. Hon, emergency caesarean sections have decreased by over 75 percent in cases where the monitor was used.

There are advances in the diagnosis and treatment of diseases. Only a few years ago an RH-positive man and an RH-negative woman were faced with a serious dilemma when they decided on the size of their family. Almost always their first baby was fine. But subsequent children were in considerable danger of developing erythroblastosis, a serious, sometimes deadly, condition. The RH factor is an inherited substance present in the vast majority of persons. Someone whose blood contains this factor is called "RH-positive;" someone lacking the ingredient is called "RH-negative." The presence or absence of the RH factor per se makes no difference in a person's health. It only causes problems if RH-positive males and RH-negative females decide to have more than one child. However, erythroblastosis, which used to produce thousands of miscarriages, dead infants and badly damaged babies, is now almost totally preventable. Immediately after the birth of her first child, an RH-negative woman married to an RH-positive man can be prevented from forming the antibodies her next pregnancy will produce, immediately after the birth of her first child, thus also preventing trouble in that pregnancy.

Even if for some reason the mother has not been treated, the danger of RH disease to the fetus in subsequent pregnancies can be easily detected early through amniocentesis, and appropriate measures can be taken. Blood transfusions into the tiny fetus in her womb can be given on a regular basis. A much less frequently used method is to operate on her uterus, free one of the fetal limbs and give a transfusion in that manner. Even after an affected baby has been born, it is possible to exchange his entire blood supply almost immediately after delivery, thus minimizing any permanent damage to his system.

The possibility of contracting German measles (rubella) early in pregnancy terrifies a great many young mothers. German measles is a harmless disease with almost no symptoms, except for a pregnant woman. If a mother gets the disease during her first thirteen weeks of pregnancy, she may have a baby who is blind, deaf, retarded, has a defective heart, or is afflicted by any combination of these conditions. When a firm diagnosis of German measles has been established during those early critical weeks, an abortion is usually recommended. Recent research has shown that some infants have been affected in a more subtle way even when the infection was contracted later in pregnancy. However, recently a vaccine was used for the first time on a nationwide basis which may wipe out the menace of German measles once and for all.

Increasingly, the computer will become one of the physician's most valuable diagnostic tools. Dr. Sidney L. Baker, a faculty member in pediatrics

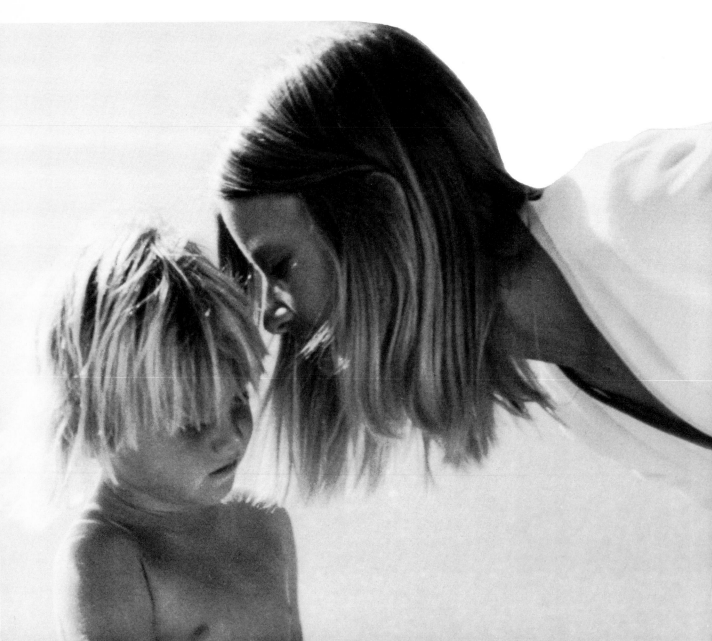

who works in the medical computer division at the Yale Medical School, predicts a brilliant future for computerized medical record-keeping. He first realized how inadequate most medical records were when he served at an isolated station in the African bush as a Peace Corps volunteer. "It was impossible to keep even minimally adequate records out there," he said. "Somewhere along the line I began to think that modern American hospitals may have a similar problem. A woman's record kept before, during and after pregnancy and delivery is sketchy at best. Of course the baby suffers from a 'lost record' for the entire nine months of his gestation period. And we know that during that period we can learn so much about him—medical facts that may be important to his health throughout his life. If we have adequate records for millions of pregnant women and unborn babies, we may eventually be able to answer all kinds of questions that puzzle us now. When a baby is born with an abnormality, we can only figure backwards. Did the mother get a viral infection early in pregnancy, and if so, what and when? What drugs did she take? When and in what quantity? If we ask her after the baby is born, the chances are she won't remember. But with a computer we can keep an almost daily record. We can do this without taking up much of the physician's time. A nurse, a social worker or a trained technician can ask the questions. Or a woman can be asked to fill out a carefully designed computerized questionnaire. Then we can correlate all this information and see some patterns in situations where previously we saw only questions and confusion.

Computers can't make medical decisions, but they can help the doctor to make his own decisions in a much more informed and intelligent manner."

Dr. Philip Sarrel, one of the new obstetricians, works with his wife, a trained social worker, to cut through some of the misinformation and emotional hangups that afflict so many young women and men who consider themselves sexually quite sophisticated. The Sarrels have recently been appointed by the University Health Service at Yale as sex counselors for Yale students. They see students individually, helping them to overcome a variety of sexual problems. In addition, courses in sexuality are offered to undergraduates and graduate students. Similar courses, some of them initiated by the Sarrels, are also taught at Smith, Mt. Holyoke and Brown. "Honest sex education is a vital part of the new obstetrics," Dr. Sarrel said.

Only six years ago, Dr. Alan C. Barnes, chairman of the Department of Gynecology and Obstetrics at Johns Hopkins, in a lecture on the prevention of birth defects, discussed the sad state of affairs into which his branch of medicine had fallen. "The fundamental problem revolves around the fact that America does not take labor and delivery seriously enough," he said. "From the point of view of the profession, we are committed to the fallacy that to be interesting one has to be adult, fully developed and preferably degenerating."

The new obstetricians are changing this picture fast. Many of the medical advances taking place at medical centers like Yale-New Haven and described in this article are not yet available in other, smaller hospitals. However, the young obstetricians who are now being trained will bring this new knowledge to their Main Street practice within one or two years.

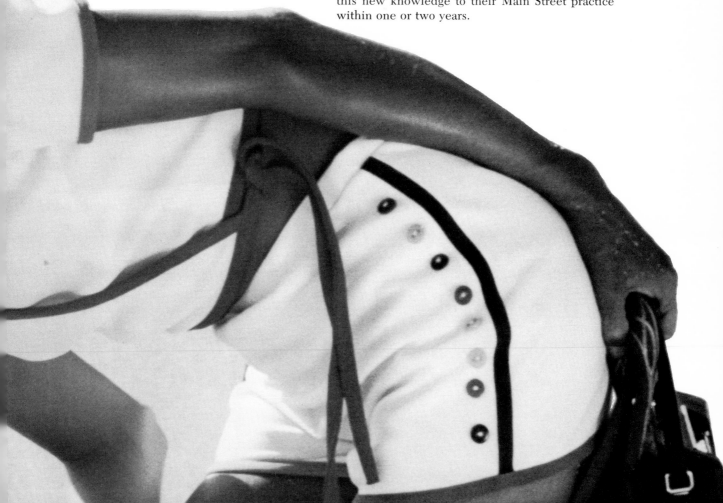

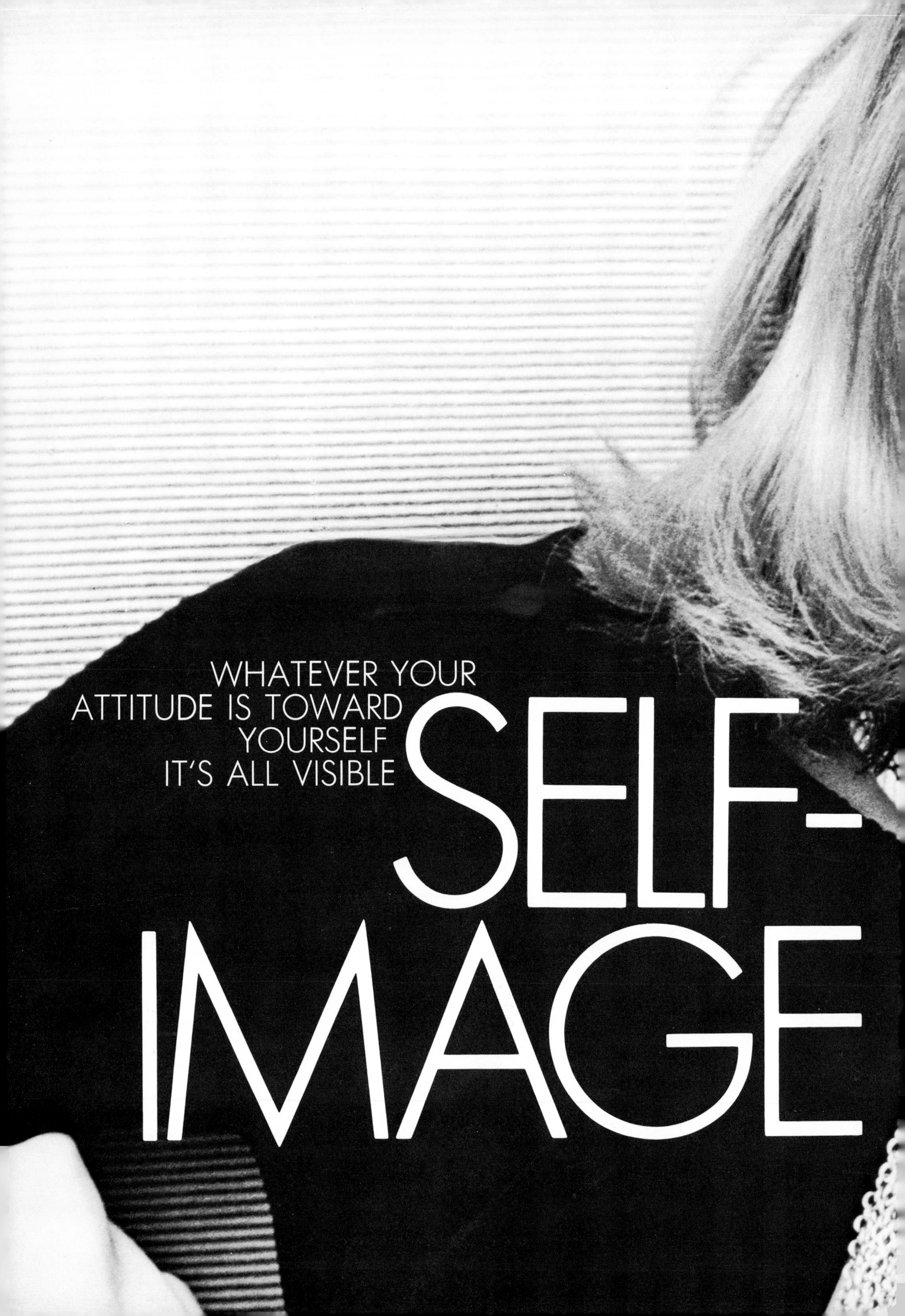

WHATEVER YOUR
ATTITUDE IS TOWARD
YOURSELF
IT'S ALL VISIBLE

SELF-IMAGE

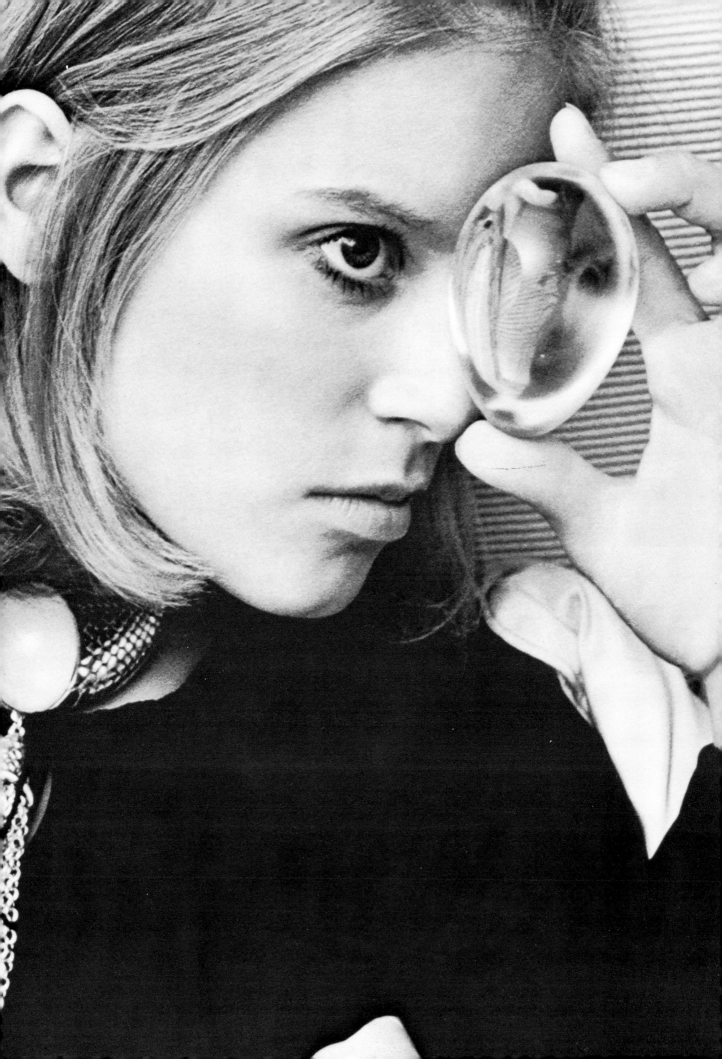

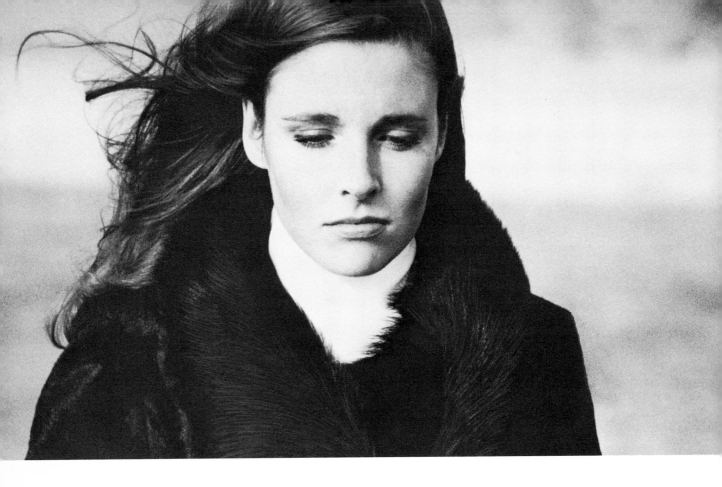

Are you the girl who
feels something like this:
"I like my face, because
it looks like me, a person
I like." Or are you
the girl who feels:
"I don't like my face
because I don't like
the person behind it, me."

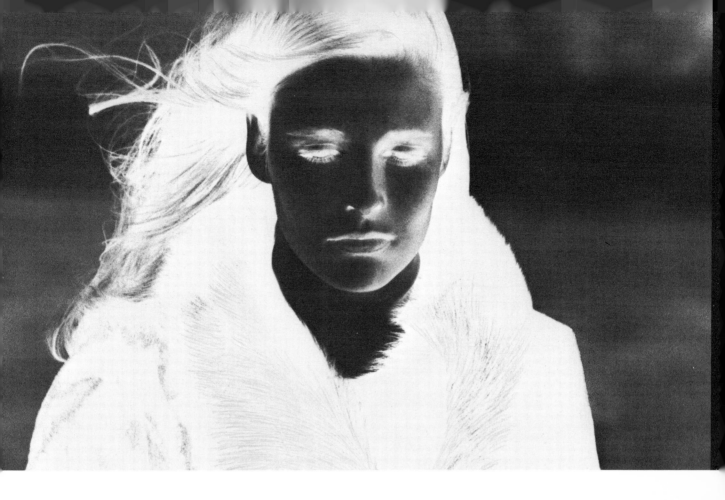

SELF-IMAGE

What you are inside shows through your height, weight, eye and hair color, the vital statistics. Whatever your attitude toward yourself is: "I don't mind my face because I'm behind it," "I wish I were anyone but me," "I'm a beauty, man, and don't forget it,"—it's all visible. When that image is poor everyone can see it uncomfortably so, when it is cloudy or phony it's going to be disconcerting to you and others, when it's good it's beautiful. So many things contribute to it—but the most important is self-knowledge or awareness. Because that is the key to any change you want to make. You can't improve either your inner view or yourself or your outer look until you are fully conscious that it might need help. That's why we start this chapter off with some psychological tests and guides geared to help you to a realistic evaluation of yourself: First in terms of whether you see yourself as others see you. Secondly to determine whether you have the self-discipline for the marriage, man, career, and family you think you want, or whether you ought to perhaps change your goals. Thirdly, to establish what kind of life style you want and if you are likely to achieve it. Fourth, what your particular illness patterns or symptoms reveal about you psychologically. After these, you'll find out how to read body language, or what your gestures and those of others may be trying to tell you; how drugs and sleep can affect people's looks; what effect scent has on you and others when you wear it.

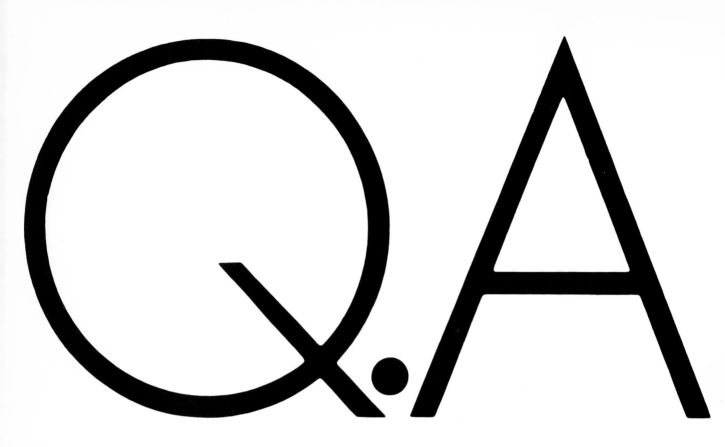

SEE-YOURSELF-AS-OTHERS-SEE-YOU TEST

First, ask a friend to answer these questions about you, putting her answers on a separate sheet of paper. Then ask a second friend to put her answers on another sheet of paper. Next, write in your own answers in the column opposite the questions on this page. Be prepared for some surprises. (You may consider yourself "a-daisy type" and impress your friends as a "rose.") Now circle every answer your friends made that agrees with your own. Add up the circles; write total at bottom of page.

What your score means

25-30: Very high score. Indicates you have an excellent idea of the impressions you create at all times. Your personality and your looks all fit together to a remarkable degree. You are not full of surprises or interesting contradictions . . . you may be disappointed in the impression you so conclusively give to others.

16-24: High score. You have a good idea of how you impress other people, probably dress in a way that reveals your personality. In this category there is room for a few surprises, e.g., a girl who is the "diamonds, roses, beauty salon" type, but prefers to drink orange juice at a party.

8-16: Average score. Your personality and the way you look are fair clues to your secret self-image, but some of the impressions you make come as surprises. (In our pretesting of the quiz, we discovered most of the surprises were pleasant—"Do I really impress you as an orchid?")

0-7: Low score. You do not see yourself as others see you. You should set about correcting your impressions.

QUESTIONS	ANSWERS	QUESTIONS	ANSWERS

She would be most pleased to receive:

(a) **a love letter**
(b) **a big check**
(c) **a literary or art award**
(d) **a beauty contest prize**   ☐

At a party she would drink:

(a) **orange juice**
(b) **red or white wine**
(c) **Scotch**
(d) **sherry**   ☐

She would rather listen to:

(a) **Beethoven**
(b) **Debussy**
(c) **twelfth-century plain song**
(d) **rock**   ☐

Ideally she should be married to:

(a) **an artist**
(b) **an advertising executive**
(c) **a professional sports-car racer**
(d) **a forest ranger**   ☐

Given $10 to spend on herself, she would splurge on:

(a) **a visit to a beauty salon**
(b) **lunch and a matinee**
(c) **a piece of jewelry**
(d) **a book or record album**   ☐

On a quiet evening at home she would:

(a) **wash her hair or give herself a pedicure**
(b) **clean out the kitchen cabinets**
(c) **read**
(d) **pursue a hobby**   ☐

She would most enjoy giving:

(a) **a party for 200 people**
(b) **a buffet supper for 20**
(c) **a dinner for 2**
(d) **a baby shower**   ☐

Her choice of jewels would be:

(a) **emeralds**
(b) **diamonds**
(c) **pearls**
(d) **jade**   ☐

She would prefer to live in:

(a) **a big city**
(b) **suburbs**
(c) **a small town**
(d) **country**   ☐

She would most remind you of:

(a) **lilies-of-the-valley**
(b) **roses**
(c) **daisies**
(d) **striped orchids**   ☐

She would prefer to read:

(a) **a murder mystery**
(b) **a best-selling novel**
(c) **current non-fiction**
(d) **a classic work**   ☐

She would bring home from the florist:

(a) **a bunch of violets**
(b) **some shiny green leaves**
(c) **a dozen roses**
(d) **a pot of geraniums**   ☐

She is:

(a) **a short person**
(b) **of average height**
(c) **taller than average**
(d) **very tall**   ☐

Given a choice, she would rather attend:

(a) **the ballet**
(b) **a football game**
(c) **a political rally**
(d) **a pop concert**   ☐

She is—more than anything else:

(a) **understanding**
(b) **intelligent**
(c) **amusing**
(d) **adventuresome**   ☐

TOTAL SCORE ☐

HAVE YOU ENOUGH SELF-DISCIPLINE FOR THE MARRIAGE, MAN, CAREER, FAMILY YOU WANT?

by David P. Campbell

Many people think that success is usually achieved through their own efforts. Bette Davis said bluntly, "There's only one way to work—like hell." Even the ancient Romans have spoken. Seneca, in the first century, said, "To master one's self is the greatest mastery." (I think, however, he was after different ends than Bette Davis.)

Psychologists cannot say with certainty why some people are strongly motivated and why others are not. The causes behind motivation—or lack of it—are complex and difficult to disentangle. However, psychologists have determined certain basic principles, and if you understand them, you will have a better chance of succeeding or achieving in the way you wish.

First, you have to decide what you want. Go through the following checklist and mark all of the things that are important to you.

True	False	
_____	_____	I want to be rich.
_____	_____	I want to be famous.
_____	_____	I want lots of leisure time to do as I please.
_____	_____	I want a husband who loves me.
_____	_____	I want a happy, closely knit family with at least two or three children.
_____	_____	I want to be talented.
_____	_____	I want to be married to a famous man who is tops in his field.
_____	_____	I want to be a popular person.
_____	_____	I want to be a successful career woman.
_____	_____	I want to fall in love often.
_____	_____	I want to be married to a husband who will spend much of his time with me.
_____	_____	I want enough authority and influence to have others working for me.
_____	_____	I want to be alone.
_____	_____	I don't want anyone ever to be angry with me.
_____	_____	I want to be free to come and go as I please.
_____	_____	I want to work in a field where I know I will have to compete with men to succeed.
_____	_____	I want to dedicate myself to others and better the world.

This checklist should make it clear to you that there are various ways to succeed, and obviously,

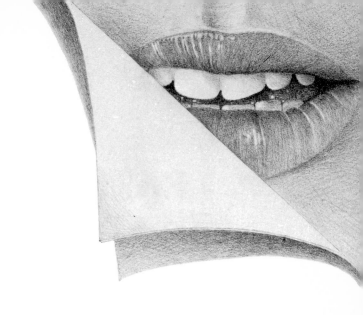

you can't have them all. If you want to be famous, then you can't be free to come and go as you please, for your public will recognize and, no doubt, annoy you. You can't be a successful career woman and expect that no one will ever be angry with you. You can't be married to a famous husband and still expect him to spend much time with you.

Choices—that's what life is all about. As Christopher Morley said, "There is only one success—to be able to spend your life in your own way."

No matter in what direction you decide to go, you must exert some effort to guide your own destiny. For example, you have to use your time wisely. Do you? Go through the following checklist to see how you fare.

Yes   No

_____ _____ Do you spend more than twenty minutes each day on coffee breaks?

_____ _____ Do you stop working each day about 3:30 or 4, telling yourself that you can't really accomplish anything in an hour?

_____ _____ Do you play cards or chess or whatever three or four hours every week?

_____ _____ Do you go shopping almost every day or every other day?

_____ _____ Do you go out with friends three or four nights each week?

_____ _____ Do you often spend more than ten minutes on a social telephone conversation?

_____ _____ Do you play almost all of every weekend?

_____ _____ If you have just finished one task fifteen minutes before lunch, do you usually avoid starting another one?

Everyone will answer 'yes' to some of these, but if you have said yes to more than three or four, then you don't appreciate the value of your time. _Fifteen minutes is important_—it's long enough to write a note to your mother, or call the library about a book your boss is looking for, or memorize five words of French, or dust off your living room bookshelves, or do fifteen deep knee-bends, or file the morning's correspondence.

Fifteen minutes in history has been long enough to start wars, lose fortunes, make babies and assassinate tyrants—so don't just sit there.

Ask yourself these questions about improving the way you use your time.

Yes   No

_____ _____ Have you ever kept a detailed account for a few days of just how you spend your time?

_____ _____ Have you ever set up a planned time schedule for completing a large task, like a term paper, and stuck to it?

_____ _____ Have you ever taken a single task that you do regularly, like making your bed, and tried to find ways to do it faster?

_____ _____ Do you have at least a rough plan for using some time each week for self-development?

_____ _____ Can you tell me, quickly without much thought, someone that you have noticed who does use his time efficiently?

_____ _____ Do you care if you waste time?

If you answered 'no' to most of these, then you are simply not conscious of time and you're probably not very efficient.

Time can spend itself. C. Northcote Parkinson, in one of his famous laws, stated, "Work expands to fill the time available." Dr. Elliot Aronson, a psychologist from the University of Texas, has done an experiment showing that this is indeed true. Two groups of students were called in and assigned the same simple task, but one group was given a stricter time limit than the other. Later, the same two groups were called in and again given identical tasks, but this time with no time limit. Professor Aronson found that the group that had had the strict time limit finished its task earlier the second time, even though there was no time limit. The second group had "learned" how to waste time. Look at your own behavior to see if you do the same thing.

Learn to use your habits to save time. You're normally not going to run your life like a crack drill team. Instead, you should, in an almost casual manner, try to mold your daily habits to work more efficiently.

Here's an example of how not to do it: You're a young wife, and one of your evening tasks is to write the checks for the monthly bills. Probably it goes something like this: You linger over your coffee, putting off starting as long as possible. You read the TV schedule and maybe watch a show. You get out the checkbook and the bills, and then remember you haven't phoned your sister for two days. Thirty minutes later you put down the phone, pick up the checkbook and open the bills. In the first one—from a department store—is a flyer for a lovely, feminine something-or-other, and you lean back and dream about what it would be like to have all the money in the world.

Finally you write a check or two—but then it's time for the evening news, and after that, TV news and Talk Show. Eventually you are frantically writing to the accompaniment of the "The Star-Spangled Banner." You have stretched thirty minutes of work over an entire evening.

A delightful book about using time wisely is *Cheaper by the Dozen*, by Frank B. Gilbreth, Jr. and Ernestine Gilbreth Carey. Their parents were both industrial efficiency experts, and the stories of how they applied these principles to raise their twelve children may help you see better ways to use your time.

The efficient use of time doesn't mean one has to be tense and always on edge. Someone once asked the father, Frank Gilbreth, Sr., why he wanted to save time—what are you going to use it for? He replied, "For work, if you love that best, for education, for beauty, for art, for pleasure. For mumbletypeg, if that's where your heart lies."

The next step is to ask yourself what you have learned to do well so far. Go down the list and check off your talents. Be honest; don't check something unless you've already done it successfully.

———— Can you play the piano or any musical instrument fairly well?

———— Can you type?

———— Can you run a 16mm sound movie projector?

———— Can you cook an authentic Chinese, French or other foreign meal?

———— Can you write a newspaper or magazine article?

———— Can you sketch clothes designs well enough to have them published in a school paper?

———— Can you weld or solder?

———— Can you play bridge?

———— Can you play tennis or golf or handball or badminton well enough to beat almost all your friends?

———— Can you write poetry?

———— Can you work simple problems in algebra? For example, can you factor $a^2 - b^2$?

———— Can you drive a car?

———— Can you tell stories to children, making them up as you go and keeping the children enthralled?

———— Can you raise flowers?

———— Can you fix a leaky faucet, change a flat tire, glue up a loose bathroom tile, retrieve a ring that has dropped into a sink trap, replace a fuse or repair a broken window?

———— Can you organize a conference of a hundred people, handling their travel, lodging and meals?

———— Can you skip rope for three minutes without missing?

———— Can you run any kind of machine more complicated than an electric toaster?

———— Can you operate a camera that has adjustments for lens aperture, shutter speed and distance?

———— Can you identify more than ten different kinds of trees?

———— Can you plan, organize and carry out a dinner party for eight, including all the cooking?

———— Can you bandage a severe cut without becoming panicky?

———— Can you waltz, polka, schottische, or do any folk dance?

———— Can you estimate distances—like how high the ceiling is in the room you are sitting now—within 10 percent?

———— Can you do simple arithmetic in your head—which is the better buy, fifteen pencils for 29¢ or twenty for 45¢?

———— Can you write a letter to a friend in French or German or Spanish or any other foreign language?

———— Can you do a flip on a trampoline or off a diving board?

———— Can you handle a small sailboat by yourself or paddle a canoe in a straight line for half a mile?

———— Can you use a slide rule?

———— Can you cut out and sew up a simple dress from a pattern?

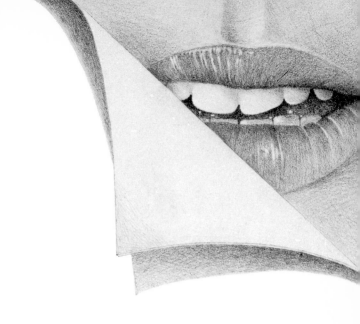

_____ Can you operate a keypunch?
_____ Can you make an omelet?
_____ Can you take someone's pulse?
_____ Can you identify more than ten different kinds of birds?
_____ Can you reupholster an easy chair?
_____ Can you send and receive simple messages in Morse code?
_____ Can you maintain an average of 150 in a bowling league?
_____ Can you swim 100 yards?

I can't tell you exactly what your score means, because some of these talents are more valuable than others. If you can play the piano well enough to appear in a public concert, that skill will take you further than any twenty of the others.

Still, it is interesting to compare yourself with others, because a wide range of talents is useful, so I'll give you a guideline. I asked several friends who I think are outstanding to fill in this checklist, and they checked about twenty-five items each. If you can honestly check that many, then you have as many skills as my talented friends. If you checked considerably fewer than that, well, maybe this list will give you some ideas of how to spend your time.

No matter what you are—student, employee, wife, at liberty—there is tremendous value in being able to do things well. First, there is the benefit of the skill itself. If you can type 60 words a minute, for example, the advantages are obvious. Baton-twirling or cheerleading may have less long-range value than other abilities, and your time may be better spent elsewhere.

The second advantage of skill is the lift that it gives to your self-confidence. There is considerable inner pride in knowing that you are more competent than others, even if it's only in flower-arranging. Psychologists have discovered that one aspect of mental health is a positive opinion of yourself, and if you know you're good, that's positive. Don't worry about being best—there will always be someone better somewhere—just try to be good.

There is a third advantage in being talented—a flat, out-and-out social one. If you can do something well, many more doors will open for you. The world likes talent, and if you're smart, you'll capitalize on the talent you have.

If you are going to guide your own life in directions that are important to you, there is another skill you must learn—living with and adapting to ever-changing conditions. Success is never static; we never find the end of the rainbow. Now, which of the following statements describe you?

Yes   No

_____ _____ "If I could only get out of school and away from home, I could solve my problems quickly."

_____ _____ "If only I had a job and my own money, I could have what I want."

_____ _____ "If I could get married and run my own home, I would never complain again."

_____ _____ "If I had a college degree, everybody would respect me and I'd have lots of friends."

_____ _____ "If only I could get pregnant and have my own baby, I'd never want another thing in life."

_____ _____ "If my baby would stop spitting up, sleep all night and let me rest, life would be continually beautiful."

_____ _____ "If only our income were a hundred dollars a month higher, we'd have all the money we'd need."

If you answered yes to even one of these, you're kidding yourself—it won't happen.

Life never stops; there are no ends, no final buzzers. But there are times of delicious success and proud achievement, and the trick is to enjoy them and not be thrown by the bleak rays of daylight over a strange, new horizon.

LIFE STYLE

WHAT KIND DO YOU WANT— AND ARE YOU LIKELY TO ACHIEVE IT?

Before the sixties only one lifestyle—work hard and move up—really prevailed for the majority in America. Now there are at least two more strong contenders: the less competitive style that aims chiefly at fulfilling the human biological and psychological needs of the sexes, for friendship, family and community; and the pleasure-principled one concerned with living this life fully without much dependence on outer-directed success goals. A person may really want the best of all three different styles, a little or a lot more of one than the other, or more of one at one period of life and less at another. The more choice, the more confusing things can become. That's why psychologist Ernest Dichter developed this test-game to help you determine which lifestyle or styles you lean to; how well it or they are working for you. There are five test parts; your answers will be analyzed on page 284.

1 GOALS

Imagine you have 40 chits that represent the amount of energy you have to spend.
How many do you use in achieving each of the goals below?

MONEY	_ _ _ _
PROFESSIONAL RECOGNITION	_ _ _ _
POSSESSIONS	_ _ _ _

Number of chits you spend
GROUP I _ _ _ _

LOVE	_ _ _ _
FRIENDSHIP AND COMMUNITY LIFE	_ _ _ _
MOTHERHOOD OR DAUGHTER ROLE	_ _ _ _

Number of chits you spend
GROUP II _ _ _ _

PLEASURE	_ _ _ _
TRAVEL	_ _ _ _
NEW EXPERIENCES	_ _ _ _

Number of chits you spend
GROUP III _ _ _ _

2 TEMPO

Each of the lines below represents a basic life tempo. If you could play your life's tune out for the next ten years, which tempo would you pace it to:
A) slow waltz; B) crescendo; C) uneven but dynamic; D) quiet, bucolic

☐ **A**

☐ **B**

☐ **C**

☐ **D**

3 FUTURE

What are your plans for the future? Check off how far ahead you are making plans in these areas:

		1 year or less	2 years	3 years	4 years	5 years or more
A	MONEY					
B	ADVANCEMENT					
C	TRAVEL					
D	FRIENDS*					
E	LEISURE/HOBBIES					
F	KNOWLEDGE					

* In terms of letting your desire for friends and community life influence your choice of neighborhood, city, town, club, etc.

4 SITUATIONS

In which of these situations would you be more emotionally involved and to what extent?

BULLFIGHT (C)
☐ a) very much involved
☐ b) indifferent
☐ c) cold

BIG FUN PARTY (A)
☐ a) very much involved
☐ b) indifferent
☐ c) cold

AIRPLANE TRIP (D)
☐ a) very much involved
☐ b) indifferent
☐ c) cold

PEACEFUL VILLAGE (B)
☐ a) very much involved
☐ b) indifferent
☐ c) cold

DESK AND LIBRARY (E)
☐ a) very much involved
☐ b) indifferent
☐ c) cold

5 MOODS

On the calendar below check your prevailing mood for each day of last week. (If an unusual problem like serious illness or a difficult personal problem occurred, skip last week and choose a more average one.) Then add up the number of days when you felt positive and optimistic, indifferent or pessimistic.

	SUN.	MON.	TUES.	WED.	THURS.	FRI.	SAT.
AVERAGE PAST WEEK	☐ optimistic ☐ indifferent ☐ pessimistic	☐ optimistic ☐ indifferent ☐ pessimistic	☐ optimistic ☐ indifferent ☐ pessimistic	☐ optimistic ☐ indifferent ☐ pessimistic	☐ optimistic ☐ indifferent ☐ pessimistic	☐ optimistic ☐ indifferent ☐ pessimistic	☐ optimistic ☐ indifferent ☐ pessimistic

Total optimistic _ _ _ _   Total indifferent _ _ _ _   Total pessimistic _ _ _ _

The first four tests determine the lifestyle or styles you have chosen. The fifth throws some light on how that lifestyle is working for you.

Test 1

This is the basic determining test. If you have more chits in Group I than in any other, you have chosen a possession- and achievement-directed lifestyle. Group I consists of cultural and outer-directed goals—professional recognition, possessions, etc.

If you have more in Group II, you belong in a self-oriented, peaceful lifestyle in which love, friendship and community commitment and family life provide fulfillment of your own human biological and psychological roles.

If you have a majority of chits in Group III, your lifestyle is based on the pleasure principle, you mean to get as much fullness out of this life as possible. You are interested largely in the inner experiences independent of the outside-goal-oriented forces.

If you are more or less equally balanced between the three groups, don't be confused. The better the balance, the more flexible and open your lifestyle is. You see the best in all of them.

Tests 2, 3, 4

The next three tests help to prove further your attachment to the lifestyle Test 1 indicated for you. Check yourself out according to the group you fit into. If you are well-balanced between groups in Test 1, you may find that on the secondary level explored in Tests 2, 3, 4, your preferences are more weighted to one lifestyle over another.

Possession and achievement-directed lifestyle: If you chose b in Test 2, this style would be reinforced. It's even more substantiated in Test 3 if you planned further ahead in a, b, f. The pattern continues if you answered in Test 4 A-a, C-a, D-a.

Self-oriented, peaceful lifestyle: If you answered in Test 2 d, you belong even deeper in this group. Further proof of this is if you planned longer ahead for d and e, and in Test 4 chose B-a, E-a.

Pleasure principle lifestyle: Your membership in this group is reinforced if in Test 2 you answered a and/or c, and if in Test 3 your life planning is the longest in category e and f, possibly also c. In Test 4 you would have checked A-a and maybe B-a.

Test 5

This reveals your general attitude to life, which in turn affects how you live it. If in the past week you checked more pessimistic days, you obviously have a rather pessimistic outlook. That outlook (pessimistic, indifferent or optimistic) naturally influences the way you work with your lifestyle.

For example: Take the achievement-oriented person who scores extremely pessimistically, say six days out of seven. She may be afraid or questioning the very goals that she's set out after, either because she has seen that material success does not automatically assure happiness, or maybe she feels inadequate to these goals she thinks she should pursue. A preponderance of positive days might mean that this person has made for herself a dynamic, achievement-oriented choice that she thoroughly enjoys and finds rewarding.

Or for instance: Someone who has chosen a self-oriented peaceful style but who marks indifferent days preponderantly is probably more passive than peaceful and tends to let life dominate her instead of her dominating it. On the other hand, if she had marked more positive days than indifferent ones, her peacefulness would be of a dynamic nature, a positive working for peace rather than a giving in to any means or domination that would provide it.

Another example: A person who leans toward

284

the pleasure principle style but marks more days pessimistically would probably be more of a "cop-out" than a real pleasure seeker. In the extreme she would be a person who appeared to love pleasure simply because she did not actively work to find anything else. Apathy toward life in this society is often misinterpreted as laziness and hedonism. A positive score of days combined with the pleasure principle style could be interpreted as a real desire to enjoy life, knowing that it might well be at the expense of achievement and money.

These are only a few variations; it would be impossible here to cover all the possible combinations. But the above examples should provide you with some technique for analyzing your own variations correctly. The most important purpose of Test 5 is to direct you to some life accounting, a kind of inventory-taking of how well your lifestyle may be working for you. If your attitude is overwhelmingly pessimistic or indifferent, you should try to reevaluate your chosen lifestyle and your attitude to see where the discrepancies are. Although the variety of lifestyles present in the seventies makes the choice more confusing, this nevertheless provides a broader measure of freedom than we have ever had before.

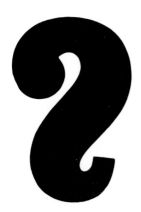

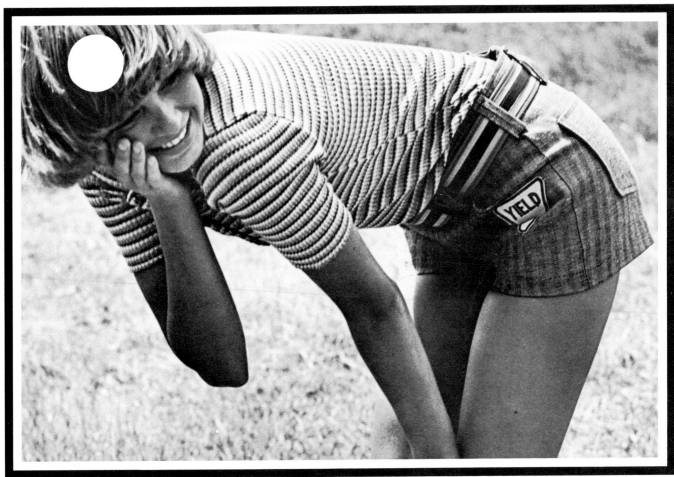

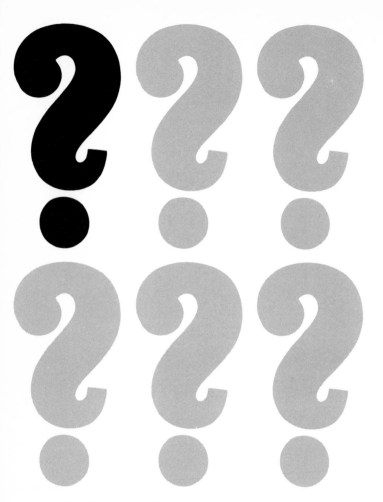

ARE YOU AGGRESSIVE? SUBMISSIVE? SCARED? JEALOUS? REJECTED? INHIBITED? HOSTILE? GUILTY?

Tell me
who you are
and
I'll tell you
where
you'll ache

by Mim Randolph Edmonds

Everyone has psychosomatic symptoms—those physical reactions that our emotions dictate, our bodies perform. Almost everyone will accept the correlation to one degree or another. Today many people can diagnose their own "psychosomatic headache" when Mother or Mother-in-law is coming to dinner, or a "psychosomatic backache" when the carpet needs vacuuming. It's all part of the modern play-psychoanalyst syndrome. But almost no one understands the why of psychosomatics, the scope of it, or the promise it holds to reduce so many of the anxiety-illnesses in this most anxious of times.

Let's start on the upbeat; it's easier to accept the positive. Happiness can bring tears. Sexual stimulation can cause an erection. Our "mouths water" when we're hungry and think about food. We "can't stop laughing." We "blush with pleasure." But we also blush with shame or embarrassment. And this brings us to the downbeat: the pounding heart and sweaty palms when we are afraid, the tightening in the stomach, head or chest when we are angry or anxious, the enervating fatigue when we are depressed. Yet, these are all common fleeting reactions, and as such, we are accustomed to them, aren't usually alarmed by them and don't even stop to think about the chemical why. We certainly don't classify them as psychosomatic illnesses. But in the purest sense they are all psychosomatic symptoms, cases of mind conditioning matter.

Now, just to catch a glimpse of the possible scope of psychosomatic medicine, take a giant step along the still-experimental, exploratory route of the science. Cancer, for example. A number of doctors—among them Dr. Arnold A. Hutschnecker, an internist-turned-psychiatrist who has studied the mind-matter interplay from both points of emphasis — believe that psychic factors play a large part in causing death from cancer. Just as our body chemistry can react to stimulation, let's say, by a step-up in the flow of adrenaline, so it can react to the wish to die by a slow-down, then a halt, in the body processes. Dr. Hutschnecker calls this the "negative state of stress."

"Cancer patients," he said, "die when they are overcome by a state of futility and hopelessness." And, by and large, these patients have a built-in affinity for hopelessness. They are, said Dr. Hutschnecker, largely passive, dependent people who have difficulty expressing hostility because of their dependency, and as their sense of hopelessness increases, so does their lack of inner will to fight disease.

Then there is the mounting research indicating that the psyche controls a child's physical growth or lack of it. Most recently, Dr. Robert Blizzard, a pediatrician, reported that this "psychosocial dwarfism," as he calls it, occurs in homes where the children are obviously unloved. When placed in another environment, he said, these children will often begin to grow; when returned to their homes, they stop.

At the extreme there is death by voodoo. Perhaps, one doctor speculated, it is death by shock, caused by the total conviction of hopelessness. Also at the extreme, but the opposite one, is the physically inexplicable recovery, the so-called "miracle" cures. Dr. Hutschnecker told of several in his experience and explained them with unscientific humility as "the will to live" — the title, in fact, of one of his books, a comprehensive layman's analysis of psychosomatics.

From a pounding heart to cancer . . . from a "lump" in the throat to dwarfism . . . from the simple to the complex. "Yet when you accept the basic premise," said one psychiatrist, "the progression is infinite."

There are still missing links in many of the intricate chains of physical reaction, but doctors have come a long way in establishing provable patterns in psychosomatics since the 1940's when the many medically unaccountable reactions to war experiences challenged the clinical book and spurred the profession to intensify research in this area. Today, most doctors will agree that emotions can cause not only temporary body symptoms but actual, sometimes permanent, changes in the body chemistry or structure.

What also proves positive is that these emotionally-caused symptoms are definitely physical disturbances. Just because they are induced by the mind doesn't mean they are in the mind. The well-meaning friend who says that an excruciating backache will go away if it's forgotten is not only doing a disservice — she's wrong. That's why most doctors treat the physical symptoms first — which in itself relieves the on-the-surface tension that makes the symptoms worse — then go on to the more complicated, underlying problem.

An equal disservice is done by the doctor who tosses off the cause of a persisting headache by just *saying* it's tension and prescribing aspirin. Unless we believe that it's tension and know the cause of the tension, all the doctor has given us is aspirin. We'll still be convinced that the headache is caused by a brain tumor; this conscious fear will mount on top of a perhaps unconscious one that caused the headache in the first place; the headache will become more persistent and we'll be caught in the spinning psychosomatic cycle.

So, understanding the emotional-physical interplay is vital. Again, let's start with the most simple reactions. What makes us blush or turn pale? As Dr. A.T. Simeons explained in *Man's Presumptuous Brain*, a mild fear (shame or embarrassment) produces a slight contraction of the arteries which raises the blood pressure; an intense fear produces a tight contraction, blocking the flow of blood. Cold feet are explained in the same way; it is indeed a circulatory disorder, but it can be caused by arteries contracting in fear. A headache, said Dr. Theodore Isaac Rubin, can be caused by repressed anger which causes the closing of a small blood vessel in the brain. The result: blood deprivation and a headache. Our nervous system, he explained, which is quite sensitive to emotions, reacts very quickly in sending messages to various parts of our body. In the stomach, the gastric juices are involved. Dr. Simeons explained: "Repressed rage and fear cause a muscular closure of the opening between the stomach and the intestines and an interruption of the gastric flow, then indigestion."

Progressing to the more complex, Dr. Simeons and other doctors, including Dr. Hutschnecker, have suggested that ulcers, rather than being caused by commonly-blamed tension, are, in fact, the result of deep guilt and anxiety. This is based on the premise that the stomach's physical reaction seems to follow a love-hate emotional pattern. Here's how it works: Equate love with food; hate with denial of food. This is a psychic hunger and of course goes back to earliest childhood when food was a visible sign of maternal love. In anticipation of food (in need of love) there is a flow of acids, but no food to utilize them. Since the need for love is thwarted, the need remains constant — and acids continue to stream, first causing irritation, finally the ulcer.

If understanding is the catalyst to acceptance of these emotional-physical interactions, then

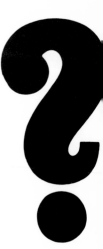

awareness is the key to cure, but a hard one to turn. So many of our anxieties are hidden, so many of our emotions are repressed. And they can range from the whisper of buried guilt to the scream of undefined fear.

The young woman account executive, for example, who *knows* that she gets a stomachache every time she has to work with a certain client isn't really in trouble. Neither is the girl who gets a headache each time her mother-in-law comes to dinner *if* she recognizes the correlation. Either may be able to solve the problem by either reasoning it away or by removing herself from the objectionable situation. Or she may have to accept the fact that, for a while at least, she will continue to have her psychosomatic symptoms (the client and mother-in-law are unmovable fixtures), but at least her symptoms won't be compounded by the fear that they are more significant than they really are.

It's when the mind doesn't understand, when the subconscious emotion hasn't reached it, that it loses control over the body and the real difficulties begin. As one psychiatrist put it: "A conscious doesn't usually create a problem; it's the disturbed unconscious that plays havoc with our bodies." And often we simply aren't prepared to accept the emotions that disturb us. We are ashamed or afraid of the cause of our anxieties and so we bury them — we don't love our husbands, we don't like our parents, we are disappointed in our children. It takes probing, often intense psychiatric treatment, to make us reveal ourselves to ourselves. But sometimes we simply haven't made the logical connection, and all that's needed is a simple explanation. "The few words a doctor may say can be much more important than the medication," said Dr. Hutschnecker, telling of a young man who had shooting pains in his stomach each morning as he reached his office. He thought he was allergic to food and that there must be something quite wrong inside. There was, but he had pinpointed the wrong part of his anatomy. Only a short conversation with the doctor revealed the young man's deep frustration with his work. He changed jobs and the pain stopped. But suppose the shooting pains started when that same young man returned home from work. It probably would not have been so easy to make him realize that his wife had become a transplant of his mother, whom he hated.

For another example: A young pre-med student had recurring headaches each time she went to biology class. She was convinced that the chemicals in the laboratory were at fault; in fact, she was afraid they were causing some permanent damage to her brain. This time, an unusually perceptive college physician led her to admit she found the young biology instructor irresistible; it was *his* re-

sistance and her repressed anger at it that was causing the headaches. But suppose this same young woman first pleaded a headache after five minutes of each class and left, finally didn't show up at all, canceling every chance of going on to medical school. It would take considerably more effort to make this girl realize that she was in an unconscious state of rebellion against her stern, inhibiting parents, who had decided when she was three that she was going to be a doctor.

Dr. Rollo May wrote in *Love and Will:* "Memory is like perception; a patient cannot remember something until he is ready to take some stand toward it."

Psychosomatic illnesses then are not only negative reactions to unpleasant situations but can also be necessary evasions of them — stalling actions until we can cope with a problem and make a decision to go on from there.

How we do this is largely a matter of personality, as is, in fact, the type of psychosomatic reaction that we have. Dr. Hutschnecker feels that "within the framework of our individual constitution, we ourselves choose the time of illness, the kind of illness, the course of illness and its gravity. Of course we do not make these choices consciously," he explained. "We do not reason ourselves into illness. The decisions are made in the unconscious court of judgment . . . they are arrived at by way of involved and turbulent argument without words, the language of the emotions.

"Also we must remember that these decisions are not irrevocable. We can and do change our minds."

In explaining the different physical reactions to anxiety, Dr. Hutschnecker divides people into two basic personality types: the aggressive and the regressive. The former follows the instincts of fight or flight; the latter retreats, seeking to evade the issue and to rely on the protection of others. Each reaction sets off its own chain of physical response. If we can fight or flee, or if we find the protection we seek, our bodies can relax and return to normal. But if the aggressive person is thwarted in his drive to act out his aggression, the regressive one rejected in his search for protection, then the physical response to anxiety continues, i.e., adrenaline or acids gush into the body. From the chemical reaction to anxiety, we can set the pattern of illness.

The aggressive personality, said Dr. Hutschnecker, is susceptible to circulatory diseases (heart trouble, high blood pressure, etc., migraines, rheumatoid arthritis, disorders of the thyroid gland and certain skin diseases and allergies). The regressive personality, on the other hand, tends toward digestive and gastrointestinal problems, also certain allergies and respiratory diseases. The young woman who feels unloved has asthma; the young man holding in his hostility toward his parents has headaches.

Of course, there is a tremendous swing in personalities between these two extremes, and within the arc it may be possible to pinpoint even more exactly who is most prone to what. Franz Alexander conducted a ten-year study at the Chicago Institute for Psychoanalysis and came up with profiles (abbreviated here) of people subject to seven emotion-related illnesses.

Asthma: feels threatened with loss of mother or mother-substitute . . . fear of alienation . . . inhibited because of maternal rejection (asthma, adds Dr. Hutschnecker, is the physical substitute for crying).

Duodermititis (skin disorders): subject to intense emotional conflict that creates a cycle—hunger for contact and love . . . exhibitionism . . . masochistic self-mutilation.

Thyroid conditions: struggles against fear, particularly of death . . . overcompensates by seeking out dangerous situations . . . accident-prone.

Ulcers: wishes to be loved . . . needs support . . . suffers frustration of dependency needs . . . overcompensates by pushing for success, accomplishment.

Hypertension: fights continuously against expressing hostility . . . inhibits self-expression . . . becomes overly compliant to suppress rage . . . when most angry will be most submissive.

Colitis: feels challenged beyond capability . . . senses hopelessness . . . lacks confidence.

Arthritis: has difficulty controlling aggressive impulses . . . usually a benevolent tyrant . . . rebellious tomboy as a child.

(For *Constipation:* read *Portnoy's Complaint.*)

This is certainly not our physical destiny. It is merely a presumed pattern of physical susceptibility when our emotions are out of control or out of mind.

There are definite signals to warn us when anxiety is becoming a threat to our health. The unconscious not only starts the destructive fires, it also rings the alarm. "Fatigue," said Dr. Hutschnecker, "is the most common sign of trouble—fatigue without physical cause, a subjective state." Another: "a diffuse state of uneasiness, a general feeling of worry, of pressure, of tension," without apparent cause. Weight gain is a warning (we overeat because of psychological, not physical, hunger). So are sexual problems—impotence and frigidity.

The expression "sick and tired" of him or that didn't spring from a vacuum. We may well be "sick and tired" in the true physical sense, though the wellspring is emotional. What do we do about it?

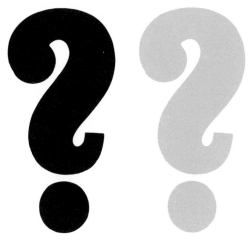

Recurring symptoms demand a doctor's attention. If he is certain there is no underlying organic cause, then be willing to search for the emotional trigger—and to see it when you find it. Dr. Hutschnecker calls this awareness a "psychological antibody." Once we learn that certain emotional responses can bring on physical discomfort, we can learn to change the response. Sometimes minor tensions can be broken easily by a hot bath, a leisurely dinner, a good night's sleep, a change of pace or a burst of honesty or anger. Some people can find and change the pattern themselves; others need help.

And help is coming from a number of directions. More and more doctors, for one, are rejecting the egotism of pure science as ineffectual in too many instances. In diagnosis and treatment, they realize, the total person must be considered. The young girl with acne needs prescribed medication, but she also needs a prescription for working out the problems that may have triggered the skin condition in the first place.

Also behavioral science is adding its techniques to those of conventional psychiatry. The theory is that we can "unlearn" adverse emotional reactions and retrain our responses without even becoming aware of the underlying causes of our anxiety. It's a short step but a proven effective one in many cases.

And what about faith—the religious cult of self-cure? "Faith is a tremendous healer," said Dr. Hutschnecker. "It can help you rid yourself of fear, doubt, general anxiety. But, subjectively as well as medically, there is an important difference between the blind-faith approach and that of psychosomatic medicine. The former emphasizes creation of a state of dependence; the latter, a state of independence which absolves us from guilt and the fear of condemnation or retribution." And this freedom from the domination of our emotions is what psychosomatic medicine is all about.

BODY LANGUAGE

HOW TO READ IT

by Flora Davis

Imagine that you're at a party and your hostess suggests a get-to-know-the-others game — *without* words. You can, she says, come up close to your partner and look him over, touch him, sniff him, hug him, use sign language — but you must not say one word.

The first thing you would learn from this experience is how limited wordless communication is. The next thing you might realize is how seldom you touch other people; how uncomfortable it is to be stared at, at close range; how disturbing to be sniffed. Eventually, you might recognize that one thing nonverbal communication does express very efficiently is emotion.

All of us communicate nonverbally. Most of the time we're not aware that we're doing it. We gesture with eyebrows or a hand, meet someone else's eyes and look away, shift positions in a chair. We assume that our actions are random and incidental. When we respond to nonverbal cues from others, we sometimes recognize those cues consciously but more often we react to them on an intuitive level.

Researchers have discovered in recent years that there is a system to body gestures almost as consistent and comprehensible as language, and so a flourishing new field for research has opened up. The general assumption: that all body movements have meaning within their specific context.

Every culture has its own body language, and children absorb its nuances along with spoken language. A Frenchman talks and moves in French. An American handles his body in a distinctively American way. Some cultural differences are easy to spot. Most Americans, observing an Englishman, would recognize that the way he crosses his legs is nothing like the way a male American does it. But it takes an expert to pick out a native of Wisconsin just by the way he uses his eyebrows during conversation.

Such regional idioms *can* sometimes be pinpointed. It's also true that men and women use the same body language in distinctively masculine and feminine ways. Your ethnic background, your social class and your own personal style all influence your body language. Nevertheless, you move and gesture within the American idiom.

The person who is truly bilingual is also bilingual in body language. New York's famous mayor Fiorello La Guardia politicked in English, Italian and Yiddish. When films of his speeches are run through without sound, it's not too difficult to identify from his gestures the language he was speaking. One of the reasons dubbed films often seem flat and unreal is that the gestures don't match the language.

Usually, the nonverbal communication acts to qualify the verbal. Casual conversation is normally quite laconic, its meaning conveyed by a few words blended in a kind of madrigal with other elements. What these nonverbal elements express very often is the emotional side of the message.

"I don't know how I know it, but I'm sure she doesn't like me," one woman complained about another. When a person feels liked or disliked, very often it's a case of "not what she said but the way she said it." Psychologist Albert Mehrabian has devised a formula to explain the emotional impact of any message: total impact = 7 percent verbal + 38 percent vocal + 55 percent facial. The importance of the voice can be seen when you consider that even the words "I hate you" can be made to sound seductive. Experiments have been done with tape-recorded voices with the sound filtered: the high register is cut out so that words are low and blurred but the tone of voice comes through. Mehrabian reports that listeners could judge degree of liking rather easily from these doctored tapes.

It isn't just feelings that are expressed nonverbally. One of the surprises is that gestures constitute almost a parallel language. Americans are apt to end a statement with a droop of the head or hand, a lowering of the eyelids. They wind up a question with a lift of the hand, a tilt of the chin or

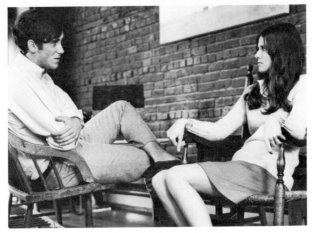

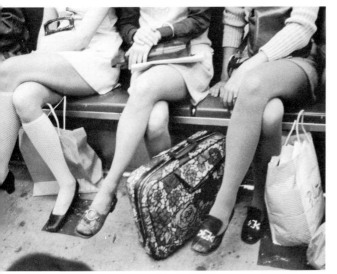

What are the possible meanings of crossing your legs?

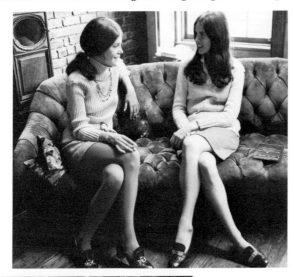

Can you tell who dislikes whom by the way they are sitting?

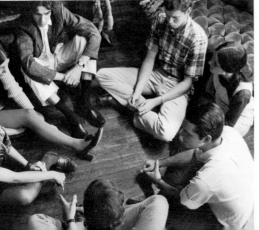

*Do you sit
in pro or
con positions in an argument?*

widening of the eyes. With a future-tense verb they often gesture with a forward movement; for the past tense with a backward one.

Experts in kinesics—the study of communication through body movement—are not prepared to spell out a precise vocabulary of gestures and probably never will be. They will not say, for example, that when an American rubs his nose it always means he is disagreeing with someone or rejecting something. That's one possible interpretation, but there are others. To take another example: When a student in conversation with a professor holds the older man's eyes a little longer than is usual, it can be a sign of respect and affection, it can be a subtle challenge to the professor's authority or it can be something else entirely. The kinesicist, recording the action with a camera and/or an ingenious shorthand system, looks for patterns in the context, not for single meaningful gestures.

The concept of meaning is tricky, since most gestures are not *intended* to mean anything. The student probably is not trying to tell the professor with his eyes that he respects, or doesn't respect, him. He is simply using the eye movement that fits the context, as he might casually use a particular word within a sentence.

Kinesics is a young science, about seventeen years old and very much the brainchild of one man, Ray Birdwhistell. Already it offers a regular smorgasbord of observations. For example, eyebrows have a repertoire of about twenty-three possible positions; men use their eyebrows more than women do; and so forth.

There's nothing here that's startling, much that seems picayune. But for the layman there's a fascination about body language, because it's so vividly *there* for anyone to see. Seeing isn't easy, though—most people find they can shut out the conversation and concentrate on the kinesics for only about thirty seconds at a time. Students of kinesics sometimes learn from video tapes, which can be played, stopped, replayed. Anyone with a television set can experiment with kinesics-watching simply by turning on the picture without the sound.

One of the most potent elements in body language is eye behavior. You shift your eyes, meet another person's gaze or fail to meet it—and produce an effect out of all proportion to the trifling muscular effort you've made.

When two Americans look searchingly into each other's eyes, emotions are heightened and the relationship tipped toward greater intimacy. However, Americans are careful about how and when they meet another's eyes. In our normal conversation, each eye contact lasts only about a second before one or both individuals look away.

Because the longer meeting of the eyes is rare, it is weighted with significance when it happens and can generate a special kind of human-to-human awareness. A girl who has taken part in civil rights demonstrations reported that she was advised, if a policeman confronted her, to look straight into his eyes.

291

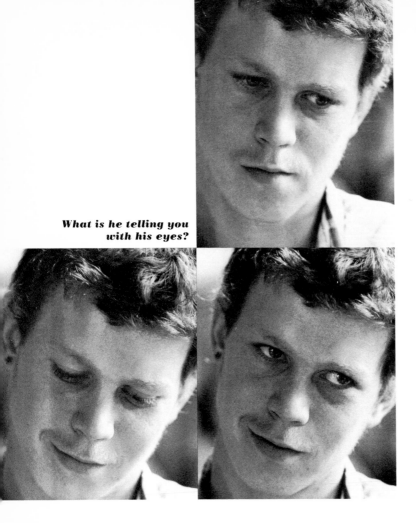

What is he telling you with his eyes?

"Make him *see* you as another human being and he's more likely to treat you as one," she was told.

Most of the time, the American interprets a lingering look as a sign of sexual attraction and scrupulously avoids this minor intimacy, except in appropriate circumstances.

"That man makes me so uncomfortable," a young woman complained. "Half the time when I glance at him he's already looking at me—and he keeps right on looking."

By simply using his eyes, a man can make a woman aware of him sexually, comfortably, or uncomfortably.

Americans abroad sometimes find local eye behavior hard to interpret.

"My first day in Tel Aviv was disturbing," one man recalled. "People not only stared right at me on the street, they actually looked me up and down. I kept wondering if I was uncombed or unzipped or if I just looked too American. Finally, a friend explained that Israelis think nothing of staring at others on the street."

Proper street behavior in the United States requires a nice balance of attention and inattention. You are supposed to look at a passerby just enough to show that you're aware of his presence. If you look too little, you appear haughty or furtive; too much and you're inquisitive. Usually what happens is that people eye each other until they are about eight feet apart, at which point both cast down their eyes. Sociologist Erving Goffman describes this as "a kind of dimming of lights."

Much of eye behavior is so subtle that we react to it only on the intuitive level. The next time you have a conversation with someone who makes you feel liked, notice what he does with his eyes. Chances are he looks at you more often than is usual with glances a little longer than the normal. You interpret this as a sign—a polite one—that he is interested in you as a person rather than just in the topic of conversation. Probably you also feel that he is both self-confident and sincere.

All this has been demonstrated in elaborate experiments. Subjects sit and talk in the psychologist's laboratory, innocent of the fact that their eye behavior is being observed from behind a one-way vision screen. In one fairly typical experiment, subjects were induced to cheat while performing a task, then were interviewed and observed. It was found that those who had cheated met the interviewer's eyes less often than was normal, an indication that "shifty eyes"—to use the mystery writers' stock phrase—*can* actually be a tip-off to an attempt to deceive or to feelings of guilt.

In parts of the Far East it is impolite to look at the other person at all during conversation. In England the polite listener fixes the speaker with an attentive stare and blinks his eyes occasionally as a sign of interest. That eye-blink says nothing to Americans, who expect the listener to nod or to murmur something—such as "mnhmn."

Let's examine a typical American conversation. Joan and Sandra meet on the sidewalk. Preliminary greetings over with, Joan begins to talk. She starts by looking right away from Sandra. As she hits her conversational stride, she glances back at her friend from time to time at the end of a phrase or a sentence. She does not look at her during hesitations or pauses but only at natural breaks in the flow of her talk. At the end of what she wants to say, she gives Sandra a rather longer glance. Experiments indicate that if she fails to do this, Sandra, not recognizing that it is her turn to talk, will hesitate or will say nothing at all.

When Sandra takes up the conversation, Joan, listening, sends her longer glances than she did when she herself had the floor. When their eyes meet, Joan usually makes some sign that she is listening.

It's not hard to see the logic behind this eye behavior. Joan looks away at the start of her statement and during hesitations to avoid being distracted while she organizes her thoughts. She glances at Sandra from time to time for feedback: to make sure she is listening, to see how she is reacting or for permission to go on talking. And while Sandra is doing the talking, Joan glances often at her to show that she is paying attention—to show that she's polite. For Americans, then, eye behavior does duty as a kind of conversational traffic signal, to control how talking time is shared.

You have only to observe an actual conversation to see that this pattern is not a precisely predictable one. None of the "facts" of eye behavior are cut and dried, for there are variations between individuals. People use their eyes differently and spend different—and characteristic—amounts of time looking at others. But if you know what to look for, the basic American idiom is there.

Just talking about eye behavior is enough to make most people so self-conscious that they suddenly don't know what to do with their eyes. But the surprising strength of these microhabits shows in the speed with which they reassert themselves the minute they're dropped out of awareness again.

A man's eye movements and the rest of his body language are more apt to provide a clue to his origins than to his secret thoughts. But it's true that there are times when what a person says with his body gives the lie to what he is saying with his tongue: Sigmund Freud once wrote:

"He that has eyes to see and ears to hear may convince himself that no mortal can keep a secret. If his lips are silent, he chatters with his fingertips; betrayal oozes out of him at every pore."

Psychiatrists working with patients respond sometimes consciously, sometimes intuitively, to nonverbal clues that signal inner conflicts. Some psychiatrists have tried to pin down these clues more precisely.

In one recent experiment Dr. Paul Ekman and Wallace Friesen filmed interviews with mental patients. Each patient was doing his best to seem calm, cool and rational, though some were still quite disturbed. Dr. Ekman and Friesen's theory—partially confirmed—was that the disturbance would be easier to deduce from gestures than from the patients' facial expressions.

People who can successfully control their faces are often unaware of what their hands, legs and feet may be doing; or else they just can't prevent signs of tension and anxiety from leaking out.

"Ted seems like the calmest, most self-controlled guy in the world—until you know about his foot," a man remarked about a business colleague. But the whole office staff knows about Ted's foot, which beats the floor constantly, restlessly, as if it had a life of its own beyond his control.

Anxiety is one emotion feet and legs may reveal. Rage is another: during arguments the feet often tense up. Fear sometimes produces barely perceptible running motions—a kind of nervous leg-jiggle. There are subtle, provocative leg gestures that women use, consciously and unconsciously.

Ordinarily we sit too close to each other to be able to observe the lower body easily. In fact, peo-ple who are forced to sit at a distance from others, without a desk or table to shield them, usually feel uncomfortable and vulnerable.

Aside from uneasy eye behavior and true facial faux pas, the best facial clue to deception is the microexpression. These are expressions or fragments of an expression that cross the face so fleetingly that they're gone—suppressed or disguised—before most people can notice them. Most expressions last half a second to a second, but the microexpression can be as quick as a single motion-picture frame, over in one fiftieth of a second. It can sometimes be caught by an alert observer, and an untrained person may react to it intuitively without being able to say just what he is reacting to. When a face is filmed and the film is then run through at a slow speed, microexpressions are easy to pick out.

Sometimes a person signals his inner emotions by his posture—sitting, for example, in a very tense way. Psychiatrist Frieda Fromm-Reichmann, to get some idea of what a patient was feeling, would imitate his posture. Recent studies by psychologists suggest that what posture often reflects is the person's attitude to people he is with.

Imagine two businessmen, Mark and Stanley, comfortably settled in a psychologist's lab. Stanley sits up very straight, hands clasping his knees, facing his companion squarely. Mark lounges far back in his chair, body twisted slightly to the right. A psychologist, observing the pair, can make several shrewd guesses about them just from their postures. The first guess: that they dislike each other. Second: that Stanley is rather intimidated by Mark, Mark not at all by Stanley.

Support for these conclusions comes from an experiment that indicates that when men are with other men whom they dislike they relax either very little or very much—depending on whether they see the other man as threatening. Relaxation was judged quite precisely within three categories. Labeled least relaxed were those—like Stanley—who sat with tense hands in a rigid posture. Subjects who slumped forward slightly—the angle was measured in degrees from the vertical—were judged moderately relaxed, and it was usually found that they liked the person they were with. Most relaxed were those, like Mark, who leaned far back and to one side.

Women who took part in this experiment always signaled their dislike with the very relaxed posture. And men, paired with women they disliked, were never up-tight enough about it to sit rigidly.

Congruent postures sometimes offer a guide to broad relationships within a group. Imagine that at the tag-end of a party the remaining guests have been fired up by an argument by postures adopted. Most of the pros, for example, may sit with crossed knees, the cons with legs stretched out and arms folded. A few middle-of-the-roaders may try a little of each—crossing their knees *and* folding their arms. If an individual abruptly shifts his body around in his chair, it may mean that he disagrees with the speaker or even that he is changing sides. None of this, of course, represents an infallible

Does the distance you stand from people reveal your nationality?

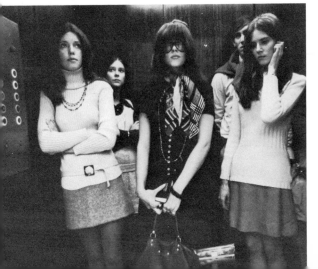

guide to group-watching. If you try to check it out, you may find several pros in the con posture and when your neighbor squirms around in his chair it may turn out to be because his leg went to sleep. But congruent postures are apparently significant enough of the time to be worth watching for.

Postural shifts sometimes parallel spoken language. Psychiatrist Albert Scheflen studied posture by filming psychotherapy sessions and found that a kind of kinesic dance took place. The individual would shift his head and eyes every few sentences, usually just as he finished making a point; would make a major shift of his whole body to coincide with a change in point of view—from that of listener or speaker, for example. Both patients and therapists worked from limited postural repertoires and produced their shifts in remarkably predictable sequences. One patient turned his head to the right and avoided the woman therapist's eyes whenever she spoke; looked directly and challengingly at her each time he answered; and then, usually, he would cock his head and turn his eyes to the left as he went off on a conversational tangent.

While children learn spoken and body language—proper postures, eye behaviors, etc.—they also learn a subtler thing: how to react to space around them.

A man's sense of self apparently is not bound by his skin. He walks around inside a kind of private bubble, which represents the amount of airspace he feels he must have between himself and other people. This is a truth anyone can easily demonstrate by moving in gradually on another person. At some point the other will begin irritably or perhaps just absentmindedly, to back away. Anthropologists working with cameras have recorded the tremors and minute eye movements that betray the moment when the bubble is breached.

Anthropologist Edward Hall was one of the first to comment on man's feeling about space. From his work the fascinating field of proxemics has evolved.

Hall pointed out that the North American demands more personal space for himself than do people from many other countries. For two unacquainted adult male North Americans the comfortable distance to stand for conversation is about two feet apart. The South American likes to stand much closer, which creates problems when the two meet face to face. For as the South American moves in to what is to him a proper talking distance, the North American feels he's being pushy; and as the North American backs off to create the size gap that seems right to him, the South American thinks he's being standoffish. Hall once watched a conversation between a Latin and a North American that began at one end of a forty-foot hall and eventually wound up at the other end, the pair progressing by "an almost continual series of small backward steps on the part of the North American . . . and an equal closing of the gap by the Latin American. . . ."

Often, North Americans can't control their own reactions to being closed in on.

"Dolores is one of those people who like to talk standing practically nose to nose," one young woman explained. "I like her and I know it's just her way, but I can't help myself; when I see her coming I start backing up. I put a desk or a chair between us if I can."

If Americans and Latins have misunderstandings, the American and the Arab are even less compatible in their space habits. Arabs thrive on close contact. They stand very close together to talk, staring intently into each other's eyes and breathing into each other's faces. These are all actions the American associates with sexual intimacy and he finds it quite disturbing to be subjected to them in a nonsexual context.

Americans maintain their distance in many ways. We actually suppress our sense of smell. Anthropologist Margaret Mead once remarked:

"In the United States, nobody has been willing to smell another human being, if they could help it, for the last fifty years."

To the Arab, on the other hand, to be able to smell a friend is reassuring. Good smells please him, and smelling is a way of being involved with another. To deny a friend his breath would be to act ashamed. When Arab intermediaries call to inspect a prospective bride for a friend or relative, they sometimes ask to smell her—but not to make sure she's freshly scrubbed; apparently what they look for is any lingering odor of anger or discontent.

When forced to share his bubble of space with another—for example, in a crowded elevator—the American compensates for the unwanted intimacy in a number of ways. He averts his eyes and shifts his body so that he doesn't face anyone directly. If forced into actual physical contact with another person, he holds that part of his body rigid. He feels strongly that this is the proper way to behave.

"I can't stand that guy," a young stockbroker remarked. "I have to ride down in the elevator with him sometimes and he just lets himself go. It's like being leaned on by a mountain of warm jelly."

Situation and mood also affect distance. Moviegoers waiting in line to see a sexy film will queue up much more densely than those waiting to see a family-entertainment movie; in fact, one suburban theater manager reported that he could get three times as many customers into his lobby for a sex comedy.

In America a man standing still or seated in a

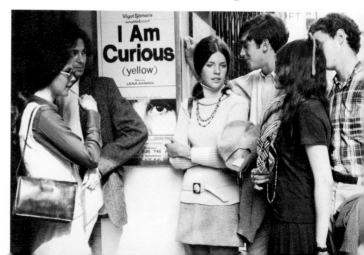

Do you queue up closer to people at a sexy film than at a family entertainment movie?

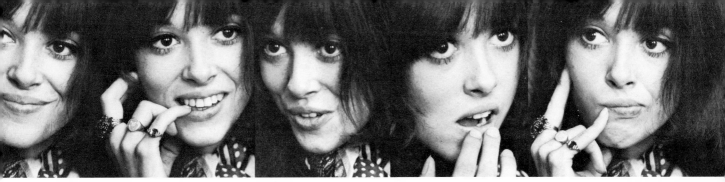

Does your eye behavior give the lie to what you're saying?

public place is assumed to have around him a small sphere of privacy, even larger than his personal-space bubble, that has to be respected. Anyone invading this space will apologize. In a nearly empty room a man does not expect a stranger to come and take a chair right next to him. If someone does, he will either put up with it or he will move to another chair, but he will not protest. Experiments have demonstrated that people rarely defend their space rights with words, possibly because they're not really conscious of the fact that they feel they have rights.

Dr. Augustus F. Kinzel, a New York psychiatrist, recently studied the "body-buffer zone" in violent and nonviolent prisoners. Placing each man in turn in the center of a small, bare room, he walked slowly toward him. Prisoners with a record of violence reacted sharply while he was still some distance away. They reported a feeling that he was "looming" or "rushing" at them. The nonviolent men let him come up quite close. Dr. Kinzel studied just fifteen subjects and isn't jumping to any conclusions until he has carried out more tests, but his experiment suggests that proxemics might provide a simple technique for spotting the potentially violent.

It's important to know how much physical space people actually need, especially in crowded city living. Animals forced to live in overcrowded conditions undergo such stress that whole populations sometimes die off.

Architects need to consider the effects of different kinds of space in designing new buildings. Winston Churchill, reacting to a postwar plan to change the intimate scale of the House of Commons, where opponents face each other across a narrow aisle, warned that: "We shape our buildings, and they shape us."

Borrowing material from both kinesics and proxemics, sociologists have also entered the nonverbal field. Their work often encompasses the verbal as well, but it is usually lumped with the nonverbal studies because the field of interest for men such as Erving Goffman is still the small behaviors of face-to-face encounters.

Taking nothing for granted, Goffman has examined the assumptions, conscious and unconscious, that underlie our everyday behavior. If most sane people didn't share these assumptions, the world would be a more unruly and dangerous place. When you walk on a public street you assume that no stranger will assault you or bar your way. In casual conversation you assume that other people will not insult you, lie to you or create a scene. People depend on each other to behave properly.

Many of our assumptions have been shaken in the past five to ten years—notably, the assumption that people will not use their own bodies to block access to a public building. Sociologists point out that wherever there are rules there is the potential for breaking rules—for making them the basis for aggression. This is all the more shocking when the rules broken are the kind that we usually take for granted.

There are other assumptions, too. We all have our territorial preserves—boundaries we don't expect people to try to cross. Personal space is one kind of territoriality, the earliest studied. Professor Goffman is concerned with other kinds, rights we assume we have: the right not to be stared at, not to be touched, the right not to be brought into strangers' conversations, the right to informational privacy—there are certain questions we don't expect to be asked. Encounter groups or sensitivity training play on these assumptions. In an attempt to teach "normal" people to live more intensely, they require participants to touch each other, perhaps even to grapple with each other, to ask intimate questions and express honest opinions, even hurtful ones. They encourage people who are usually total strangers to share the trappings of intimacy in the hope that real, deeply emotional—if temporary—relationships will result and that in the process each participant will learn something about himself. Those who join a grope group, as encounter groups are sometimes called, are expected most of the time to *do*, rather than to talk, for the theory is that by the time we are adults we have learned to hide our feelings behind a screen of polite words—hiding them so well that often they are inaccessible even to ourselves.

Which brings us full circle, back to that nonverbal party game with its emotion-charged undertones.

George du Maurier once wrote:

"Language is a poor thing. You fill your lungs with wind and shake a little slit in your throat, and make mouths, and that shakes the air; and the air shakes a pair of little drums in my head . . . and my brain seizes your meaning in the rough. What a roundabout way and what a waste of time."

Communication between human beings would be just that dull if it were all done with words; but actually, words are often the smallest part of it. So it's fun for a time to put them aside and to become aware of the rest of what goes on when people meet face to face.

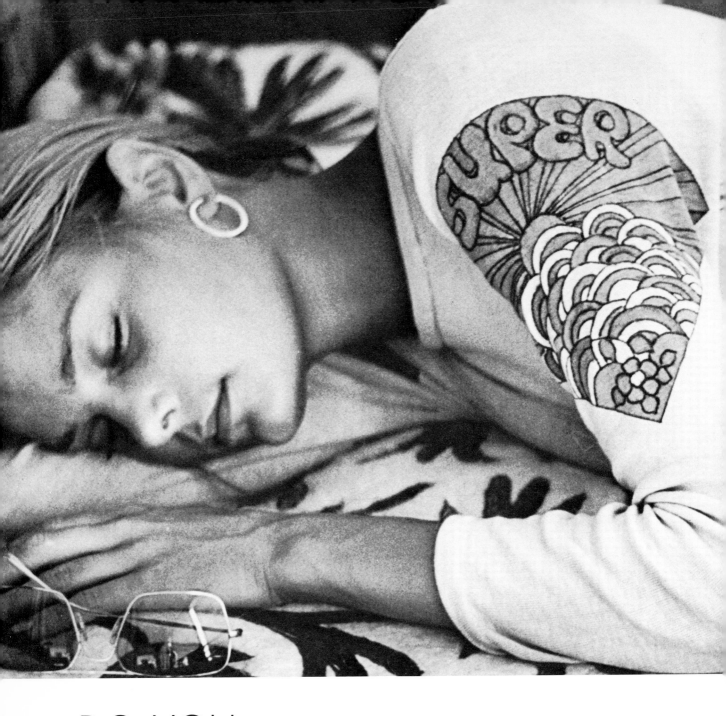

DO YOU EXAGGERATE YOUR LACK OF SLEEP?

by Flora Davis

Are you afraid of sleep because it means losing control of self?

Do you retreat into sleep when life gets to be too much?

Or are you just a poor sleeper or a temporary situational insomniac?

The pillow has turned unaccountably lumpy. The blankets just won't stay put. You've been lying in bed for hours, waiting to go to sleep, but it seems as if you've forgotten how, for your mind churns on relentlessly. You don't know what to do about it. You probably don't even know what kind of insomnia you have—temporary, situational, imaginary, fear—which of the many kinds that an estimated one half of all adult Americans suffer from at one time or another.

We spend a third of our lives asleep, yet to most of us sleep is a mystery and therefore so is insomnia. Many people assume that sleep is simply oblivion. But scientists now know that the sleeper

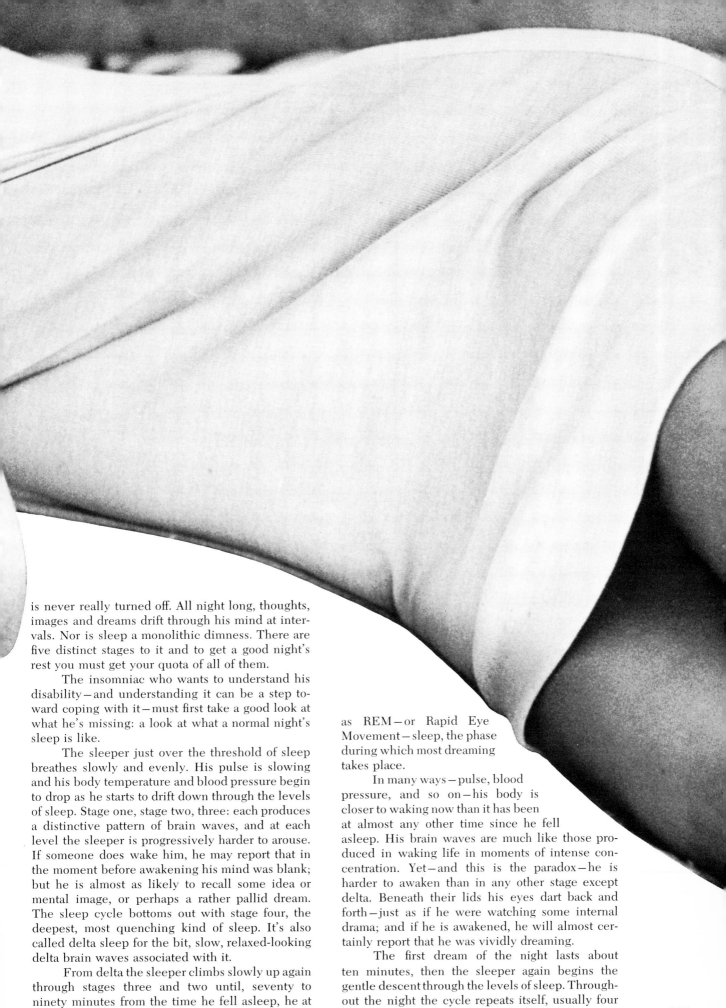

is never really turned off. All night long, thoughts, images and dreams drift through his mind at intervals. Nor is sleep a monolithic dimness. There are five distinct stages to it and to get a good night's rest you must get your quota of all of them.

The insomniac who wants to understand his disability—and understanding it can be a step toward coping with it—must first take a good look at what he's missing: a look at what a normal night's sleep is like.

The sleeper just over the threshold of sleep breathes slowly and evenly. His pulse is slowing and his body temperature and blood pressure begin to drop as he starts to drift down through the levels of sleep. Stage one, stage two, three: each produces a distinctive pattern of brain waves, and at each level the sleeper is progressively harder to arouse. If someone does wake him, he may report that in the moment before awakening his mind was blank; but he is almost as likely to recall some idea or mental image, or perhaps a rather pallid dream. The sleep cycle bottoms out with stage four, the deepest, most quenching kind of sleep. It's also called delta sleep for the bit, slow, relaxed-looking delta brain waves associated with it.

From delta the sleeper climbs slowly up again through stages three and two until, seventy to ninety minutes from the time he fell asleep, he at last enters the fascinating, paradoxical stage known as REM—or Rapid Eye Movement—sleep, the phase during which most dreaming takes place.

In many ways—pulse, blood pressure, and so on—his body is closer to waking now than it has been at almost any other time since he fell asleep. His brain waves are much like those produced in waking life in moments of intense concentration. Yet—and this is the paradox—he is harder to awaken than in any other stage except delta. Beneath their lids his eyes dart back and forth—just as if he were watching some internal drama; and if he is awakened, he will almost certainly report that he was vividly dreaming.

The first dream of the night lasts about ten minutes, then the sleeper again begins the gentle descent through the levels of sleep. Throughout the night the cycle repeats itself, usually four or five times in all, and as it does, proportions

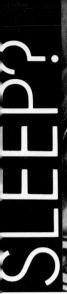

within it change. The sleeper gets most of his delta sleep the first and second times around, and as morning approaches, spends more and more time in the REM phase. His last dream period may fill sixty minutes of a ninety-minute cycle, and toward morning he may simply drift from REM sleep down to stage two and back up to REM sleep again.

How do we know all this about sleep?

Since 1952, when the REM phenomenon was first discovered, scientists have been studying sleep in special bedroom-laboratories. The sleep lab at New York University, for example, has a pair of bedrooms very much like small dormitory rooms except the walls and doors are burlap-covered—an aid to soundproofing. Subjects usually come to the lab at about their normal bedtime, get ready for bed, and then are decorated with electrodes—tiny metal cups—stuck onto brow and scalp with collodion. Each cup is attached to a bright-colored wire which plugs into a panel on the wall above the bed. The electrodes pick up shifts of electrical current within the brain and eye muscles, producing a "write-out" in a monitoring room outside. There, on fully half a mile of graph paper, the subject's sleep is mapped, penned in parallel rows of squiggles: one row for brain waves, one for eye movements, perhaps others for blood pressure or temperature.

"Every individual has his own distinctive sleep pattern," Dr. Leo Goldberger, associate director of New York University's Research Center for Mental Health, explained. "This pattern is so regular that, once we become familiar with it, we can usually predict what he will do next—when he will roll over, or enter his next REM stage. If he feels depressed or anxious, this may show up as a change in the pattern—for example, in stage four sleep the pen that has been tracing out those big, relaxed delta waves may suddenly start to scribble furiously."

"Sleep is the best cure for waking troubles," Cervantes once wrote.

Unfortunately, it isn't always that simple. Many people take their troubles to bed and their sleep is like a dark mirror, reflecting the stresses of their daytime lives. Too many of them believe that the solution to their problem is just a sleeping pill

away. But in the last ten years sleep researchers have begun to investigate abnormal sleep. The answers aren't all in yet, but the ones that are challenge many of the old assumptions about insomnia. They tell us what a sleeping pill can do and what it can't. They reveal that there are actually several different kinds of insomnia and that one of the commonest kinds is the imaginary sort.

What you are determines how you sleep. And how you sleep, the particular kind of insomnia you have, should determine the way you cope with the problem. Before we consider ways of coping, though, let's look at a few of the different varieties of insomnia.

Situational insomnia: One of the commonest kinds of insomnia is the sort apparently caused by a specific stressful situation. One woman described it this way: "Six months ago I was fired from my first job and suddenly I had the most awful insomnia. Night after night I was awake until three or four in the morning. Finally a friend suggested that I try her sleeping pills. They worked, so I got a doctor to prescribe some for me, and I really thought I had the problem licked."

For a month this young woman took a barbiturate every night. Then she found a new job and stopped taking the drug. But on her first night without it she was awakened several times by nightmares. The second night the same thing happened. Frightened by this new and unexpected problem, she went back to taking the barbiturate. The nightmares immediately stopped, but sleeping pills were now a necessity for her.

What she didn't know was that nightmares were a predictable result of the drug's withdrawal. Most sleep-inducing drugs do not produce a normal night's sleep. What's more, if you take them for long enough, they will continue to distort your sleep for weeks after you have given them up.

Though sleeping pills have been in use for years, their precise effect on sleep was discovered only recently. Two West Coast researchers, Doctors Anthony Kales and Allan Jacobson, ran a series of experiments in which they dosed subjects with various drugs. They compared the normal sleep of the subject with his drugged sleep and went on to see what his sleep was like after the drug was withdrawn. They found that barbiturates and most other sleeping drugs suppress both the delta and REM stages in ratio to the amount of the drug and the length of time it is given. Tranquilizers and stimulants have the same effect. In one Kales and Jacobson study, volunteers who took a barbiturate for just twenty days didn't get back to normal sleep patterns for a month after the drug was discontinued, and these subjects reported having had ugly dreams.

The dreams were undoubtedly tied in with REM rebound, a reaction familiar to sleep scientists. People who are deprived of their REM sleep—in the laboratory it's usually done by repeated awakening—show a steadily mounting need for it. When they are finally allowed a normal, uninterrupted night's rest, their REM quota shoots way up, as if they were making up for what they lost. People deprived of REM sleep for eight to ten days or longer become quite irritable and anxious.

Imaginary insomnia: Not all insomnia is real. Most insomniacs exaggerate their difficulty, and some even see a problem where none exists.

One middle-aged woman, who consulted a doctor with a request for sleeping pills, complained that she hadn't been sleeping well for months. She slept, she said, only about six hours a night and she kept waking up in the night.

Part of her problem was that she was so sold on the idea that she must get eight hours' sleep a night that when she realized she was getting only six, she was ready to believe that she was a chronic insomniac. Actually, sleep requirements vary widely. Five hours a night or even less are normal for some people, while others regularly need ten hours or more. Differences show up even immediately after birth, when some newborns sleep twenty-three hours out of the twenty-four, others for as few as ten.

Middle-of-the-night awakenings were what really convinced this woman that she had insomnia. In her case, the awakenings were due to the natural aging process. Sleep patterns change with age. Children spend the first several hours of the night sunk deep in delta sleep, and while it lasts they are almost impossible to awaken. Beginning at adolescence the delta stage is cut back, diminishing until it almost vanishes in middle age, sometimes as early as the forties.

Imaginary insomniacs exaggerate their own lack of sleep. It's easy to confuse the lighter stages of sleep with wakefulness, to feel that you haven't slept at all even though you have. Lab subjects awakened in stages one, two or even three often maintain that they haven't yet slept. Furthermore, the mind tends to fuse together repeated awakenings in the night: you tell yourself you heard the clock strike every hour and conclude that you haven't slept at all, when actually you have simply been awakened several times by the clock.

Poor sleepers: Sleep scientist Lawrence Monroe has done a study of this problem, comparing the sleep of people who said they slept well with that of people who said they didn't. He found that the poor sleepers dropped off in about fifteen minutes in the lab, although most of them estimated that they usually lay awake for an hour; however, good sleepers took only about seven minutes. The poor sleepers woke twice as often during the night. Physiologically, their bodies stayed closer to waking levels than those of good sleepers: their pulse rate was faster; body temperature higher; and they tended to thrash around more. They woke in the morning with their temperatures still at a nighttime low. Temperature for the good sleepers began to climb a good hour and a half before waking. Mood and alertness seemed keyed to the body-temperature cycle: a person feels best and is most alert when his temperature is at its daily high.

As a group, Monroe's poor sleepers were more neurotic and prone to psychosomatic illness than his good sleepers, but there is no way to be sure whether they slept badly because they were neurotic or were neurotic because they so often slept badly.

Early-morning insomnia: Another sort of insomniac is the person who comes-to regularly in the predawn hours.

"Ever since my fiancé and I broke up, I awake every morning at five A.M.," said one young woman. "It's not even light outside, but there I am, wide awake and feeling hideously depressed."

Poor sleep, unpleasant dreams and early morning awakenings often go with depression. Sleep scientists, studying the sleep of people depressed enough to need medical help, have found that they usually don't get nearly enough delta sleep and they are easily nudged by noise into lighter, more fragile stages of sleep. It's possible that early-morning noises and the light of dawn are more disturbing to these people than they are to most.

Treated with an antidepressant drug, depressed patients sleep better and are less easily awakened by sounds. Sometimes a sudden increase in delta sleep, noted in the sleep lab, is followed the next morning by a vast improvement in mood.

Fear insomnia: Children sometimes have trouble falling asleep because of a fear of sleep itself. One college student recalled: "When I was a child I was terrified of sleep. So many nights, just as I was dropping off, I'd suddenly become aware that I was going, that the real world was slipping away from me and I was about to be overwhelmed by strange feelings and the weird images in my head. The worst times were when I'd suddenly feel that I was falling."

That sensation of falling—almost everyone has it occasionally—is a perfectly normal phenomenon. Called the myoclonic jerk, it happens during sleep onset and is caused by a tiny burst of electric charges going off all together in the brain.

The child or adult disturbed by sleep onset is usually happier if he is not cut off from all stimulation at bedtime. A dim light, a radio playing softly and—for the child—toys in the bed provide comforting, real-world ties.

Dream-deprivation insomnia: A very few insomniacs stay awake because they are afraid to

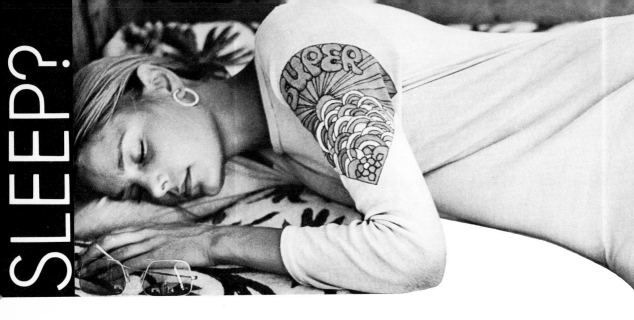

dream. One man said: "I've been having such nightmares lately—really gruesome—that I start getting tense as soon as I get into bed, and then it takes me ages to drop off. I've come to dread sleep."

Scientists recently discovered that there are actually two kinds of nightmares. The kind that happens in REM sleep is simply an unpleasant dream. But a very few people have nightmares during delta sleep and these are profoundly disturbing, terrifying dreams. The victim wakes from them feeling very disoriented and usually can recall little about his dream. It has been suggested that the delta nightmare takes place in an aroused state that is not really sleeping, nor is it alert wakefulness.

Few people become really disturbed by their own nightmares—probably few have the delta kind—but some people may be, on an unconscious level, unwilling to dream, for there is a variety of insomnia in which the sleeper keeps waking up just as he passes into REM sleep, as if to prevent himself from dreaming.

Most dreams are not nightmares, but it's the REM nightmares we're most apt to remember. Usually, a dream evaporates almost as soon as it is over. The sleeper wakened just a few minutes after a REM period has ended probably has already lost the ability to recall his dream. Yet some dreams stay with us quite clearly. Mostly, they are the last dreams we have just before awaking in the morning, or the unpleasant dreams that shock us awake.

Dream research indicates that it is actually kinder *not* to awaken a person who is obviously having a bad dream, since if he is able to go on sleeping, he will probably not remember the dream the next morning. That frightening feeling of paralysis that sometimes comes over you in a dream—when you want to run or scream but can't—happens because in REM sleep the body goes completely limp. The head of a dreaming cat drops to the floor; the dreaming man lies like a tossed down rag doll. Sometimes if a sleeper is awakened suddenly from a dream, the feeling of paralysis persists—frighteningly—for a few seconds.

Studies of dream content suggest that the dreams to be frightened of are not the violent or grisly ones. People who have attempted suicide have reported dreams, before the attempt, that were chillingly barren: the dreamer, alone, might be sitting in a desolate, rocky place, performing some meaningless, rhythmic act such as banging his fist on the ground. Later, just before their suicide attempts, these people stopped recalling dreams at all.

Insomnia is not the only sleep problem. There are, for example, hypersomniacs, who retreat into sleep whenever life gets to be too much for them. They sleep too much, have a lot of trouble waking up, and their sleep is not refreshing. Usually, the underlying problem is depression.

Now that we've considered how some kinds of insomnia work, it's time to ask: What can be done about it? I put the question to Dr. Allan Jacobson, director of this country's first sleep center, which was opened at Cedars-Sinai Medical Center in Los Angeles early in 1969.

When an insomniac comes to the center for help, Dr. Jacobson first does tests to make sure there is no medical cause for his sleeplessness. Hypothyroidism, for example, can cause insomnia. Next, imaginary insomnia must be ruled out. For insomnia that is both real and severe, Dr. Jacobson usually recommends a combination of psychiatric help and sleep therapy—treatment with drugs. He doesn't use barbiturates at all except in cases where the patient has become addicted to them; then he will sometimes continue the drug for a while, withdrawing it gradually.

There *are* new sleeping drugs that induce a nearly-normal sleep, proved out in the Kales and Jacobson studies. The same studies indicated that one older drug, chloral hydrate, disturbs sleep patterns very little if taken in the doses usually prescribed. "But there is still no perfect sleep drug," Dr. Jacobson warned.

The question most apt to puzzle the average insomniac is: How can he tell whether his disability is severe enough to need psychiatric treatment? Gay Gaer Luce and Dr. Julius Segal, in their fascinating book *Insomnia: The Guide for Troubled Sleepers,* suggest criteria. The concerned insomniac might ask himself:

Has his sleep change been a dramatic one?

Has the problem lasted for quite a while?
(One sleep scientist suggested that in cases of severe insomnia, a week is a long enough period to wait before getting medical advice.)

Could the insomnia be simply a function of the way he lives?

Many people unwittingly interfere with their own sleep. Coffee and cigarettes affect sleep. Strenuous, unaccustomed exercise in the evening can distort sleep, though daytime exercise may improve it. Alarming experiences before bedtime—televised or real-life ones—disturb sleep. Alcohol causes mental slowdown and drowsiness in some people, but too much of it reduces REM sleep in the early part of the night.

The fourth and perhaps most significant question is: *Is the insomnia accompanied by daytime problems such as chronic fatigue and lethargy, lapses of memory or attention, poor coordination, irritability?*

For persistent insomnia, especially if it is accompanied by these daytime problems, you should consult a psychiatrist. Emotional problems are almost always at the root of insomnia. In the long run, then, psychotherapy is the best answer, since it gets at the cause of the problem. However, it is still no *guaranteed* cure. In one case it helped the patient enormously, caused sweeping changes in his life, while alleviating but never really curing his insomnia. On the other hand, when scientists studied poor sleepers, they found that those who'd had therapy showed almost normal amounts of REM sleep, while those who'd had none scanted their REM time.

Many insomniacs, convinced that theirs is a short-term problem, consult not a psychiatrist but their family doctor. If the doctor simply prescribes a sleeping pill, the patient should protect himself by asking whether it is a drug which will give normal or nearly-normal sleep, as demonstrated by sleep-lab tests. If it's not, he should rely on it only for a few days at a time.

For the kind of insomnia that appears to be just a reaction to a particular stressful situation, the smart thing to do is to try to ride it out. Dr. Howard Roffwarg, a New York psychiatrist and sleep scientist, suggests that, instead of reaching for the pill bottle for help, the temporary insomniac give his body a chance to work out the problem by itself. One can get by for a few days on very little sleep. Eventually the need for sleep becomes so urgent that in most people it becomes irresistible, and given some resolution of the emotional difficulty, normal sleep patterns are soon restored. The insomniac who *must* stay alert during the day is probably better off over the short term taking stimulant drugs than sleeping pills. However, the stimulant must be taken first thing in the morning, because the effect lasts twelve to sixteen hours. The object is to have the stimulant wear off the next night in time for you to succumb to sleep.

Some insomniacs have been cured by hypnosis. How well hypnosis works depends largely on the patient's susceptibility. One out of every five people can't be hypnotized at all: one in five is very easy to hypnotize; and the others can be hypnotized to some degree.

Another kind of exercise that sometimes helps is the progressive relaxation technique developed by Dr. Edmund Jacobson. He believes that muscle tension usually accompanies insomnia, possibly exaggerating it, and that total body relaxation does not permit the kind of racing, worrying mind that keeps one awake. He taught patients to work over all the muscles of their bodies in sequence, first tensing, then relaxing. It takes practice, but most people can learn to relax their bodies at will.

But for the occasional, mild bout of insomnia, the old-fashioned remedies are probably still the best. You can try a high-protein dinner and then milk at bedtime—both contain amino acids, which have been shown to have a soporific effect. Add a dull book, a warm room and the comfort of bedtime rituals: checking the frontdoor lock twice, tucking a hand under the pillow in a particular way—we never stop to think how reassuring these little habits are.

If all else fails and you are really wide awake, not just floating gently in the lighter stages of sleep, then you can always get up and use the time to get something done.

Sometimes it helps to realize you have company. Luce and Segal wrote: "On any night in history in any city of the world if the wakeful had risen from their beds and left their houses, a great crowd would have poured through the streets."

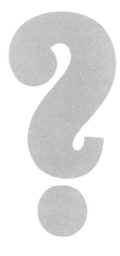

ALL OF US SHOULD KNOW MORE ABOUT THEM

by Ellen Switzer

Recently, Anne, a twenty-year-old student, visited her college psychiatrist with a problem. Her fiancé was taking almost daily injections of a powerful amphetamine. His whole personality was changing from trusting, gentle and shy to antagonistic, aggressive and suspicious. He insisted that the rather slapdash paintings he had recently taken to turning out were great works of art and that a hostile "art establishment" was conspiring to discriminate against him. Sometimes he accused Anne of aiding and abetting the conspiracy. He also had abrupt changes in mood. There were days when he was elated and unrealistically optimistic, when he painted furiously for hours at a time, without food or sleep. Then there were days when he was too depressed to get out of bed. Anne, who had heard enough about "speed freaks" to be worried, told the doctor that she had tried to get him to give up the drugs. "I've begged, I've cried, I've threatened to break the engagement . . . but nothing has helped. Once I took the drugs and flushed them down the toilet. He got so angry that I thought he'd hit me. What can I do?"

Susan, who visited the same psychiatrist, had a slightly different problem. She was about to lose her boyfriend because she refused to accompany him on his LSD trips. "John says that he just can't communicate with someone who doesn't share his world," she said. "He tells me that I'm afraid and

inhibited and that if I don't change, he'll drop me for a more liberated girl. But the whole idea of taking LSD scares me to death. Am I really a coward?"

The psychiatrist had little encouragement for the two girls. He told Anne that for the moment, at least, the drug obviously meant more to her fiancé than she did. Speed is not physiologically habituating. A speedster crashing down from his high may get so depressed that he takes another dose just to feel normal. Trying to get rid of his drug supply wouldn't help, as she had already discovered. Neither would tears or threats. "We have always told wives of alcoholics that begging, nagging and pouring liquor down the drain only drive their husbands to the bottle faster," he said. "The same is true for the intensive drug user."

He advised Anne to encourage her fiancé to get medical help if and when she felt that his drug habit was beginning to bother him too. If such suggestions just made him angry, she should seriously consider breaking the engagement, since the prognosis for a confirmed, intensive amphetamine-user is pessimistic. "There are usually progressive personality changes such as the ones you have already noticed, and they may be irreversible," he said. "There also is the possibility of permanent brain damage. And as the hippies put it, 'Speed Kills.' An overdose can cause death and so can an illness aggravated by the user's poor physical condition."

To Susan he suggested that her young man probably had a very serious personality problem which might have been the cause of his taking LSD in the first place. Why was he trying to blackmail her by threatening withdrawal of his love into an experience that clearly terrified her? Why was he so insistent that he could form no lasting relationship with a girl who did not share his drug-oriented world? Had he, perhaps, turned to LSD because he could not bear a close involvement with another person without feeling threatened? The psychiatrist advised Susan to take a cold-sober look at her whole relationship with this young man.

Such once-removed drug problems are coming to the attention of college counseling services, mental health centers and private psychiatrists—the problems of nonusers whose life situations are strongly affected by drugs. The use of the various "pop drugs" is so much a part of the current culture that almost anyone under thirty will probably be confronted with a drug-related problem at some time during his life.

Acting Commissioner Ernest A. Shepherd of Connecticut's State Department of Mental Health, who is also Associate Commissioner for Alcohol and Drug Dependence, feels that the whole subject of pop drugs is so emotionally charged that many people either overreact or underreact to the problem. This results in official and unofficial behavior that aggravates the problem, rather than solving it. Politicians, citing figures on pot-smoking among college students, start talking about "the deterioration of moral fiber among America's youth." Police chiefs in small suburban communities have declared "drug emergencies" when a few marijuana cigarettes were found in high school lockers; yet for years they ignored widespread use of sleeping

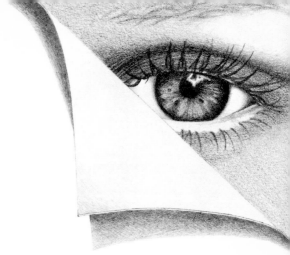

pills and amphetamines among respectable middle-class housewives. In spite of rising drunken-driving accident rates, no one has declared an "alcohol emergency." Some parents have been so appalled when they discovered that a son or daughter was smoking pot that they have called the police and demanded that the offender be arrested. All of this is overreaction.

On the other hand, there has been a notable lack of concern about the fact that over 90 percent of all barbiturates and amphetamines found in the black market in the United States were manufactured legitimately. In many states, up to the present time, manufacture and sale of the high dangerous hallucinogens (like LSD) are considered much less serious offenses than possession of marijuana (which is still classified falsely as a narcotic along with heroin). All this is underreaction.

It is important to have as much knowledge as possible about drugs, their use and misuse. The following questions are those most frequently asked in student counseling and mental health centers and psychiatrists' offices. The answers are a summary of facts and advice most frequently given by experts in the field working with drug-users and those who are involved, either directly or indirectly, with the drug subculture.

Why do people take drugs in the first place?

"The desire to take medicine is perhaps the greatest feature which distinguishes man from animals," wrote the nineteenth century physician Sir William Osler. People take drugs because they expect the pill, the capsule, the injection or the cigarette to make them feel better. Few drugs promise to cure any disease. However, they do alleviate unpleasant symptoms. The patients who swallow the cold capsule know perfectly well that no one has yet discovered a cure for the cold, but they do expect, temporarily at least, to get rid of their headaches and stuffed noses.

Mind- and mood-changing drugs alleviate a different kind of symptom: psychological discomfort, such as boredom, depression, anxiety and shyness. A study, "Students and Drugs," by Dr. Richard H. Blum of Stanford University, indicates that most students start using a drug out of curiosity. If the drug does nothing to lessen a psychological problem (or if there is no problem in the first place), the user either discontinues it or takes it only occasionally—about once a week. Alcohol is used in a very similar manner. Most social drinkers don't become alcoholics, but six and a half million have, almost three times the number estimated to be heavily dependent on pop drugs. Most people who smoke an occasional marijuana joint don't become potheads either. But some have, although marijuana, unlike alcohol which produces both physical and psychological dependence, can cause only a psychological one.

Most students are introduced to a drug not by the pusher—who lurks around the corner—but by a friend. Whether a drug becomes a habit depends on any number of unpredictable factors. A good rule of thumb might be that if any drug (including alcohol) makes the world seem attractively warm,

loving and pleasant when without chemical assistance it seems continuously bleak, lonely and dull, the time has come to throw out the drug. The temptation to escape from psychological discomfort into pleasant unreality may become irresistible.

The same is true of drugs like tranquilizers, sleeping pills or amphetamines that have been prescribed. Many physicians, perhaps unwisely, trust their patients' good judgment sufficiently to give open-ended prescriptions for mood-altering drugs. An open-ended prescription, however, is not automatic permission for open-ended use. If life without the drug becomes difficult, it's time to tell the doctor. He may want to change the prescription or stop it altogether.

I have a friend who takes a drug once a week. Is there any sure way to tell whether he may become addicted or habituated?

The answer to that question is probably "no." Psychiatrists used to talk a good deal about "addictive personalities." Now they don't use the term very often. Dr. Max Pepper, professor and chairman of the Department of Community Medicine at St. Louis University School of Medicine (and also a psychiatrist), said that just about everyone has the potential to be addicted to something. The overweight girl who can't stay on a diet is addicted to eating. The man who can't stop calling the office four times a day during his vacation is addicted to his job. Millions of people are addicted to cigarettes, even though they know that smoking can produce cancer, heart disease and any number of other serious ailments. Then there are those six and a half million alcoholics.

It is very difficult to pinpoint a drug-prone personality. However, Dr. Blum's study provides some guidelines. In comparing the "occasional" pot user with the "intensive" one, he said that "intensive more than less-intensive users . . . come from unsettled (highly mobile) families, are totally uninterested in athletics, academic- or career-oriented activities, are opposed to their fathers' and mothers' political stance . . . intensive users are also more dissatisfied with their coursework, find life worse than expected . . . and feel like outsiders in various groups, such as family, student body and the nation." The more dangerous and exotic the drug chosen by intensive users, the more pronounced these characteristics become. Also, 99 percent of intensive users drink alcohol and 94 percent smoke tobacco. (As an interesting sidelight, intensive users also drink a great deal of coffee, some tea, few soft drinks and no hot chocolate.) It appears from this that the occasional drug user who is generally pessimistic, easily hurt, finds it difficult to form close relationships with other people and has family problems had better closely watch his step. He might well turn into an "intensive" user, and from there go on to addiction or habituation.

I have a friend who seems to be headed toward a serious drug problem. What can I do to help?

No amount of preaching, crying, nagging or threatening will persuade a habituated user (or probably even an intensive one) to stop. Probably no amount of logical argument will help much either.

Tell a speedster that his drug can cause permanent brain damage, and he'll answer that this is just "an establishment lie." Tell a confirmed LSD user that his trips can lead to a very serious psychosis, and he'll tell you that is just a theory dreamed up by hostile psychiatrists "who are probably crazier than I am." Tell a potential barbiturate addict that he may become hooked on the pills (if he isn't already), and he'll tell you that he can stop taking them anytime he wants to . . . just as many alcoholics insist that they can stop drinking anytime.

The only really helpful thing that you can do is to get the problem drug user to seek medical and psychological help as quickly as possible. That won't be easy either. "Drug users get pleasure from their drug," said Dr. Herbert Kleber, a psychiatrist on the Yale Medical School staff and director of the drug dependence unit of the Connecticut Mental Health Center. "As long as the pleasure outweighs the pain of drug-taking, few habituated users want to give it up. Only when the drug has made them acutely uncomfortable are they sometimes ready to accept help."

Alcoholics Anonymous, one of the few organizations that has helped confirmed alcoholics, operates on a similar theory. Only when the alcoholic has really "hit bottom" and is ready to admit that he has a problem he cannot solve by himself is he willing to accept help.

No psychiatrist can force a patient to change his ways. The patient will only be able to benefit from the counseling he is able and ready to accept.

Why do friends who smoke pot or take LSD always try to pressure me to join them?

Dr. Blum's study indicated that the intensive drug user is frequently suspicious of the non-user and of the whole straight world. There may be a number of reasons for this. The user may feel guilty about his drug involvement (although at the same time he may boast about it), and the non-user aggravates these guilt feelings. On the other hand, he may feel his own special world is so much more exciting than the real world that he wants to share it.

Again a comparison with alcohol use is appropriate. In the movie *Days of Wine and Roses*, the alcoholic husband insists that his non-drinking wife join him in his before-, after- and during-dinner drinking. He tells her that he can't relax with his martini while she sips ginger ale. Eventually, she gives in to the pressure and becomes an alcoholic herself. At the end he is cured . . . but she cannot stop. In the same way the occasional user may "turn on" a friend, who becomes habituated. Pressuring someone else to try a drug is assuming enormous responsibility.

Is there a completely harmless drug?

The answer to this is "no," but only because any chemical substance can be harmful to some people. This is especially true for women in their childbearing years.

Of course some drugs are more dangerous than others. Heroin is addictive and so are barbiturates. Amphetamines are habituating and may cause brain damage and death. LSD can cause severe emotional trauma via a "bad trip" and even a psychosis that must be treated in a mental hospital. Early research findings also indicated that the drug caused some chromosome breakage. Although later findings did not bear this out, the whole question of the relationship of LSD to birth defects has not been answered conclusively. Combinations of drugs are more dangerous than the same drugs taken individually. The mixture of barbiturates and alcohol can be deadly.

However, usually when someone asks, "Are all drugs dangerous?" he is really asking about marijuana. The same answer applies: no drug is harmless to everyone, and some that are harmless for the majority can be dangerous for a minority. However, the dangers of pot have been vastly overestimated, partly due to the continuing efforts of the Federal Bureau of Narcotics (now called the U.S. Bureau of Narcotics and Dangerous Drugs). In 1937, marijuana was not even an illegal drug. That year, for legal purposes, it was lumped in with heroin as a "narcotic." This is medically and legally wrong. Marijuana is not a narcotic; it is a mild hallucinogen and euphoriant. In spite of overwhelming evidence to the contrary, the Bureau stuck to its position. Posters were printed that told the pot smoker that his habit caused "Death, Insanity and Murder." These posters have become collector's items and often decorate the pads of pot-smoking students. Today, probably in reaction to overemphasis on danger, the supposed "harmlessness" of marijuana is exaggerated. Some experts believe that the dangers of pot are about equal to those of alcohol, which no one considers a totally harmless drug; others say that we know so little about the effects of pot that any comparison is misleading.

Very little information is available on the long-term effects of pot. No conclusive research has been done on any correlation between marijuana and birth defects. We don't even know whether continued use of marijuana cigarettes can cause lung cancer, since we don't know exactly which chemical causes the cancer after prolonged use of regular cigarettes.

However, whatever may or may not be the medical dangers of pot smoking, the legal dangers are real. In most states marijuana is still treated by law as a narcotic, and conviction on charges of possession alone is considered a felony. In 1969, a twenty-year-old model student and track star was sentenced to twenty years in jail by an eighty-year-old judge for possession of a small amount of pot. He has recently been pardoned as a result of an appeal, but not until he had spent more than six months in prison. Even a much less drastic punishment, such as a one-year suspended jail sentence on a felony charge, may bar a person from any number of professions, including, in many states, law, teaching or government employment.

Pot smokers frequently point out that many people drank illegally during Prohibition. But there is one major difference. Only the manufacturer and seller of liquor went to jail, not the user. Almost every expert in the drug field thinks the marijuana laws should be changed to conform more to the reality of its widespread use. However, few would support legalizing it outright without any controls. After all, we have some fairly stringent controls on the manufacture and sale of alcohol and cigarettes.

Will drugs help me to learn more about myself, to become more creative, to get rid of my inhibitions?

Again, the answer is "no," although, perhaps, a more qualified no. In many tests with marijuana and amphetamines, the participants have been convinced, while under the influence, that they were doing original and creative work. What they actually produced did not bear out their convictions. There are, of course, individual people of demonstrated ability who have experienced spurts of creativity under the influence of stimulants. Some have used marijuana, many, many more alcohol (but only because it's been around longer). And, of course, Samuel Taylor Coleridge wrote "Kubla Khan" under the influence of opium. But it's safe to say that although narcotics and other stimulants may promote creativity for short bursts in certain talented individuals, they cannot produce it where it does not exist already. And if used consistently, they ultimately deaden creativity entirely. You don't need statistics: just read some accounts of the struggles of some of our major writers with alcohol. Or ask an old newspaperman. Drugs are no different.

As to the medical good uses of drugs, LSD has been used experimentally in the treatment of severe alcoholism, and did seem to be helping the alcoholic to see himself and his problems more clearly. But most of the experiments have been discontinued, because the dangers of the drug seemed to outweigh the benefits. It might be possible for a person on an LSD trip to learn something about himself that he might not have known without the drug. But often, what he learns is destructive and may be the precipitating factor to an emotional breakdown. Perhaps Dr. Blum sums it up best of all: "The promise of transfiguration is inherent in psychedelic drug use," he says. "But there isn't an erg of work, a microgram of love, or a degree of motivation in all the psychoactive agents that exist. These qualities exist in people; they are in no way "contained" in the drugs themselves.

DRUG GLOSSARY

AMPHETAMINES

Pop names: speed, crystal, crank, meth, bennies, dexies, Christmas trees, "pep" pills, black beauties, ups.
Ingredients: chemical compound.
Specific effect: stimulation of central nervous system.
Medical use: treatment of depression and narcolepsy, appetite suppressant.
Dangers: psychosis, high blood pressure, death by overdose, physiological habituation.

BARBITURATES

Pop names: goofers, goof balls, downers, red devils, red birds, yellow jackets, yellow birds, green dragons.
Ingredients: chemical compound.
Specific effect: depression of central nervous system.
Medical use: treatment of insomnia and epilepsy, sedative.
Dangers: physiological addiction, death by overdose; especially dangerous in conjunction with alcohol.

LSD

Pop name: acid.
Ingredients: lysergic acid diethylamide.
Specific effect: produces intense hallucinations, changes user's sensory perception of environment.
Medical use: none (has been used experimentally in treatment of severe alcoholism and to alleviate fear and depression of the dying).
Dangers: psychosis, "bad trips," accidents and death due to faulty judgment, psychological habituation. Possibility of genetic damage, still being investigated.
Drugs with similar effect: mescaline, peyote, psilocybin and other chemical products more potent than LSD such as: DMT, MDA, STP and DET.

HEROIN

Pop names: H, horse, junk, skag.
Ingredients: derivative of opium poppy.
Specific effect: depression of central nervous system, respiratory sedative.
Medical use: none (although other opiates such as morphine and codeine are used as pain killers.)
Dangers: physiological addiction, death through overdose.

COCAINE

Pop names: coke, snow.
Ingredients: natural (leaves of the coca bush found in Peru and Bolivia) or synthesized (chemical compound).
Specific effect: stimulation of the central nervous system.
Medical use: ingredient in local anesthetic.
Dangers: habituation, predisposition to violence.

HASHISH

Pop name: hash.
Ingredient: the resin from the flower of the Cannabis plant, a more concentrated form of marijuana's active ingredient.

MARIJUANA

Pop names: pot, weed, broccoli, grass, hemp, tea, mary jane, boo, joint.
Ingredients: leaves of the female hemp plant, Cannabis sativa.
Specific effect: alters perception of reality.
Medical use: none.
Dangers: possibility of psychological habituation, very rare psychosis. Experiments on long term use and genetic damage still in progress.

Drugs with similar effect:

THC

Pop name: none.
Ingredient: a chemical synthetic of the active ingredient in the Cannabis plant.

EVERYTHING YOU DIDN'T KNOW ABOUT DEODORANTS

Few things excite a quicker sense of a women's appeal than the perfume she wears . . . and nothing undermines that appeal more easily than an unpleasant body odor. For some women this is a serious, unnerving problem, but for most it really doesn't need to be. It's what most women—and men for that matter—don't know about body odors that causes most of the trouble. So let's start right off knowing that it is underarm odor that is the real offender, usually not all-over body perspiration.

When and how often

There are few cases of underarm odor that can't be controlled by careful hygiene and an effective deodorant. Double back over those two key words "careful hygiene." Under normal conditions that means one soap and water washing and one application of a deodorant every twenty-four hours. If that's not enough, try two applications of a deodorant every day—once in the morning and once at night. You'll get better results from your deodorant if you put it on when you're at rest, or just going to be—for instance, about fifteen minutes after you've showered and are going to sleep. Don't apply it directly after your shower or bath, on the possibility that the following theory which some experts hold is correct. They believe that after the bath, having hydrated your skin and closed off the pores that lead to the perspiration ducts, the deodorant cannot permeate beyond the skin surface. Provided you are going to go to sleep, and use only one application of deodorant a day, the night is a better time to apply it than the morning. In the morning, you're probably perspiring a little from the effort of getting up, you have to get to class or a job or get breakfast for your family, you are heading into a day of stress. The deodorant at that time has to work, as it were, upstream, while the glands are pouring out perspiration. When you're resting, your glands are less active and there's less resistance to the deodorant. The cleaner your skin the better because anything you have on it tends to activate the odor, but this does not mean that every time you apply deodorant you must bathe first. That's only necessary once a day. The more frequently you apply a deodorant the more effective it is going to be. But when you first start with an antiperspirant, it takes four days of application to build up maximum protection. You can get some reduction of perspiration and odor on the first day but not full strength until you've used it once a day for four days. After that if you discontinue using the antiperspirant, you still get what the scientists call "a measurable inhibition up to fourteen days."

Deodorant vs. Antiperspirant

All deodorants reduce odor; some also reduce perspiration. The deodorants that reduce perspiration are called antiperspirants and those that reduce only odor are called only deodorants. Sometimes you'll see both billed on one label. Don't let it confuse you. That's just the manufacturer's way of letting you know you're getting your money's worth. The obvious advantages of the antiperspirant are the cutting down of perspiration and the lessening of possible damage and staining to your clothes. If you are not a heavy perspirer, a just-plain-deodorant-type deodorant may be sufficient, a very effective killer of bacteria that cause underarm odor.

Not the heat but the emotion

It is important to realize that underarm odor is activated not by temperature, but by emotion. It could be 110 degrees or 50 degrees, the amount of perspiration produced by the apocrine glands in the underarms remains the same. The reactors to temperature are the eccrine glands located all over the body, and subject to emotional stimulus too. Both the apocrine and eccrine glands produce perspiration but eccrine perspiration is an odorless water and salt combination, while that of the apocrine glands is a cloudy liquid with proteins and fatty acids in it that bacteria like to feed on. It is the decomposition of these materials by bacteria that causes underarm odor. Eccrine perspiration doesn't nourish them, so they stay away from it and create no odors. If, however, eccrine perspiration is kept enclosed, as in socks and shoes, an odor can form: but it is not caused by anything in the perspiration itself but by bacteria decomposing the dead cells that rub off the surface of the foot skin so easily. Actually it doesn't require much stress or emotion to activate the underarm glands. An exacting conversation can be enough. Taking an exam or having an argument with a friend can increase most women's perspiration measurably. So if you know you're going to be under particularly stressful conditions on a particular day, and you have a body odor problem, the most effective thing to do is repeat your deodorant during the day. It's simply enough to go into the women's room or your own bathroom, take your dress or sweater off, and roll on, spray on or whatever. You can improve the effectiveness considerably by doubling the application. It's not important to wash at that time—once a day is enough.

"If there were one thing I could do for the women of the world . . ."

said a deodorant research man, "it would be to convince them that they need a deodorant as much in the winter, if not more, as in the summer." That's because in the winter the underarm area is not only covered up with clothes but people tend to bathe less frequently, and this provides very snug conditions for the breeding of the bacteria that cause body odor. In the summer, underarms are exposed to air and water, both of which contribute to the reduction of odor. Actually, the amount of perspiration produced by the apocrine glands is the same all year round, but the sales of deodorants peak in July and go down in January. It is a matter of complete misconception by women and men.

Some more big misconceptions

If you believe any of the following things about deodorants, *don't* for the following reasons:

1. It is unhealthy to stop underarm perspiration.—It is perfectly true that people can die of anhydrosis, as the girl in *Goldfinger* did when they painted her gold, but the underarm area is too small to affect general health.

2. You have to switch deodorants because you become immune to them.—There has never been a case of such immunization determined. What probably happens to someone who thinks she has become immune to her deodorant is simply that she noticed once or twice that it failed her. It may have failed her before under certain emotional situations but she didn't happen to notice. No deodorant is perfect or protects fully under all conditions. You must make sure to apply it more frequently under situations of super-stress. There are some people who are zero responders to certain materials—aluminum and zirconium salts in deodorants. They don't get protection from deodorants when they first start using them, so obviously they don't get immune. They have just always been nonresponders.

3. All perspiration smells bad.—Perspiration itself is odorless. Bad-odor perspiration is made that way only by the reaction of bacteria on materials in it or surrounding it. Kill them and you kill odor.

Irritations

Every time you see an underarm irritation it isn't caused by your deodorant. It could be from any number of other things: the chemicals in fabric finishes and dyes, the way you shave, even a sensitivity to your own perspiration. Or it may stem from more serious diseases. To help prevent underarm skin irritation, shaving correctly is one of the best things you can do. You need a blade just as sharp and fresh as a man uses every morning for his beard because when you use a blunt blade you are dragging layers of skin off with it, opening up your underarms to the stinging feeling you often get from a deodorant after shaving, and worse still, to irritation from rubbing by your clothes and to infection. If you have an acid-skin condition, you are likely to get an irritation from deodorants. In that case, stop using the deodorant and switch to another type—cream, roll-on, stick or whichever you haven't been using. Some deodorants are less acid than others. Acid does make for a strong deodorant but everyone cannot take it, just as everyone can't use aluminum chloride, a very strong deodorant that many models buy at the druggist's—15 to 20 percent strength—to use when they are working under the lights. It has been used since 1880, but not everyone can stand it. The cause of irritation may also be the particular perfume in a deodorant. This does not mean that you will respond the same way to another perfume in another deodorant; again, the solution is to switch. Then, too, some people are sensitive to the chemical salts that are in antiperspirants but not to the ingredients in an aerosol deodorant. Whatever your sensitivity, if the irritation keeps up, definitely see your doctor.

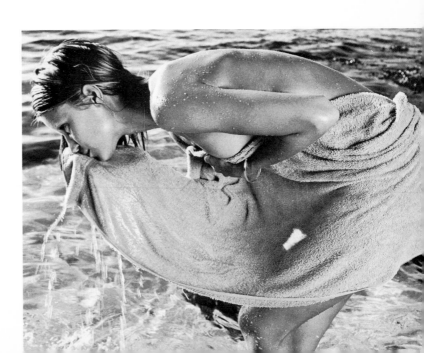

SCENTED DOS AND DON'TS

A man or a woman's sense of smell seldom operates on its own, independently of the other senses. It is always in a state of delicate balance between sight, sound, memory, desire and a mass of psychological associations, conscious and unconscious. But the instrument of that delicate balance, the human nose, is so strong that it is estimated it can detect a millionth of a milligram of scent—and we can be turned off or on by that power as effectively as by something a person says, does, or the way she looks. Particularly Americans can, because we are more finicky about scent than many other nationalities. That's why this four-page briefing in scents that you wear—their dos and don'ts, their possible effects, how to evoke feelings with them, where to put them, how they can heighten or detract from pleasure. And since there are some thirty thousand scents known to man, let's start with this narrowing-down:

Don't put perfume on at the last minute before you rush out of the house; allow it to set for at least ten minutes until the body chemistry develops it to its best advantage. Keep your scents from extremes of temperature which may upset their balance. Suit your scent to the season and occasion—light for summer, office, home; heavier for winter, evenings out, etc. Use more perfume in winter because it doesn't have as much staying power on cold days as on warm summer ones. Heat heightens scent, so if you're going to a crowded cocktail party, be sparing with yours. Put on more perfume if you're going outdoors, where the air carries it off faster than indoors, where it lasts longer. . . . Don't save perfumes forever. If you hoard them, you're likely to find they've evaporated or spoiled when you finally do decide to enjoy them. . . . Don't put scent directly on furs: it can stain them. . . . Use more fragrance if your skin is dry because it does not retain scent as long as oily skin. . . . Don't restrict yourself to just one signature perfume which everyone knows is you. Change scents, collect them. The nose develops something of an immunity to fragrances and responds less to one that it's been exposed to over and over again. . . . Put empty scent bottles in sweater, lingerie or ribbon drawers—just as you use sachet—to get the most from the remaining scent. Drop a bit of fragrance in the rinsing water of your lingerie. Spray cloth clothes hangers with a light scent and spray your hem linings, handkerchiefs, scarves (if they don't stain easily). Spray closets, too, with scent just after you've cleaned. Fragrance on the lining of your purse is a pleasant surprise everytime you open it. When you're deciding on a new perfume or scent, wear it around

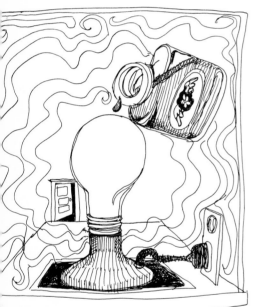

To diffuse a favorite scent throughout a room, put a drop of it on a light bulb before you turn it on. The heat will make it more effective and lingering.

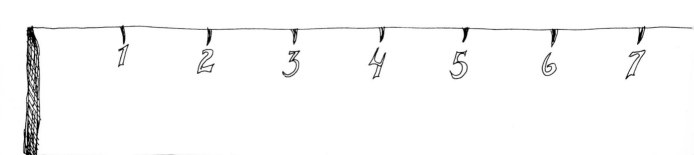

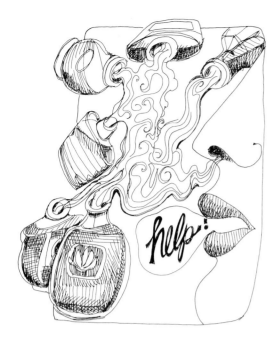

Don't, when you go to pick a new scent, try on everything at the counter. Three are the most your nose can possibly handle at the same sampling without losing its ability to distinguish.

the store for about ten minutes and see how you like it before you make a final judgment. Scents change after they have been on the body for a time. The alcohol evaporates and the fragrance begins to blend with your own skin's oils. Your skin must have no traces of other odors, other scents, when you try a new perfume. It should be thoroughly clean. In hot weather, cologne keeps your hands cool and dry because the alcohol content helps to evaporate perspiration. In summer, spray air conditioners with cologne to scent and freshen the air. Pressing clothes on an ironing board that's sprayed with scent allows them to pick up just a delicate hint of scent. For parties, put perfumed candles about the rooms; they will evoke all sorts of sensual, scented feelings and fantasies.

If you can't get the stopper out of a new bottle of perfume, take a glass tumbler and gently tap the stopper all around the sides. Or you might run hot water over the neck of the bottle. To scent hair, drop a teaspoon or two of a fragrance in the rinsing water after your shampoo. Scented bath powders and talcs not only scent you but keep your skin fresh and help prevent chapping by absorbing moisture. A scented bath is a great pickup before going out in the evening, or before going to bed it can put you into a relaxed, languid mood. Fragrant bath and body oils have the double advantage of being skin treatments: they help smooth and soften skin. Keeping scented soaps in lingerie or clothes

drawers makes double use of their scents. If you've failed with looks and words up to now to stir or attract someone you want to, give this old Kipling line a chance to prove itself: "Scents are surer than sounds or sights to make your heartstrings crack."

When you travel be sure to pack the aerosol version of your chosen scent. Keep linen, sheets, towels, pillowcases lightly scented with either a spray fragrance or sachet. If you have a garden, dry some of the flowers with the strongest scents and keep them in a little open bowl in your linen closet. To quickly revive bangs that have gone limp and oily, instead of shampooing your whole head, try stroking the bangs with a wad of cotton dampened with cologne or toilet water. The alcohol in the fragrance will take up some of the excess oil. To make your scents last longer, to double their impact, match them up. For instance, have a cologne or toilet water or perfume with its own particular scent repeated in your soap and bath oil. . . . When you go to buy a scent, know the difference between perfume, cologne and toilet water. Perfume is the most concentrated and lasting, therefore the most expensive. Toilet water and cologne are names often used interchangeably in the United States and contain the same fragrance notes as the perfume but in a lighter concentration. Do touch up your scent during the day. . . . And finally, since the sense of smell, remember, seldom operates independently, make that connection between nose, ears and voice sweeter by wiping your telephone with a cloth dampened with fragrance. The person on the other end may even be able to detect a new sweetness in you.

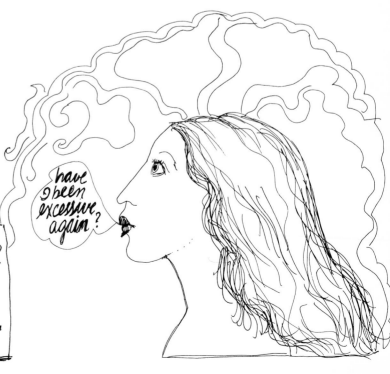

Don't assault people with perfume. If it's noticeable over twelve inches away, it's too noticeable and you have been heavy-handed.

INDEX